Praise for *Creating Healtt*

T. Colin Campbell, Ph.D., author of *The China Stua,,* ... ...
far reaching nutritional study to date, endorses *Creating Healthy Children:*

"Karen Ranzi has written a most important book, *Creating Healthy Children,* that is
must reading. The scientific evidence is now clear that a plant based diet means optimal
health, and the sooner young people are started on this diet, the better. The story line in
this book is personal, professional and very, very sensible."

T. COLIN CAMPBELL, PH.D.; Jacob Gould Schurman Professor Emeritus of
Nutritional Biochemistry, Cornell University, Ithaca, NY

"*Creating Healthy Children* is a valuable compilation of research and findings on
different aspects of children's health. Karen Ranzi is an honest researcher and a dedicated
mother, and I envision this book being embraced by all loving parents seeking optimum
health for their children. Karen's bold suggestions, sincerity, passion, genuine style and
interjection of personal anecdotes make this book a valuable read."

VICTORIA BOUTENKO, award-winning author of *Green for Life* and *12 Steps to Raw Foods*

"*Creating Healthy Children* is a superb, long-needed 'how to' guide for parents desiring
to succeed with the raw-health lifestyle. Karen covers all the intricate aspects of natural
parenting with uncommon insight, sensitivity and depth, as only a well-experienced,
effective teacher and mom could. Her unique background with the Natural Hygiene health
science program and continuum parenting education have afforded Karen the expertise to
write this comprehensive book and to be a leader in the natural health field.

The best feature of this book is how, in personable, heart-centered terms, Karen
portrays a balanced picture of how to work at mastering the natural parenting process
and make it a pleasurably nurturing lifestyle for the entire family, one with reverberations
which radiate out to the local community. Her treatment of the integration of the raw
food diet and homeschooling is most authoritative, compassionate and practical.

Is the author's teaching approach valid? No doubt! I have heard some of Karen's
warm, embracing lectures, met her, her husband and their two exceptionally healthy,
well-poised teenagers at their home and will attest Karen is a superb teacher, loving
mother and holistic thinker. Moreover, the parents I've known who've applied the same
basic principles Karen teaches have reaped similar results—the poised, bright, happy
and healthy children and close family bonds are beautiful to behold.

Indeed, this book demonstrates how to create healthy families, and it uplifts our
unhealthy society in wonderful ways. Karen deserves our heartfelt thanks, and the book
deserves a thorough read by all."

DAVID KLEIN, PH.D., publisher and editor of *Vibrance Magazine,* author of *Self-Healing
Colitis and Crohn's Disease* and Director of Colitis & Crohn's Health Recovery Services,
and co-author of *Your Natural Diet: Alive Raw Foods.*

"I have read stacks of books on the benefits of living foods and, over the years,
have incorporated much of this knowledge into my lifestyle. When I had my first child

at age 38, I wanted guidance from a fellow mom who'd 'been there, done that'—who understood my desires to provide the healthiest environment, internally and externally, for my son William—not just to survive but *thrive!* What I love most is that although Karen has studied under the best of the best in living foods and natural hygiene, she relies on her maternal instinct and personal experience to sort through all the data and varied opinions to determine what's best for her and her family—and encourages others to do the same. I found this approach refreshing and inspiring. It's clear that Karen is sincere and passionate about her mission of Creating Healthy Children!"

KELLI D. ANDERS, owner of What's Your Why? Ltd., Baltimore, Maryland

"The greatest gift we can give our children is the gift of health now and long into the future. *Creating Healthy Children* offers all of the tools you'll need to create not only healthy children, but also healthy families. Karen's holistic approach is essential and refreshing as she writes from personal experience. I recommend this book to parents, parents-to-be, grandparents, aunts and uncles, child caregivers, and, of course, kids. Reading this book will be vitally rewarding to your children's health...and yours too! Kudos to Karen."

SUSAN SMITH JONES, PH.D., author of *Be Healthy~Stay Balanced* and *The Healing Power of NatureFoods: 50 Revitalizing SuperFoods & Lifestyle Choices to Promote Vibrant Health*

"For more than fifteen years, Karen Ranzi has been a prominent force in promoting healthy living through proper feeding. She has raised a beautiful, healthy family despite the fact her young boy was extremely ill. I have been a personal witness to the boy's full and complete recovery from what doctors called 'incurable disease.' She is knowledgeable, intelligent, experienced and a TRUE student of the principles of health, a rare find in today's world. I highly recommend her book."

MATTHEW GRACE, author of *A WAY OUT: Dis-ease Deception and the Truth about Health*

"I've known Karen for many years and have sent all my clients with questions about raising healthy children to her. This book is a must-read for everyone who has children and wants to learn how to bring them up healthier. There is so much wisdom in it Karen has compiled over the years; it belongs in every home and library. I'm excited the world can now learn and apply Karen's program that really works!"

PAUL NISON, author of *The Raw Life, Raw Knowledge, Formula for Health* and *The Daylight Diet*

"Karen Ranzi's comprehensive, thoughtful and lovingly produced book *Creating Healthy Children* provides a wealth of valuable information and insight for mothers and mothers-to-be who are planning to raise their families on the raw/live food diet.

One of the few resources available, by a mother who has actually done it with amazing results. This book is honest, real and I highly recommend it."

RHIO, author of *Hooked on Raw* and host of *What's NOT Cookin' in Rhio's Kitchen*

"Before reading Karen Ranzi's book, I thought I was all done with kids—and glad of it! I understand why people want to go raw for its anti-aging benefits, but I always thought it would be a real challenge to raise raw kids. Karen Ranzi made it seem easy and fun. The book *Creating Healthy Children* is full term pregnant with parent-child wisdom. It should be priceless to its target audience since I was reading it at 50 and wishing for an offspring just to exercise her expert advice and experience the joys of raw parenthood."

TONYA ZAVASTA, author of *Your Right to Be Beautiful, Beautiful on Raw, Quantum Eating: The Ultimate Elixir of Youth,* and *Raw Food and Hot Yoga*

"I believe that reaching and teaching our young people about health and the human body is our foremost task as educators and healers. That is the focus of my work now, and Karen Ranzi's *Creating Healthy Children* offers great support for this grand task. I suggest we all embrace her ideas for ourselves and our families."

ELSON M. HAAS, MD, Founder and Director,
Preventive Medical Center of Marin, California
Integrated Medicine Practitioner
Author of *Staying Healthy with Nutrition* and many other books

"With her generous spirit, vast knowledge of nutrition, reassuring manner, and years of experience as a mother and counselor, Karen Ranzi is a treasure for families wanting to embrace wellness. She has helped me transition my young daughter, who was diagnosed with ulcerative colitis, to a vegan diet with fantastic results: she's symptom- and medicine-free!"

ALICE MARIE, New York City

"The raw food lifestyle made me a living example of what is possible—to literally bring oneself back from the very edge of life. And this is only in the last decade. It took me 35 years to figure out the hard way what real health is. For most of those years, I was so congested with mucus I could hardly breathe. I was literally choking to death. My heart was suffering from the lack of oxygen. My brain couldn't think straight. Nobody, not even doctors, knew the cause was mainly from what I was eating. If I, or my parents, knew as a child what I know now, I would be Superman now. This is the first thing they should teach parents and children before anything else. If you truly value life and your children's wellbeing, please take this seriously! The decisions you make right now affect everything else for the rest of your life and especially that of your children. The change starts right now with you and this book."

MARKUS ROTHKRANZ, Filmmaker, Artist, Raw Food Promoter

"*Creating Healthy Children* is a must read for anyone planning or striving to raise a healthy child. Karen's in depth research and personal experiences cover the very important issues facing the modern day parent."

DR. CRAIG B. SOMMERS, N.D., C.N., author of *Raw Foods Bible*

"In *Creating Healthy Children*, Karen shares the true story of her family's raw food way of life and offers practical tips for incorporating more fruits and vegetables into your diet. True food for thought for all of us who want to improve our health and vitality."

VICTORIA MORAN, author of *The Love-Powered Diet*, *Fit from Within*, *Creating a Charmed Life*, and *Shelter for the Spirit*

"An outstanding expert on raw foods—Karen's easy to follow instructions and recipes are extremely helpful. She provides an excellent approach for motivating your children to live a healthier lifestyle."

CHRISTIE KELLOGG, Certified Raw Food Chef and mother, North Carolina

"*Creating Healthy Children* is a must-read book, highly essential for every parent and every child. This book is the first of its kind on raising truly healthy children, containing information not easily found elsewhere. In addition to the excellent nutritional information, the benefits of long-term nursing, holding and sleeping with your child are explained in detail for all parents to understand. I strongly recommend you read this wonderful book for the superb health of your child and your entire family."

DR. WALTER J. URBAN, Research Psychoanalyst, registered with the Medical Board of California, The Founder and Director of the Energy of Life Institute in Costa Rica, and author of *Do You Have the Courage to Change: The 12 Reasons Why People Don't Change and How You Can;* and *Integrative Therapy: Foundations of Holistic and Self Healing*

"During a time of confusion concerning my son's health issues, Karen was a beacon of light for us. Her clear, direct advice was exactly what I needed to continue on my conscious parenting path. Karen is insightful, experienced, supportive, and quite knowledgeable on issues related to children, family and societal dynamics."

JOHANNA ZEE, RN, NHP, C.PH.D.

"I don't have the words to thank Karen. Even though I already knew introducing more raw foods to my diet had gotten rid of my migraines from which I suffered ever since childhood, and took care of other health issues, I had many questions about how to better feed my 4 year old daughter. Not only did Karen have answers for every one of my questions, she was always positive and supportive about everything I was going through. Just knowing she and her kids have been eating raw foods for years and stayed healthy is comforting and assuring. I used to give only Cheerios and a piece of bread to my daughter for breakfast, but she now eats baby carrots, broccoli, half an avocado, almond butter and fruits instead. She is still a very picky eater, but I've learned how to choose more healthful food for her. Even my big meat eater husband has been eating more vegetables these days. Karen has transformed my family's diet which has improved our health, and I can't thank her enough!"

YUKO LAU, Walnut Creek, California

"Live raw food and green smoothies along with fasting about 35 hours weekly have given me the fountain of youth. I'm getting younger and younger. This truly is a remarkable journey and I must thank you, Karen, for being an integral part of it. Life truly is a gift to be savored with joy."

ARNIE WEINTRAUB, New York

I received this note when I returned home after presenting my seminar "Creating Healthy Children" in Michigan in May 2004.

Dear Karen,

Thank you so very much for coming to Michigan and speaking in Lansing. We enjoyed meeting your daughter and her two friends. We truly appreciate your message. For my husband and I personally, you reaffirmed and made us feel more confident about our life choices. We have been planning to homeschool Austin and your words really reaffirmed our decision. Your story on all the issues such as raw food, breastfeeding, homeschooling, vaccination, circumcision, etc. were so right on with our beliefs, and it was so good to hear your talk. Austin is 4 years old and I still nurse him, and Chris is so supportive. We, too, end up in different beds because Chris is a light sleeper, while Austin and I sleep in another room, which just works for us. One thing you brought back into our consciousness is the skin-to-skin contact. Austin loves skin to skin contact from both of us. So thank you for what you do! We know the Raw Parenting and other topics you discussed are a subset of the Raw Food Movement, but we are so glad your voice has emerged to focus on these issues. Please know we are forever grateful for your journey to Michigan and your message. You and your message will stay with us forever. I really believe your lecture and words of wisdom need to be heard by many. You are healing the planet with your talks. When I heard your talk, it gave my inner voice strength. It gave me energy and renewed my enthusiasm. We applaud you, Karen, and your mission on this planet, Earth, of reawakening parents to their instincts.

BETH BECHTEL, Lansing, Michigan

"I was diagnosed with breast cancer in November of 2004. I had a mastectomy in January of 2005. It was evident I needed to make some life changes, but I didn't know where to start.

I went to a holistic doctor for a complete physical and was shocked to find out my cholesterol was extremely high at 364. The time for change was not later.

I was very afraid for my life, and called my good friend Karen Ranzi and said "Help!" I was stressed out and scared, and getting started seemed so overwhelming. It was Harvey Ranzi who said to me, 'If you want to get well, remember it's so simple.' With Karen's support, little by little, I changed my outlook. It just took lots of encouragement. It was okay to make mistakes. I went to a few raw food meetings and liked what I saw and heard. I bought 90% organic produce, and found when I ate the old way, it no longer tasted as good, and I didn't feel the same. That helped me to stay on track. With new recipes and delicious raw food, I see major differences. My cholesterol went down in just a couple of months to the 220 mark, and after just 9 months it went down to 202, and it will continue to drop. What's not to like about feeling good and getting well with lots of delicious food.

Karen, I thank you from the bottom of my heart for saving my life."

WENDY POLLER, Woodcliff Lake, New Jersey

"As a new mom choosing to raise her baby on living foods, I was discouraged by how few resources were available for support and learning. The few materials I did find didn't place nutrition in the context of attachment parenting or any other parenting style. Karen Ranzi is helping to fill that void. Learning Karen has maintained a living food diet since 1994 and raised two healthy children on it was extremely encouraging. Not only was she able to provide me with well researched nutritional information and resources, but she shared practical 'mom' tips, tried and true from her own parenting experience (like how to make simple foods in a hurry!). I came away from our conversation feeling supported and with new ideas to try."

KAREN REZAI, Lafayette, California

"With the rise of childhood obesity, childhood asthma, childhood type II diabetes, attention deficit disease, and many others...could we be in an epidemic, a pandemic threatening our children, our very future as humans on Earth? With the profound nutritional and lifestyle changes elucidated by Karen Ranzi in her monumental book, *Creating Healthy Children,* I have seen each of these catastrophic diseases reversed as well as juvenile arthritis, childhood onset heart disease, and the biggest fear...cancer. There are simple and livable answers.

There is a light emanating from this tragedy of childhood sickness—not only can we help our kids who are afflicted with these hideous diseases, but we can prevent them from ever occurring. Yes, there is hope when there are no real answers anywhere else other than palliating the symptoms or numbing the pain. Hope is right here in these pages of *Creating Healthy Children.* In an age of junk food and chemicals, computer games and inactivity, are we shortening our children's lives, undermining their self-esteem, and making it harder for them to cope? The facts are there, lifestyle will affect the lives of every child, more than education, status, or talent.

Dr. C. Everett Koop, renowned pediatric surgeon and former United States Surgeon General, once said, 'Except for smoking, obesity is now the number one preventable cause of death in this country. Three hundred thousand people die of obesity every year.' Obesity, where it all starts, is reversible and preventable. And it is on the rise in our children. The World Health Organization says that natural foods and lifestyle can definitely reduce our chances to be plagued with heart disease, cancer and diabetes. If the human race is to survive, it is obvious we need to do some things differently, and we need to start with our kids.

Karen Ranzi has simplified the science for parents to understand. Most importantly, Karen has given us secrets to entice our children to healthier choices. *Creating Healthy*

Children is showing us the answers of how to insure our kids' future as well as our own. Karen Ranzi answers questions we did not even know to ask but need to know. It is all here, in enough detail to truly understand how to get our children and us out of the downward spiral, and to embrace living healthfully. Karen does not overpower us, with details, yet she gives us all we need to uplift us to true health. Do we not want the best for our kids? This is the book to show us the way."

Dr. Timothy Trader, Ph.D., N.D.

Dear Karen,

I went to your in-home workshop last spring, and spoke to you about the variety of symptoms my 6-year old son had developed (allergy, chronic sinus issues, facial tics, post nasal drip, cough). Our naturopath had diagnosed him with intestinal yeast and said he needed a long term regimen off sugar, wheat and dairy.

I just wanted you to know your workshop was very, very helpful. I was so overwhelmed, but I kept thinking about what you said: "Just start with fruits and vegetables." That's what we did — green smoothies every day, cutting out most gluten and dairy, and all processed sugar. Within weeks, we saw noticeable improvement (so did his Kindergarten teacher). For a child who had missed 25 days of school in 5 months, he was not sick at all from May through September. It has been difficult to keep him on his regimen going back to school — but his teacher has been very, very cooperative about keeping junk food out of her class. And all of this has gotten me involved with my local Board of Education and heading the district's Wellness Committee to improve the foods the children in school are eating.

So...I just wanted to let you know, I am a big advocate of what you are doing.

Karen Burka, New York

Dear Karen,

Thanks so much for coming to Warwick to speak to our Holistic Moms chapter. You are a wonderful speaker; we found your experiences inspiring! I think it's especially interesting your father was your nutritional "guide" in life. That is so rare; usually, it's us moms who lead the way in that department! Again, many thanks; you'll see many of us at your upcoming classes!

Love, Ginny
Coordinator, Holistic Moms Network

CREATING HEALTHY CHILDREN

Through Attachment Parenting and Raw Foods

Karen Ranzi

Forewords by
Serafina Corsello, M.D. and
Ruza V. Bogdanovich, N.D., Ph.D.

Disclaimer

This book is about understanding and abiding by the truths in life through raising healthy children—creating a good life and education for them. It was written with the intention of providing families with information about the raw foods lifestyle and motivating them to implement it. The ideas presented have been tested with excellent success by the author and her family as well as by the other families featured in this book. By adopting a raw foods lifestyle and attachment parenting values, we are going back to our roots. This is quite unusual for our current society. Raw foods are not being forced on anyone. Some families may choose to increase only the percentage of raw foods in their current diet.

The information contained herein is not intended as a diagnosis, cure or treatment for any disease or ailment. Because an initial cleansing and detoxification reaction can often occur as a result of a simpler and cleaner diet, parents and all readers are advised to properly educate themselves and seek advice from a qualified medical doctor or health professional when needed. The author does not accept any liability or responsibility for any loss, injury, or damage, or any adverse consequences that may be encountered from following any information or suggestion in this book.

Editor: Joel Brody

Book Designer: David Ruppe, Impact Publications

Indexer: Tamar Raum

Published by:
SHC Publishing
P.O. Box 13
Ramsey, NJ 07446

Printed in Canada.

Library of Congress Cataloging-in-Publication Data
       Ranzi, Karen.
          Creating healthy children : through attachment
       parenting and raw foods / Karen Ranzi ; forewords by
       Serafina Corsello and Ruza V. Bogdanovich.
          p. cm.
          Includes bibliographical references and index.
          ISBN-13: 978-0-615-33150-8
          ISBN-10: 0-615-33150-5

          1. Parenting. 2. Health. 3. Parent and child.
       4. Attachment behavior. 5. Raw foods.   I. Title.

HQ755.8.R36 2010   649'.1
                         QBI10-600001

Dedication

I dedicate this book to my wonderful loving father,
Sol T. Horowitz, who inspired me to be passionate in caring
for my wellbeing and that of those I love. My father felt a
great interconnectedness among all beings, and he instilled a
deep compassion in me for the animals who share the Earth.
Sol was the strong support system in my life, teaching me to
question, and always to remain faithful to what I believe to
be the truth. I will always be grateful to have had this most
dedicated father in my life. His support continues to
inspire me throughout the writing of this book.

Table of Contents

Foreword to
Creating Healthy Children
by Serafina Corsello, M.D.

In medicine, the science of today is the garbage of tomorrow. It should suffice to cite the leeches of mainstream medicine of the seventeenth and eighteenth centuries and the chains for the mentally ill of the nineteenth century, sanctioned by the "scientific consensus" of the time. Faced with such a discrediting record, I welcome the courage of those who resort to good maternal instincts combined with the collective wisdom of millennia of trial and error which in different cultures has assembled safe and non-toxic ways of facilitating natural healing.

This approach to degenerative diseases—the diseases of our time from arthritis to cancer, has a far superior record for safety and efficacy compared to the approach of allopathic medicine which aims at obscuring symptoms rather than dealing with the causes. Any honest, patient-centered physician would attest to this truism. Fortunately, despite the effort of big Pharma to persecute its proponents, natural healing is gaining momentum because in the end, truth always prevails.

Hippocrates, the greatest Ancient Greek physician codified his approach around two basic statements: first, "Do no harm!" second, "Let your food be your medicine!"

Until the discovery of fire, our ancestors survived the harshness of the environment using their animal instincts, and by consuming berries and herbs they gathered during their incessant roaming. The advent of farming created abundance but brought with it the danger of repetitive food intake. Mini farming communities began to observe reactions and responses to various foods and other substances that became the basis of their medical wisdom which was passed down without interruption for millennia.

Now we have the so called scientifically unimpeachable "double blind studies" that should protect us from the unwanted side effects of synthetic drugs, but instead, very often, these so called safe drugs have had to be pulled from the market and declared dangerous to our health. When one puts together side effects of medication, therapeutic errors, exposure to hospital super infections, and surgical and medical errors, this so called scientific medicine has emerged as the number one cause of death. I, as most people who have lived into their seventies, have had the misfortune of personally experiencing some of the destructive effects of pharmaceutical medicine governed by the Midas touch rather than the love of humanity. Like Midas, they will eventually perish because of their greed. These observations are beginning to erode people's trust, even those brainwashed by the well-positioned propaganda of big Pharma.

For the past two generations however, most people have been totally disconnected from the wisdom of their ancestors and would have nowhere to turn were it not for dedicated people like Karen Ranzi who has assembled a superb amount of well-researched information to validate the wisdom of the past and the healing power of nature. If everybody took to heart the prenatal and post natal advice on child nutrition and child rearing Karen suggests, we could revolutionize the world. If a few of us do it, I hope it will inspire others.

Healthy children are happy children. Happy children make for balanced adults, less prone to be litigious—the fewer litigious people, the fewer wars. Can you imagine such a world? It will only be possible if as many women as possible begin their children's care from the womb and use this wonderful book as a step by step guide.

I see Karen's book coming out at the right time and the right place, playing a role of catalyst that could spearhead the "quantum evolution" we are all hoping for. I hope to live long enough to see it, and if not, to have my grandchild live it.

Karen gives us all the information necessary to make this "quantum peaceful revolution" take place. This book contains references and knowledge gathered from some of the most brilliant minds of our time, many of whom I've had the fortune of knowing personally.

One only need read what she advises, question her when in doubt, providing the questions stem from honest doubt and curiosity and not from second hand dogma. Karen is open to challenge which she meets with humility and open-mindedness. These are the attributes of real teachers. The great healers of humanity were all supreme teachers.

And finally, I can't wait to send this book to my daughter, to congratulate her and reaffirm her good instincts in child rearing, even when faced with skeptical opinions. No doubt this book will enrich her already sound instinctual knowledge with so much information about diet and unnecessary medical interventions.

My grandchild, fortunate indeed with her start in life, ultimately will be the beneficiary of such enrichment and, hopefully, she will become a future proponent of good, sound ways of living in harmony with nature.

ॐ

Dr. Serafina Corsello began on the path of natural healing methodology in 1972. In 1992, Dr. Corsello was one of twenty-five physicians chosen by the National Institute of Health to formulate the guidelines of the Office of Alternative Medicine, now known as the Center for Complementary Alternative Medicine (CCAM). Dr. Corsello has written *The Ageless Woman,* a compendium of her lengthy experience in anti-aging medicine. She has also written many articles and chapters for books by other authors. Dr. Corsello has lectured extensively throughout the United States, Europe, and the Caribbean and in November, 2007 was a featured speaker at the First Swiss Medical Symposium in anti-aging medicine in Geneva, Switzerland.

Foreword
by Ruza V. Bogdanovich, N.D., Ph.D.

While reading this book, you must forget what you've been taught so you can remember what you've really always known deep within—your true nature. Once in touch with it, you can now correct your mistakes. Karen Ranzi will show you how, step by step.

Today we are taught very early in life to think and act from the scientific point of view, believing Nature is not good enough and science is more important. Throughout our school years, and later on the job, we're taught to produce or sell products that unknowingly cause harm to our fellow humans, and to all living beings, as well as to our very mother Earth in the process. Time and again we have seen in the long run, scientific research has proved to be wrong because it wasn't in accordance with Nature's laws. Classically, big interest groups have used, and still use, "science" as a means to foist their money-hungry schemes on the unsuspecting masses. Man-made laws are devised to benefit special interest groups, organizations and bureaucrats, placing great burdens of suffering on innocent consumers, especially our children. The boomerang theory has now come into effect, and we are suffering deeply. Can we still turn it around? Time is of the essence, and Karen's book is past due and desperately needed.

Karen clearly demonstrates Nature's way is best because in Nature there are no rewards or punishments, only consequences. For many reasons explained in this book, we are not aware of the consequences and our loved ones are forced to suffer needlessly from the very beginning, even before conception.

Reading this book will lead you to a true understanding of Nature—her immutable, permanent laws, in accordance with life itself. Now, with Karen's simple and beautiful explanations, heartfelt words, her love and hands-on experience as a parent and teacher, you will see how easy it is to implement Nature's laws.

The new generation of conscious children will help turn this "un-natural" world around—and what a job they have ahead of them! This book is so vital for this reason alone. Once aware of its message, we don't have to make the same mistakes again. Now, we can get it right the first time, but only when we've learned the truth that we and Nature are one.

What will it take to wake us up? What will we do when we really awaken? Yes, we have all been hurt, the Earth, the meek, the innocent, and our children. We have no choice but to wake up and take action. Since you have also been hurt, what can you do to help? Your best efforts are needed now. I urge you to take a deep look at the gifts Karen is giving you.

Robert Bly puts it this way: "The gold comes to the place where the injury was and is…" I find this to be a truly amazing concept—the idea that the human being's wound and genius are located at the same place. It is from the spot where we were wounded that we will give our main gift to the community and the world.

In this awesome labor of love, Karen Ranzi truly covers every subject imaginable for humankind's wellbeing, from the very start—naturally! She searched and researched it, experienced it with her own family and friends. She has involved so many views from the most brilliant minds in the field of natural medicine, education and life in general. I wish for everyone to have this information before starting a new family, and for those who want to do it right from wherever they are now and in accordance with Nature's laws. It truly can be done right now, wherever you are on the path of raising a family of future-conscious winners who will lead the world to peace, love, abundance, health and joy. And, it is all in this book.

When I first started to read Karen's manuscript, I felt that I was reading an encyclopedia of life choices that followed the most natural ways with the least resistance and suffering. I could just imagine the time and energy spent on this labor of love and the collections of the variety of data from natural doctors and parents, including their mistakes. It is mind-boggling.

This book should be available for every new parent-to-be, as well as for doctors, teachers, schools and universities, so the important things can be brought to light before many mistakes are made.

Karen is walking her talk and will walk you through it step by step. So much valuable information is in this book. You could go to college and not learn any of this information because they don't teach it there. All the websites, phone numbers and addresses are available in this book for every branch of wellbeing. You can explore it all more deeply now, as well as meet many enlightened souls who dared to be themselves and one with Nature.

Even though there are many raw food nutritionists who disagree on the subject of what nutritional combinations should or should not be taken, when, how and why, Karen reasons with them and follows Nature's way to simplicity and truth. She has been experimenting on this path for decades and raising her family by experiencing it all. That alone is worth millions because there's nothing like perceiving the truth through hands-on natural experience.

All the information about homeschooling brought tears of joy to my eyes because we homeschooled our two sons also. We listened to our hearts and not what others told us we should be doing. Today our sons are following their own hearts on Nature's path, helping others with love and peace. One of the main reasons we homeschooled was we didn't want to have our children vaccinated, and we wanted them to learn the truth about Nature, history, science, biology, economics, and to depend on Nature's laws and themselves and not on institutions of any kind.

We have to understand that the most brilliant minds never went to school, and they are brilliant because no one clogged them up at early ages with lies and misconceptions. We all teach ourselves by experiencing and feeling life when we are ready. Not every child is ready when the teacher thinks so. Being forced to learn nonsense and things one will never need is an absolute waist of time in addition to learning false information that will prevent the brain from being logical and making the right choices. "The teacher appears when the student is ready," and the student is also the teacher, if the teacher is open. I learned more from my students than I did in college.

One fact most miss is the reason schools are mandatory. They exist not to teach us the truth, but to control us from an early age. We learn throughout our entire lives by experiencing new events, and on a daily basis by feeling it all.

Karen, I applaud you for the vaccination information. Again I had to weep because of all the suffering we went through when our son Jesse got paralyzed from a polio vaccine, when the doctors wanted to remove the ligaments in his legs and to have him bound to a wheelchair. We were told: "If you do not trust your doctor, whom are you going to trust?" Daa..! What about Mother Nature? She is the real doctor, the only one that actually heals when we get out of her way completely.

As nothing endures unless it is of use in the world and in the economy of Nature, life does not occur without life. Every part of the body is dependent on the whole. Be wise, read and re-read this book, and do use it as you would use the encyclopedia because this is the true one. You will have good consequences because correcting oneself is correcting the whole world. Being the example is all it takes. "The Sun is simply bright. It does not correct anyone. Because it shines, the whole world is full of light. Transforming yourself is a means of giving light to the whole world." We are One, and each one is a part of the whole.

Indeed, the next step is up to you, dear reader. You can help your children to see the light by seeing it and truly being it yourself. Karen will show you how.

"Plunge, plunge into the vast ocean of consciousness, let the drop of water that is you become a hundred mighty seas. But do not think that the drop alone becomes the ocean. The ocean, too, becomes the drop." – Rumi

I love you all from my heart, the Universe.

જી

Ruza V. Bogdanovich, N.D., Ph.D. is the co-founder of The Cure Is in the Cause Foundation, a nonprofit organization dedicated to public awareness and understanding of natural healing processes. She is an internationally renowned lecturer, a consultant on raw food nutrition, and the author of *The Cure Is in the Cause* and *Love Your Pet, Let Nature Be the Vet*.

Acknowledgements

I'm especially grateful to my wonderful and gifted friend and editor, Professor Joel Brody—known as the "Renaissance Man" because of his profound interest and knowledge in so many fields. Working on my book with Joel has been a truly rewarding and ceaselessly educational experience.

To my book designer, David Ruppe of Impact Publications, I appreciate your dedication and good taste in the thousands of choices you've made in bringing this book to its satisfying fruition. My gratitude goes to Tamar Raum. With your analytical and organizational skills, you wrote the most complete, detailed, and well-organized index.

To my friends, authors Rhio, Victoria Boutenko, Dr. Ruza Bogdanovich, and Tonya Zavasta, thank you for reading my book and giving me your valuable time and suggestions.

Thank you to Dr. Ruza Bogdanovich and Dr. Serafina Corsello for the time and effort you put into creating brilliant forewords for *Creating Healthy Children*. I would like to thank Barbara Harper for her warm, welcoming preface.

To my extraordinary grandmother, Celia Horowitz, whose intimate rapport with Nature imbued her with raw food knowledge far ahead of her time—her influence came clearly into my thoughts when I became a mother, particularly when my son wasn't well.

I'm filled with gratitude for my lovely yet tragic mother whose death in 1980, as I was just completing college, inspired the beginning of my quest for health. I always felt my mother was deprived of a good life because of the tragedy of the Holocaust, and finally, when she was talked into accepting illogical medical decisions that inevitably ended her life at a young age.

To my children, Gabriela and Marco, you're my gifts from God, and I've learned very valuable lessons from you. Gratitude to my beautiful daughter, Gabriela; I still remember all the love, support and enthusiasm you gave me when I was transitioning the family to raw foods many years ago when you were a child. You asked many questions and trusted your mom's decisions. You wrote "Raw Rules" everywhere. Then, later, as a teen, you displayed honesty and clarity when constantly insisting the choice of the raw food lifestyle needs to be one's own—not imposed by one's mother. I thank my son, Marco, who as a toddler led me to understand the only way to heal was through a healthful lifestyle, and for his emotional cries at the young ages of 3, 4 and 5, imploring not to be separated from his mother. To my husband Harvey, I know how difficult it was for you to deal with the many changes I made to our family's diet and lifestyle, starting in the mid 90s. Thank you for your love, for your willingness to learn foods and vaccines do affect our systems, and for encouraging me to write this book. I'm also grateful for my sister Barbara's continuous unconditional love throughout the years. I am very proud of Barbara for the wonderful work she is doing as the head of her town's environmental committee. I send my love to my mother-in-law in Colombia, Araceli Vallejo de Ranzi, who now drinks green smoothies daily, and my brother-in-law and sister-in-law in Switzerland, Mauricio and Claudine Ranzi, who have an abundance of fruits and vegetables available when we visit them in their gorgeous surroundings.

I would like to express my gratitude to my mentors, those who were great inspirations to me on my raw food journey, and those who permitted me to quote their brilliant writings, abounding with wisdom. I have immense love and respect for all of you: Dr. Timothy Trader, Rhio, Dr. David Klein, Dr. Ruza Bogdanovich, Tonya Zavasta, Dr. Gabriel Cousens, Professor Rozalind Graham, Dr. Douglas Graham, Paul Nison, Matthew Grace, Victoria Boutenko, Dr. Roe Gallo, David Wolfe, Dr. Fred Bisci, Viktoras Kulvinskas, Dr. Brian Clement, Ana Inez Matus, Dr. Vivian V. Vetrano, Dr. Ritamarie Loscalzo, Susan Schenck and Brenda Cobb.

I would especially like to thank Dr. T. Colin Campbell, Dr. John McDougall, Dr. Joel Fuhrman and Dr. Neal Barnard for their excellent research and graciously permitting me to quote from their writings in the field of vegan nutrition.

I am very grateful to all those who wrote articles or accounts of raw food family journeys for this book: Laurie Evans, Carole Blane, Robert Lichtman, Victoria Boutenko, Roger Haeske, Hygeia Halfmoon, Dr. Vivian V. Vetrano,

Dr. Rick Dina, Dr. Gina Shaw, Esther van der Werf, Diana Heather, Beata Barinbaum, Carol Iwaniuk, Kathy Raine, Francesca Repass, Professor Rozalind Graham, Beth and Steve Corwin, Nancy Durand-Lanson, Jingee and Storm Talifero, Shannon Leone, Laura Sutton, Amy Schrift, Eric Rivkin, Yemaya Kimmel, Shawn Kimmel, Erika, Sue Ann James, Miko Nelson, Laura Meyer, Sue Nackoney, Rick Philip, Sarah Parker, Kristi Shafer, Luke Swift, Jaylene Johnson, Dr. Ruza Bogdanovich, Andrea Nison, Jenny Silliman, Karmyn Malone, and Dana Stewart.

Thank you to everyone who permitted me to quote his or her books and articles, to those creative chefs who shared their recipes for the kid-tested recipes chapter, and to those who wrote reviews of the book. Space does not permit me to thank everyone by name, but I am grateful to all of you.

Special gratitude is due to my dear friend Donna Perrone for bringing together the raw food community in New York City.

I thank my friends Tom Coviello, Aldo Aragao, Cheryll Lynn, Scott McNabb, Stephen Parker, David Giardina, Carol Pessin, Vickie Hatcher, Dafna Mordecai, Kevin Shuker, Ohbeeb Cavalcante, Robert Dyckman, Roger Haeske, Alan Berger, Gail Zikri, Laurie Jordan, Hope Stanger, Mary Maher, Diane Scallo, Robert Spector, Catherine Moon Rubin, and Arnie and Michael Weintraub for the fun we've had together and for your willingness always to share information and ideas on the raw food lifestyle and other topics.

Additional special gratitude goes to my dear friends, Linda and Scott Murray. Linda, my longtime devoted friend and roommate, got rid of her three fur coats and switched her diet from standard to vegan. Scott and Linda, I'll always be moved by your open-mindedness and love of animals that led to your activist work.

Special thanks go to longtime friends who have given me unconditional support: Sharon DeLaura, Steven Corwin, Amy Schrift, Victoria Jordan, Chantal and François Sciboz, Liliana and Michael Popp, Mark and Carolyn Gizzi, Pia Jacangelo, Jackie Lilienthal, Wendy Poller, Cathy DePaola, and Carole Bollini.

Gratitude is also due to farmer Guy Jones, who so beautifully and meticulously plants and harvests the finest local organic produce at his Blooming Hill Farm in Blooming Grove, NY, only a half hour away from my New Jersey home. With his year-round produce, I can eat organically, seasonally and regionally.

And finally, to the wonderful mothers who have inspired me to follow my heart when it came to raising my children. Thank you to Sandy Rzetelny who passionately guided me to becoming a more nurturing mother, helping me to recognize maternal instincts that had been buried within me. Thank you to these devoted mothers and special friends in my life who have followed attachment parenting principles. You are all my mothering mentors: Carole Blane, Lynne Lisa, Laurie Evans, Joy Cohen, April Schoenherr, Nancy Durand-Lanson, Beth Corwin, Cynthia French Delson, Ellen Forman, Rabia Nagin, Sandra Griffiths, Jane McGirty, Wendy Blair, Mary Ann Baiyor, Susan Mogren, Debbie Eaton, Vanessa Anton, Francine Lucidon Reichman, Lynda Elie, Sarah Adams, Sonia Idelsohn and Gina Ironside.

Lisa Heyman was a leading influence regarding my decision to unschool my children. Her lively, fun, loving and nurturing mothering example, always responsive to the needs of her children, caused me to examine my own parenting practices. Through her beautiful guiding light, I realized what was really important were my expressions of love and respect for my children.

My admiration goes to Mother Nature. If we look to Her, we will understand "The goal of life is living in harmony with nature." (Zeno – 335-263 BC).

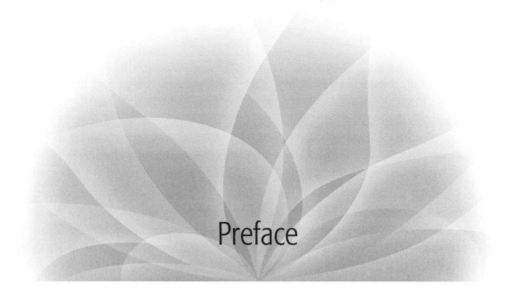

Preface

Karen Ranzi has created a much needed source book for parents already living a raw food lifestyle who need more information about the nutritional needs of pregnancy, lactation and early childhood and for those who are curious about how to increase the percentage of raw foods in their diet and shift to a more balanced lifestyle throughout their parenting journey.

As I have traveled widely and experienced life in many different countries, food and fellowship are at the heart of every culture. Understanding there is a connection between diet during pregnancy and long-term health, even into adulthood, helps us see the far reaching implications of pregnancy nutrition. What a pregnant woman consumes while growing a baby can lay down the health and genetic code for that new human being, predisposing that person to ailments such as heart disease in later life. The health of our children is of great concern today as we are exposed to an ever more toxic environment.

During my second pregnancy, I maintained a raw food diet under the guidance of my husband, who had studied with raw food expert, Viktoras Kulvinkas. The result of that pregnancy was the healthiest of my three children, and my son, now 23, has never been ill, other than a few colds. My two other children have had their share of health problems such as allergies or allergic reactions. I found keeping a raw food diet was difficult for me, especially since I didn't have a guidebook or the scientific evidence and rationales. It was certainly not the norm back in the 80s. Karen's book is just the guidance that would have been wonderful to consult. I went off of raw foods because it required a lifestyle commitment, and I just did not have the support for it. Now, as I'm older, I eat a much more balanced diet and continually incorporate more and more raw foods.

As I raised my children, many people encouraged me to explain why I wore them, slept in the same bed, and nurtured them as intelligent people, instead of empty vessels I had to fill up. I discovered that what I thought I had to teach my children about the world, they were really teaching me. I didn't know my style of parenting was someday going to have a title, an international organization and millions of supporters of what I already knew and practiced. Attachment parenting was natural, second nature, and the only way I could approach nurturing and caring for my children.

Karen Ranzi has used her own experience raising her children in an attachment parenting lifestyle to now put into words and stories what I was not able to do. I'm so thankful someone has linked the natural diet of raw foods and the attachment parenting lifestyle. Both prove nurturing and sustaining for those who choose to follow. Thank you, Karen, for being bold enough to share your experience so the world can benefit from your understanding of the impact of parenting and dietary choices.

Sincerely,
Barbara Harper, RN, CLD, CCE
Author, *Gentle Birth Choices*
Founder, Waterbirth International

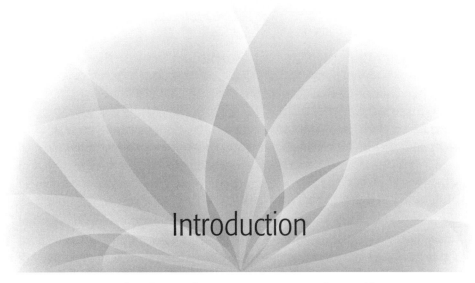

Introduction

"Be the Change That You Want to See in the World."

GHANDI

I feel two compelling reasons to write this book on raising healthy children. My first is to expose the dramatic life-changing difference raw vegan foods can make during pregnancy, lactation, and in raising the healthiest children possible. The second reason revolves around security and trust, and the strong inner knowing of one's true place in the world, developed only by the close skin-to-skin attaching relationship between mother and baby.

I believe all parents and parents-to-be should study the physiological and emotional needs of their children, and learn how to care for them in a way that meets those needs. Taking care of these needs will bring health and excellence in all areas. The problems children face in today's world are largely the result of misguided and uninformed parents. Trillions of dollars are spent annually on drugs, hospitals, nurses and physicians, showing the vast extent of disease and suffering. There are a growing number of physicians who realize the importance of a healthful diet and lifestyle but continue to treat symptoms without looking for their cause. Most doctors have not been trained in nutrition and health but solely to test, administer drugs, and perform surgery.

It's tragic the civilized world has developed an eating style that causes children so much suffering — both now and for the rest of their lives. We have followed a medical way of looking at pregnancy and childbirth which often leads to a couple being more concerned about the mother's recovery from surgical delivery instead of naturally focusing on nursing the baby. The many "experts" who talk about avoidance of spoiling children by insisting they sleep alone have conditioned mothers and fathers to emotionally detach themselves from their children, going against their own parental instincts.

While writing this book, I was advised to keep it strictly to the topic of raw foods for children, but I don't see how I could possibly separate the emotional needs of babies and growing children from their biological and physiological needs. Only all of these integrated factors will lead to a fully healthy, evolved being. I felt it was most important to present all aspects of raising a fit and well-adjusted child.

It is my passion to disseminate valuable information about a healthful family lifestyle so children can have the benefits of living their lives without illness, and have the strongest possibility of realizing their true potential. We don't always have control over much that goes on in our physical world. Water and air pollution affect us every day, and the daily stresses of life are detriments to our health. The only things we have complete control over are what food we choose to put into our bodies, what we use on our skin, the amounts of sleep and exercise we get, and the love and emotional support we give ourselves and our children.

One third of the United States population is reported to be severely overweight due to the standard diet. It is unfair to children that parents are so uninformed about how to care for their young. Thousands upon thousands of children are allowed to become obese because their parents feed them fast foods. We need to bring people back to Nature by guiding them to observe how other species thrive. I truly wish I had all the information I'm now presenting in this book, before having my children. The food we put into their bodies, and the love and care we give to our children as they grow from infancy, should nourish them for a beautiful disease-free secure lifetime.

I am not a doctor, but I have seen quite clearly through my studies and observations, health is created when we take control of it. My own children have been healthiest when eating predominantly raw foods, and my observations of raw pregnancies and raw vegan families have provided me with information pointing to the necessity of staying on this path.

What is raw, alive vegan food, and why eat more of it? Eating all or mostly greens, fruits and vegetables is the simplest way to establish and maintain optimal health and weight. Uncooked greens, fruits, vegetables, nuts and seeds are also called "live" (rhymes with thrive) foods because they have all of their enzymes intact. Live foods don't contain the toxic chemicals created by high cooking temperatures, and their vitamins, minerals, phytonutrients and fiber remain whole. Complete nutrition, undamaged by fire, helps to prevent disease, reduce weight and increase energy. Fresh natural food also keeps its delicious flavor. Everyone can make improvements by eating more raw food. It's especially important to eat a fresh green salad if eating a cooked starch or protein meal. If you think it's too time-consuming to prepare raw food recipes, simply eat a bowl of colorful organic berries. Raw vegan food can be that simple—the original and ultimate fast food.

One of the main objectives here is to help families to increase the amount of natural, live foods in their diets, no matter what their diets now contain. There is absolutely no pressure to eat raw food exclusively. I think a raw food diet done haphazardly can be harmful to one's health, and this will be elaborated on in later chapters.

There are also many other important aspects to health not to be overlooked. Over many years, I've learned focusing on food alone is not sufficient. Time outdoors each day, a relaxed positive attitude, plenty of exercise and enough sleep should also be top priorities in a healthy lifestyle.

I am so grateful to be able to present the information in this book which I believe will best benefit your growing children. I have included what I have studied and learned from mentors, research and many years of experience. I have also asked others to contribute articles with valuable information about raising healthy children. And I am so excited about the section on raw family journeys. These are all people whom I contacted and questioned, asking them to include their special stories imparting their life experiences.

This is a book about consciousness, about raising our awareness of our surroundings. With intent and mindfulness, we can nurture our children through feeding them fresh plant foods drawn from the earth and treat them with the ultimate respect they deserve as human beings—our only hope for the future, so they can grow up to be strong, secure, and aware individuals.

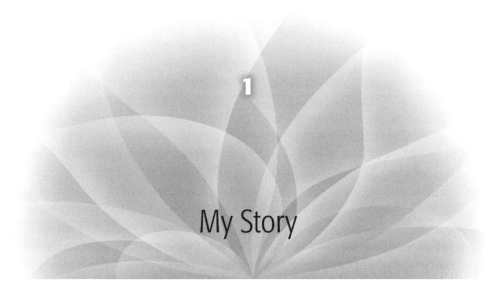

My Story

"Incomparable is the joy that Man finds in this world of a thousand wonders when he lives in communion with Nature."

<small>ZOROASTER (THE GREEK NAME FOR THE PROPHET ZARATHUSHTRA)</small>

I was brought up in a family with my vegetarian father, Sol, and my mother, Naomi, who ate the animal foods so popular in the 1950s and 60s. My paternal grandmother, Celia, who often lived with us, was a vegetarian who believed in and practiced Natural Hygiene and the raw food diet. In the 1920s while in her early thirties, she was extremely ill, suffering from severe asthma and emphysema. She was hospitalized, and the doctors gave her six months to live. There were no medical cures for asthma and emphysema at that time. A brother of hers wrote to her from Michigan, advising her to become a vegetarian and gradually to move toward a raw food diet. She was able to get Professor Arnold Ehret's *The Mucusless Diet Healing System* and one of Dr. Herbert Shelton's early health and nutrition books, and began her journey to a healthier life. Grandma Celia shocked her doctors and lived another forty-five years.

My mother had promised my father to raise my sister and me as vegetarians, but because of her beliefs in the standard diet on which she was raised, she gave us meat when my father wasn't home. She had been raised on a high protein animal food diet and was afraid her daughters would risk deficiencies without meat. My father was disappointed and upset when he found out, but my sister and I continued on the S.A.D. (standard American diet). I remember being frequently ill as a child and often taking medication. I also remember giving the pediatrician a very difficult time while he was administering the vaccinations to

1

me in his office, so he came to our home and chased me around until he and my mother could pin me down and he could jab me with the needle.

I recall the many arguments about food and medicine between my mother and grandmother. My grandmother would talk with me privately, telling me how important it is to eat fruits and vegetables, and how we as humans are not meant to eat animals or anything that came from them. Grandma told me, "Medicine will only hurt you and will not cure any ailment or disease." She sometimes spoke in more detail, but I, unfortunately, ignored and forgot most of what she said. My grandmother, and even my father, seemed fanatic and eccentric to me when I was eight or nine because they ate differently, never went to doctors or used medications, and had unique thoughts and opinions about how the body worked. And they had a respect for animals and Nature no one else seemed to have! They felt strongly about our relationships with the other creatures sharing this world, and this love has always remained strong in my heart. The following poem was written by my grandmother, Celia Horowitz, early in the twentieth century:

> Will the world ever efface the stain
> Caused by the blood of animals slain?
>
> World progress is apt to reach a stage
> When a slaughterhouse will be an outrage.
>
> Oh 'man' whenever the blood of animals you spill
> Remember the commandment of "Do Not Kill."
> Unthinking man discard that horrid knife
> With which you take for food a creature's life.
>
> Juvenile delinquency would be easier to erase
> If parents would learn how their children to raise.
>
> Vegetables and fruits are the food for man
> Carcasses of animals shorten the life span.
> The nutritional value of natural food
> Will keep one healthy, and it tastes so good.
>
> If humanity would only adapt a code
> Of "Do Not Kill, and Shed No Blood,"
> Then, fear of war would entirely cease
> And the world would enjoy everlasting peace.

Kindness and friendliness should be ordinary
Gestures of human behavior.

If nutritional ways you earnestly seek,
Just read the following lines with care —

Good food
Good activity
Good air
Good water
Good sun.

Grandmother Celia wrote a book of quotes and poems, many of them pertaining to health. Here are several of her quotes:

"Health depends upon proper nutrition for the body and mind."

"Broad-mindedness; a person who is broad-minded possesses a capacity of vision and understanding. Most of the time, he arrives at right conclusions. He thinks deeply and constructively about all matters confronting him and the world. He reaps a mental harvest to his satisfaction."

"Health-mindedness; a person who practices health-mindedness nourishes his body and mind with proper nutrients. He selects natural foods, fruits and vegetables (excluding animal foods) for his diet. He is always interested in health-knowledge and also in any knowledge that leads to progress."

"Miracle medicine keeps on changing almost as frequently as ladies' fashions."

"Anxiety produces a destructive influence upon the physical, mental and spiritual states of human beings."

"The process of cooking destroys many a natural nutrient, so essential for health and wellbeing."

"People nowadays do not die natural deaths; they kill themselves by refusing to abide by the laws of nature and health."

"If health is your constant companion, this companionship will make you immune to innumerable diseases that plague the present-day world."

"Health, strength and eternal truth
Are the embodiment of nature's way.
Anyone who bears nature's torch
Is the greatest martyr of today."

"Love and truth are two of the greatest and highest realities in existence.
Within their framework the force of divine power revolves."

I give gratitude to my grandmother, Celia, and my father, Sol Horowitz,
for providing me with these truths which created my passion for the healthy
lifestyle, and for this very religious connection I feel toward Mother Nature. My
grandmother wrote the following little poem for me on my third birthday:

Greetings, greetings, Karen dear,
On your birthday of your third year.
May happiness be your guiding light,
Making your life gay and bright.
Should you chance to walk on Nature's road,
Health and strength will be your reward.
All in all, have a joyful day,
And continue to bloom like a flower in May.

Your loving grandma,
Celia Horowitz

My father taught my sister Barbara and me to carry even the tiniest of creatures outside without harming them. I grew up with this respect, or *Ahimsa*,
the ancient Sanskrit word for not to harm, for all of Nature. My father would
sit outside in the backyard for hours observing and feeding the squirrels. I
have never seen squirrels so trusting of a human being as they were of him.
They sat next to my dad, eating directly from his hand. Animals just seemed to
know my dad was a vegetarian, a deeply spiritual person who always believed
in the interconnectedness of all creatures on this planet.

At age 17, it suddenly hit me that I also believe in this interconnectedness
of all creatures, and yet I was consuming animals. I became a vegetarian because
of my growing moral convictions we as humans did not have a right to kill and
eat other creatures. Although I was certainly saving animals by becoming a
vegetarian, I was not interested in achieving superior health, and lived mainly
on a junk food vegetarian diet which consisted mostly of processed and refined
foods. Throughout my teenage years and even later, I was laden with physical

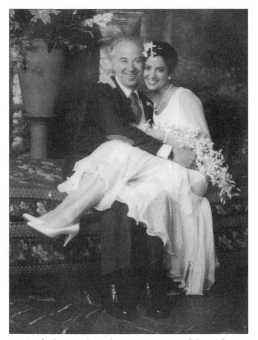

My father Sol and me on my wedding day, June 28, 1986

problems: cystic acne, gynecological problems, indigestion, Candida, chest pains. When I visited dermatologists and asked if food could be causing my skin disorder, I was told I could eat whatever I wanted, and my problems were totally unrelated to food. They even said I could eat as much refined chocolate as I desired and it would have no effect on my skin. I endured painful hydrocortisone shots in my face and very toxic medications (such as a dangerous drug called accutane) for twenty years. Later when I became a raw foodist, those twenty years of aggravating, painful skin eruptions were completely relieved within a few months. Then I remember thinking how those particular doctors didn't understand how the body works.

In my twenties, I became an animal rights activist, and participated in hundreds of demonstrations against the leg-hold trap, animal experimentation in laboratories, the fur industry, and the fast food industry. The moral aspect of vegetarianism, my love of animals, was very important to me. It wasn't until after my mother died in 1980 that I began to have some interest in the health aspect of vegetarianism. Through my pain at having lost her at an age when she still had so much more to live for, I began to go over her life in my mind and her decisions which led to her death.

My mother died when I was just out of college, in my early twenties. She believed in a doctor, a gynecologist, who convinced her she would feel young again if she had a hysterectomy. She decided to listen to this advice when at the same time my father was telling her not to get a "major operation for minor symptoms"—she couldn't keep up with him when they went for walks because her bladder had dropped, so a hysterectomy was the wrong operation anyway. She decided to listen to the doctor and go through with the hysterectomy. There were complications during the hysterectomy, and my mother became a complete invalid, having to go to a convalescent home after the hospital. The impact of the surgery caused a heart attack soon after, and within another six months my mom died. I feel sure her heart was weakened by her SAD diet, and the operation then triggered the heart attack. When we brought her home, the hospital reported they could no longer help her, that only 18% of her heart was operating. During the six months that followed, I watched my mother suffer terribly while hallucinating on the many drugs she was taking.

I still feel pain when I remember one of the last things she said to my dad before she died was she wished she had taken his advice and not had the surgery, and also wished she had been a vegetarian. Since my mother was a survivor of the Holocaust and had already endured such difficult times, I was in a state of denial and depression which I later realized was because of my feelings her life was cut off so undeservedly.

It wasn't until many years later that I became interested in achieving good health, and this desire was sparked by the pregnancy with my first child, Gabriela. Before giving birth to this beautiful little girl, I had planned to work full time and have someone else care for my child during the day. I am thankful I fell so deeply in love with Gabriela, I listened to my maternal instincts about wanting to be present for her and raise her myself.

While pregnant with Gabriela, I began to study vegetarian cooking and nutrition at the Natural Gourmet Cookery School in New York City. During that first pregnancy and for a short while after Gabriela's birth, I continued to eat dairy and eggs. I ate a lot of processed food, and thought if I bought organic processed food at the health food store, it would be good for me. I didn't realize not all the food at the health food store creates health. Gabriela had colic and got frequent colds and coughs. As an infant, she woke up irritably in the middle of the night, sometimes needing to be carried and rocked for a couple of hours before settling down again. I wonder now if the food I was eating had made my breast milk difficult to digest, causing the colic and fussy behavior. Just before my second pregnancy, I became a vegan and gave up all animal products. I continued with cooking classes, practicing a predominantly macrobiotic diet consisting of whole grains and beans, tofu, cooked vegetables, oils and seaweed, also still including some whole grain pasta, whole grain breads and rice cakes. I thought I was eating so healthfully until my second child, Marco, was born. I had gained 35 pounds during my second pregnancy, and Marco was born at 8 lb. 14 oz. When I gave birth to him, he presented with shoulder distosia, as his head was out but his shoulders could not be released. As a result, I was given an episiotomy, and the midwife panicked in birthing him. Had I only studied about healthy live food nutrition during pregnancy, I would have learned that to insure a speedy, safe, and smooth delivery, the mother should not gain an excess of pounds, and a lighter infant weight is desirable for an easier childbirth.

At five weeks, Marco was so sick with mucus and croup, we were admitted to a hospital in New York City. He had excessive mucus and respiratory difficulty, and I was too frightened and confused to try handling it at home. Marco slept in an oxygen tent at the hospital and cried for me, but the doctors refused to let me nurse him. The only thing that relaxed him slightly was placing my thumb in his mouth. I wanted to get into the bed with him, but I was not allowed. Marco had so much mucus, he came very close to death in the hospital, and I felt lucky to bring him home after four days. But the next three years were a nightmare, as Marco developed chronic allergic rhinitis which resulted in constant ear and throat infections and asthmatic symptoms involving difficulty breathing and wheezing. After three years of frantically running to allopathic and alternative physicians (pediatricians, family physicians, allergists, naturopaths, osteopaths, homeopaths, chiropractors, Chinese herbal medicine doctors, etc.), I felt frustrated, stuck and very frightened for my child. At night, we would frequently run to the shower to give Marco relief from his difficulty in breathing. I would sleep with him on top of me as I was afraid of losing him at night. I tried food elimination diets to determine a dietary cause, but the respiratory problems continued. I had started feeding Marco solids later in his first year—banana, sweet potatoes, and whole grains, but then discontinued solids for a while because of his illness. At this difficult time in our lives, I reflected on my own past and thought about my grandmother Celia, about her talks with me concerning health, medicine, and natural foods. It seemed clear to me that I needed to search for people who were living a raw foods lifestyle to see if this could heal my son. I eventually found a woman in Connecticut named Jo Willard, who had a radio show and wrote a quarterly journal called Natural Hygiene Inc. I traveled to Stamford, Connecticut for seminars by Dr. Scott of Ohio and a doctor of optometry who believed in the raw food diet. This led me to a raw food support group in New York City called COHR (Coalition for Health Re-Education), founded by Matthew Grace. This group became a strong support for me. I attended every Monday evening to receive information and support to practice the raw food diet at home.

I transitioned my children to a mostly raw diet (close to 100%—they ate cooked vegan food occasionally on the weekend with their father or at New York EarthSave events we attended), and within a year my son Marco was healed of all the ear and throat infections, allergies and asthmatic symptoms.

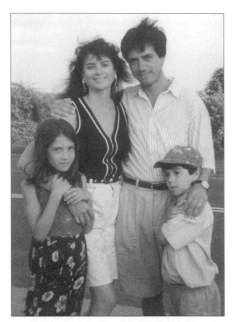

Gabriela, Karen, Harvey and Marco Ranzi in Montauk, Long Island, 1996

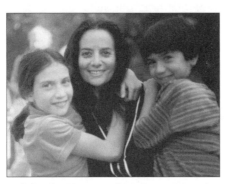

Gabriela, Karen and Marco on Marco's birthday, May 3, 1998

The experience of his healing was astonishing to me, that the painful chronic ear infections my child endured had dramatically come to a halt in under a year's time. At that time, I regretted I hadn't learned about the benefits of live foods even earlier, as I recalled the agony the ear infections, allergies and respiratory problems had caused. When he had been tested for allergies, the tests revealed he was allergic to most foods, all pollens and weeds and all animal hair. I was informed he could not have an animal in the house. When we switched to eating fresh, natural, vegan foods, Marco's allergies completely disappeared. He was no longer allergic to animal hair (we got a dog and a rabbit) or pollens of any kind. Because he was not eating wheat or dairy (the casein in dairy and the high gluten in wheat are the worst hindrances to digestion), and was eating simple, digestible uncooked fruits and vegetables instead, his body was cleansing and healing. I felt an amazing revelation and sense of personal empowerment when I discovered I no longer had to depend on running constantly to doctors, and could actually create health in my children with my own knowledge.

Much later, Dr. Timothy Trader told me people are allergic to protein, either in food or in airborne particles, and an allergic attack is very dangerous, similar to going into anaphylactic shock. The change in diet eased Marco's burden and allowed his body to heal. Because of the change in nutrition, his internal body was stronger and capable of dealing better with the pollen and other outside forms of allergens. I learned so clearly from our experience that when the internal body is clean, infection is avoided. I haven't had the flu or other illness for many years. Others living on natural fresh foods have the same experience. The real cause of infections is not germs. Instead, it is because of an internally unclean body. Our children played together with ill children but never "caught" their sicknesses.

Unfortunately, I feel when my infant son was in the hospital for asthmatic complications, the Dexatron in the IV caused the decay and deformity of his primary teeth. A pediatrician later expressed antibiotics and drugs in infancy can cause this problem, and it may have been my processed food consumption during pregnancy that exacerbated it. Two years following Marco's transition to fresh fruits and vegetables, his permanent teeth came in fine.

I nursed Gabriela for four and a half years and nursed Marco for six years. I had read and heard that breastfeeding protects children from allergies and all sorts of other problems. I learned differently for myself, as I feel my son was not able to digest the components of my former diet given to him in my milk. I totally believe breastfeeding is one of the most wonderful gifts a mother can give her child, both for nutrients and for emotional bonding. However, I know now the food the mother eats while pregnant and nursing can have a positive or negative effect on the child's wellbeing.

The benefits I personally received from the change of diet included the complete cure of my lifelong acne condition, improved digestion, the end of gynecological problems, and my Candida symptoms vanished. My skin now felt soft and smooth, and the pimples I tried to cover up for so many years were gone after only three months on raw foods, and never returned again. My menstrual cycle which had always been extremely erratic suddenly became like clockwork, every 28 days. I no longer experienced painful cramps and heavy blood flow. I actually began to enjoy getting my monthly period, which began each month without any discomfort and lasted only a few days. The fatigue I used to experience every day by 5 p.m. was replaced by energy and a zest for life. Recently, when I entered the menopause years, I experienced none of the traditional symptoms. After I stopped eating at 5 p.m., I began to sleep extremely well at night.

One horrible negative experience we did suffer involved dental problems from eating too much dried fruit when we switched diets, not realizing how they very quickly wreak havoc on the teeth. Dried fruit is very sticky on the teeth. Much of the packaged dried fruit found in supermarkets and health food stores is cooked. Pitted dates are often machine pitted and then steamed. In order to be packaged, they need to be dried. There are a few reputable companies, such as The Date People, that have truly raw dates which are not dried. Organic dates with pits that come in bulk are often uncooked. Nevertheless, brush your teeth after eating them! They can be minimally used in smoothies and sauces, but stay away from eating dried fruit by itself. (Dehydrated tomatoes actually become less acid-forming as their water comes out with some of the hydrogen ions.)

Gabriela and Marco often came with me when I led "Accent on Wellness" meetings in New York City. Gabriela wrote "Raw Rules" all over the board. We (Gabriela, Marco and I) were interviewed by author and television host Matthew Grace on the Manhattan Cable TV show "Accent on Wellness" about our diet, the benefits and difficulties (which for us were the social pressures). The children and I created many beautiful raw food dishes together and raised two raw food dogs, one of which recovered from severe hip dysplasia through the raw food diet. We attended raw food potlucks in New York City and got the support of many others who were following the diet because they believed it led to improved health, a better world environment, and a more peaceful state of mind. It did come with its pressures and difficulties for the children later on, and I'll discuss this later in the book. Some raw food families have been able to avoid or limit these pressures and difficulties.

As children, Gabriela and Marco loved preparing raw food meals together at home. They often prepared these healthy meals in their "raw food restaurant," creating their own menus, and my husband and I were the customers who ordered and bought their creative dishes.

We were filmed by a crew of producers and cameramen for television's "Nickelodeon Kids' News" in February 2000, as the children prepared a raw meal. The raw food diet was not discussed on the program, but our family was obviously eating differently from the other vegetarian family interviewed for the segment. They were lacto-ovo vegetarians, eating dairy (cheese lasagna for dinner) and eggs. Marco and Gabriela were creating a raw food menu (avocado boats stuffed with avocado and tomato, and a layered cashew and tomato dish)—all viewed nationally! The producers and camera crew were all extremely inquisitive about our raw food diet.

Over the years of embracing a raw food diet, some people have called me a "fanatic," telling me I should eat cooked foods in moderation, and I should relax and be less disciplined about my diet. The truth for me is I am convinced fresh foods provide optimum nourishment, and I lost my cravings for cooked foods many years ago. Therefore, moderation makes no sense to me. It's really very simple and relaxing to live this way and takes no discipline at all. However, it's important to do the raw food diet properly, or it can cause health problems just as does the standard diet. During the first years of a raw food diet, I ate excessive amounts of nuts, seeds and avocados, thinking as long as it was raw food, I would be fine. However, in the light of research by vegan doctors, Dr. Joel Fuhrman, Dr. John McDougall, Dr. T. Colin Campbell and Dr. Neal Barnard, I understood that to avoid health problems, the vegan diet should be low in fat. The low fat vegan diet could easily be applied to fresh raw vegan foods, focusing on lower consumption of nuts, seeds and avocados.

Many life experiences have led me to studying, researching, and participating in numerous seminars with mentors in the field of raw food nutrition since 1994. During these years, I have improved my raw vegan diet to what feels the most health giving while providing me with the most energy.

In the years after I became a raw foodist, I brought my food with me wherever I went. As I was thrilled with my delicious food, many people asked questions and some of them also turned to raw foods for health and healing. The following is an article I wrote for *Living Nutrition Magazine*, Volume 13, Page 9, (2002) titled "Discovery":

"Since I became a raw foodist nine years ago, I have seen many changes in my life. I homeschool my children in Bergen County, New Jersey, and we are part of a homeschool support network called Tri-County Homeschoolers. We get together frequently with other homeschool families for classes, projects, field trips, and socializing. In the past several years, I have enjoyed wonderful relationships with many of these open-minded people, and I feel my example and my willingness to answer various questions about health and nutrition, has led a number of my friends to the raw food lifestyle. Many of them had already been vegetarian, but felt becoming a raw food vegan was too much of a stretch for them.

Initially, friends looked at me strangely when I showed up with my own food, either fruit or salad, at our get-togethers. Some of them even called me a 'fanatic.' But over time, their curiosity was sparked, prompting them to inquire about the benefits of my lifestyle. They wanted to know how this simple way of living could help them in their own lives. They shared their problems with me: obesity, chronic fatigue, frequent colds, high blood pressure, skin and respiratory problems, and allergies. I did not want to advise them unless they were truly receptive to the information.

As time went on, some of the exotic and more unfamiliar fruits, such as cherimoya or white sapote, also caught their interest. They would ask such questions as 'What is this funny-looking fruit you're eating, and does it taste good?' I would offer them a piece, letting them discover the deliciousness of such fruits.

After several years, some of these friends have become raw foodists and are enjoying the numerous benefits this diet provides. It is so nice to have a gathering where raw foods are plentiful.

When my father became ill a few years ago, he approached me with the idea of trying a raw food diet as an alternative, in the hope it would help his condition. At the time, he had a severe life-threatening respiratory problem. He had been vegetarian for most of his life, 79 years, but was not eating mostly raw foods. When he switched to raw foods during his illness, he saw a remarkable improvement. Then a few years later, prompted by a diagnosis of glaucoma, he was close to a 100 percent raw food diet for several months. It seems the raw food lifestyle helped to reduce the pressure in both eyes, and he was able to avoid the medication. His opthalmologist was amazed and called him 'the miracle man.' Most of the time, my father ate raw foods during the day and a steamed potato and vegetables for dinner.

It is amazing to me that my dad, whom I always looked up to for his opinions, was now calling me whenever he had questions related to nutrition and healing. I've come to realize just how powerful is the example of one sincerely pursuing the natural, healthy way of life."

In the end, however, my father died in an opposite way from how he lived his life. In January of 2005, he had a seizure during which he broke his hip. We were unsure of what caused the seizure. Following the hip operation, my father was very weak. He was having problems with urination as well. Upon my suggestion, he worked with Dr. Timothy Trader, N.D., Ph.D. who tried to guide him toward a temporary diet of melons, water and green juices. My father immediately began to gain more energy, and was improving during the three weeks he stuck with this program. Then Dr. Trader attempted to get him off one of the medications he was taking, a leading brand medication to facilitate urine flow. His legs swelled in reaction to the medication circulating in his bloodstream. A family member panicked at this reaction and decided he should return to the hospital. I was amazed when my father went along with the decision to go back to the hospital, and made it clear to me that I shouldn't say anything further. Because of the love I have for my family and the choice I made to respect my father's decisions, I accepted that they weren't willing to listen to my suggestions at this point. At the hospital, his blood was taken, and a high white blood cell count was observed. From what I have learned about the human body, the white blood cell count increases when the body is encountering foreign invaders. My father had anesthetics and other medications to which he was not accustomed in his system. At the hospital, they decided this increased white blood cell count might be walking pneumonia, so they put him on intravenous antibiotics for pneumonia. My husband Harvey and I watched in horror as the nurses brought cough medicine into my dad's room when he didn't have the slightest hint of a cough or any congestion at all in his lungs. We asked them to leave, and we told my dad we didn't feel he had pneumonia. Although he had always used natural methods of healing, my dad had decided to go the medical route now and did not want to hear my views. I felt completely helpless as I watched the pneumonia antibiotics lead to a stomach infection which turned into colitis. Then fear tactics were employed as my father was told he would die if he didn't take an extremely powerful antibiotic for the colitis. I knew very well it would be the drug that would kill him. He was talked into taking that terrible drug, which led to blood clots in the legs, and then my father's body shut down. He was literally paralyzed from his chest down. At that point, the doctors and the hospital told him there was no longer anything they could do to help him. My father was so depressed he didn't want to live any more, so hospice was brought in to help him to prepare for death. I had never heard anything like this before. A person who is still quite alive and should be focusing on doing everything possible to make progress is now being talked into how to die. I was grief-stricken and shocked, as my husband and I were trying to fight to save my dad's life. As soon as he got home, I pushed for dad to work with Dr. Trader again. Dr. Trader had not given up on him and felt he could still make progress, but it would take much longer after all the medication he had been under, maybe six months to a year or longer. This time as there was nothing else medically to try, I got the support from my family to fly Dr. Trader in from California. However, when he arrived, my dad was so weak and so unmotivated that he was unwilling to try any more. He did not follow Dr. Trader's recommendations. He was becoming very dehydrated, and did not follow instructions to drink significant amounts of water. He deteriorated rapidly in the next couple of months, and died on August 2, 2005.

I later learned from author and lecturer Tonya Zavasta about the catastrophic result that can occur if a vegan takes the drug Coumadin, a drug prescribed for my father (who was vegan) to prevent blood clotting. The following warning is printed in Tonya Zavasta's book, *Your Right To Be Beautiful*:

> Warning! Coumadin (warfarin) is a drug often prescribed after surgery to prevent blood clotting. The raw food diet includes a number of leafy green vegetables (broccoli, Brussel sprouts, kale, and cabbage) which are high in Vitamin K. This vitamin assists blood coagulation and stops bleeding naturally. According to The People's Guide to Deadly Drug Interactions, Coumadin can interact with a diet abundant in these vegetables with

deadly results. Not all surgeons are aware of this situation, so be sure to bring it to your doctor's attention if you must have surgery while on any vegan diet.

If the dosage of drugs doctors routinely prescribe for the average person is given to patients on a clean vegan diet, the results could be disastrous.

The unnecessary death of my father Sol, a man who respected all of life, was a great loss to me. A saying by Albert Schweitzer reminds me of how my dad lived; it was engraved on his gravestone:

By respect for life, we become religious in a way that is elementary, profound and alive.

I lost both my mother and my father to operations and medications—the third greatest cause of death in the United States after heart disease and cancer. It's called iatrogenic disease—induced unintentionally by the medical treatment of a physician. Never in my life would I have thought my father would die in this way. It fuels my passion even more to help people understand the simple truth about health and healing.

My tragic family experiences have taught me to take charge of my own health, and to help others to heal naturally and to manifest health in their own lives.

Following the years of looking at natural solutions to many of life's problems, researching nontoxic answers, our daughter Gabriela has embraced the concept by pursuing her passion for helping the Earth through environmentalism. She was chosen for an internship called "Change It," working with the directors of Greenpeace and Seventh Generation in Washington, D.C. The "Change It" program involved teens passionate about changing the world through environmental leadership. Now in college, Gabriela is majoring in Global Environmental Studies because she wants to do meaningful work to improve her world.

My children have grown up with very important information on how to live their lives to the fullest potential, if they so choose. Although as teenager and young adult, they experience the everyday pressures to conform and have sometimes chosen to, they know the difference between foods that harm the body and foods that nourish.

—Karen Ranzi
www.SuperHealthyChildren.com

2

The Health of Mother and Father
Prior to Conception

"If you want to have an effective, loving experience of family, you must learn to be patient and to not let the little things drive you crazy."

DR. RICHARD CARLSON AND KRISTINE CARLSON,
AUTHORS OF *DON'T SWEAT THE SMALL STUFF*

The health of the mother and father prior to conception is of utmost importance and is truly connected with the health of the child-to-be. Although we've all inherited genes from our ancestors who may have eaten depleted, enzyme-deficient foods, we have the power to make major changes for future generations by embarking on a path to a more natural way of living. If family members have died of cancer, heart disease and other illnesses, we often fear the illness is hereditary, but this does not have to be so. What we eat and how we live our lives can have a huge impact on our health and the health of generations to come. Ideally, both future parents should be eating mainly raw vegan foods. According to how much our bodies have adapted to unhealthy habits, it can take weeks, months, or years of eating more healthful foods to feel the true benefits.

After aspiring mothers and fathers have enjoyed at least three months on raw foods, a brief period of fasting would be beneficial. This fast should ideally take place at least a few months prior to conception. When fasting on water alone for more than a few days, I recommend a visit to one of the many fasting retreats or fasting directors in the United States or abroad (See pages 429 to 430). Supervision is crucial when doing a fast for longer than three days. I don't recommend doing lengthy water fasts without supervision because every individual has a different history, and it would be important to benefit from the expertise of an experienced fasting supervisor to avoid problems that may arise. Fasting on water is a way to regain health, detoxifying old unhealthy debris from the cells. When the body is not busy digesting food, its energy can be used for healing. Adequate rest and sleep during water fasts are imperative.

I went to a wellness center in Maryland for a two week water fast in April of 2004. I had thought my two week fast would be a totally relaxing vacation since I had gone on several water fasts for periods of 3 to 7 days (although I continued many of my daily activities during these fasts), and I was a raw foodist for over ten years at the time of the fast. It turned out my prediction was incorrect. Since I decided to get as much bed rest as possible, I went into a very deep phase of fasting. I felt nauseated for the entire fast, my head pounded every night, and I lost 22 pounds during the two weeks. I was extremely weak and slept only one of the thirteen nights. I also tasted old medicine on my tongue during this fast. I had thought after being on a raw food diet, my body would have already detoxified old medicines. Now I believe as long as we are eating solid foods, we cannot completely detoxify from previous medicines or the long-term consumption of unhealthful foods.

After the two week long water fast, an unexpected benefit came powerfully to my attention: it was no longer possible to bite my fingernails. Compared to the soft, pliable, easily broken fingernails I used to bite since childhood, I was now enjoying their transformation into strong, hard, healthy nails.

When the body is not digesting solid foods, its energy can be used for healing; and when digestion is made easier by juicing or blending leafy green vegetables, healing is further facilitated. This is why I recommend potential parents embark on a supervised fast or period of green juicing or blending for at least a couple of weeks prior to conception. A week or two of drinking only water and green juices would give the digestive system a much-needed rest. There are green juice cleansing retreats in many locations in the United States and abroad, listed on pages 429 to 430.

The accumulation of heavy metals is a serious problem for followers of the standard diet, particularly if animal foods, especially fish, had been eaten. Victoria Boutenko has discovered regular consumption of green smoothies that liquefy the greens into their most absorbable form helps to eliminate the accumulation of heavy metals.

Both parents-to-be should secure sufficient sleep to maintain health. Recent research links lack of sleep to health problems like obesity, diabetes, the common cold, and even cancer. Lack of sufficient sleep may spoil a person's chances for a long and healthy life (read the article "Sleeplessness in America," by Susan Brink, in U.S. News & World Report, October 16, 2000). In an article, "Sleep Your Way to Health," in Living Nutrition Magazine, Volume 13, 2002, Professor Rozalind Gruben-Graham points out, "During sleep, a recharging takes place of our low voltage electrical current, known as nerve energy. This is the energy upon which the nervous system depends in order to function. There is also an acceleration of healing and repair, known collectively as anabolic processes. Other vital processes that are accelerated during sleep include detoxification and elimination. Any symptoms of bodily distress indicate the need to minimize energy expenditure and maximize sleep."

At a time when a woman wants to conceive and enjoy a healthy pregnancy, restful and reenergizing sleep is as important as eating raw vegan foods and getting adequate exercise. I have found it is important not to eat anything for at least four hours prior to going to sleep for the night. On the nights when I have eaten anything close to bedtime, I often don't sleep as well because my body is focusing on digestion instead of sleep. And this can result in the need to get up to go to the bathroom one or more times, also disrupting the sleep cycle. When eating late in the evening, the body will focus on digestion all night. Most of the body's energy will be used for digestion, and in the morning one is tired and lacking energy. For the best quality sleep, go to bed as early as you can before midnight.

Of major importance for parents choosing to have a raw pregnancy, homebirth and raising children in the raw foods lifestyle is spousal support. A relaxed, happy and supportive relationship is one of the most important aspects to a successful pregnancy and childbirth, and to a happy and healthy family life. The father's care has a great influence on the mother's wellbeing. When parents differ in their belief systems in these areas, it creates a huge stress factor and much anxiety. It is crucial that parents-to-be discuss their plans for pregnancy, childbirth and raising children so both are on the same page in these areas. Fathers, who help in preparing meals, and show care for mother and baby, help to create a healthy family. The maternal instinct is very strong, and mothers who are respected in their attachment to their babies will feel happy, relaxed and loved. Many men in our contemporary culture expect women to go back to work soon after birthing. Women who stay home to raise their children are often looked upon as "doing nothing" because they're not contributing to the family income. Men who decide to set their priorities toward the happiness of wife and children, supporting the mother's instinct to remain close to her children as they grow, will enjoy the close relationships attachment parenting brings. In order to have a loving family experience, patience and understanding on the part of both parents are paramount. Parents who focus on the small details of life, such as a messy house, will deny their families a loving, calm and relaxing environment that is so important to the health and security of growing children.

As children grow into communicative beings, it's important to include them in family meetings to discuss their views and respect their opinions in family decisions. Mealtimes should be occasions for enjoyment and relaxation with little or no talk so food can be properly chewed and digested. Emotionally charged topics should not be initiated at mealtime, and if children are playing and not hungry, they should not be coerced to the table. There are plenty of opportunities for family bonding outside of mealtimes. The happiness of the family as a whole should take priority, and most especially, the needs of the children. Before conception, the parents need to be in agreement concerning their children's nutritional needs. Their objectives for raising a family with a non-coercive lifestyle must also be taken into consideration.

Smoking, alcohol, drugs, caffeinated products, and refined foods will all create risks during pregnancy, birth and afterwards, so it's best to eliminate these toxic, albeit well-advertised products, long before pregnancy. Smoking has been linked to infertility, erectile dysfunction and impotence. Even second-hand smoke can do tremendous physical damage. Smoking cigarettes kills more than a million people every year. For further information on all of these poisonous products, refer to books *The McDougall Program for Women* by Dr. John McDougall and *Disease-Proof Your Child* by Dr. Joel Fuhrman.

Good health is the most important element for a successful childbirth. Foods which digest quickly are best—fresh foods are supreme, particularly fruits and green leafy vegetables. The human body needs bio-active water, amino acids, glucose, enzymes and chlorophyll, which can be supplied most adequately in a diet of fresh fruits and vegetables, and some soaked and/or sprouted nuts and seeds. Fruits provide us with fuel for energy while green leafy vegetables supply us with an abundance of minerals, especially calcium. Cooked food is toxic, therefore it is stimulating, and this stimulation wears out the adrenal glands. On a raw food diet, the adrenal glands get the rest they need in order to function well. Only unheated foods contain enzymes which aid digestion. In his book, *Enzyme Nutrition*, Dr. Edward Howell discusses the negative effect heat has on enzyme activity, revealing the body then has to use up its own digestive enzymes.

Many vegan women have told me they feel it's important to consume legumes, especially during pregnancy. When I ate cooked beans many years ago, I was frequently gassy and constipated. I sometimes took Beano, a digestive aid to help with these problems. Since switching to raw foods, occasionally I've eaten a small amount of soaked and sprouted lentils or mung beans with leafy green salads, and these problems didn't occur. In his book, *Eating for Beauty*, author and superfood proponent David Wolfe reveals: "The Pythagoreans, like the Egyptians who preceded them, abstained from eating beans. They held beans to be unclean. Beans (legumes) contain course, irritating proteins that cause inflammation. Beans (including peanuts) naturally contain a host of alkaloid toxins. These protect the beans from animals that would eat them in the wild. Several of these compounds are toxic cyanogens, such as cyanide."

Soybeans, especially the fake meats, can cause thyroid problems as well as significant problems with women's hormones. According to author and lecturer Paul Nison, "There is evidence soy can be a factor in causing breast and ovarian cancer in women because of the high amount of estrogen found in soy products. In men, it can lead to problems with sperm count." In his book, *Rainbow Green Live-Food Cuisine*, Gabriel Cousens, M.D. gives five reasons for not recommending soy products as food for mother or baby:

1. Soy is Kaphagenic—damp and cold;
2. Soy has an excess of copper, manganese, aluminum and estrogen;
3. Because 70% of soy is genetically modified, it is one of the top ten allergenic foods;
4. Soy is not meant to be used as a regular food, as it is highly processed and denatured;
5. Soy is high in estrogen and may be hormonally unbalancing. This includes all soy products: tofu, tempeh, soybeans, miso, soy sauce, soy milk. Soy products have been linked with thyroid and prostrate problems.

Drs. Anna Maria and Brian Clement, directors of the Hippocrates Health Institute in West Palm Beach, Florida, comment on soy and soy products: "Its high estrogen levels further compound the environmental estrogens that the body uptakes, helping to expedite mutagenic concerns."

Current research studies present evidence that soy is unhealthful. After years of massive advertising in favor of soy products over cow milk, we are realizing from more recent research, the soy industry, like the dairy industry, has major commercial interests in the promotion of their products. The serious implications for eating food containing soy are evident in the article, "Newest Research on Why You Should Avoid Soy," by Sally Fallon and Mary G. Enig, Ph.D. (www.westonaprice.org). Here are excerpts from that valuable article:

> Soy can produce severe gastric distress, reduced protein digestion and chronic deficiencies in amino acid uptake. Soybeans are high in trypsin inhibitors, causing enlargement and pathological conditions of the pancreas, including cancer. Trypsin inhibitors are also known growth inhibitors, and when these antinutrient soy products were given to weanling rats, they failed to grow normally. The high phytate content of soy- and grain-based diets prevents the absorption of calcium, magnesium, iron and zinc, the soybean containing one of the highest phytate levels of any grain or legume studied, causing enlarged organs in test animals, particularly the pancreas and thyroid gland, and increased fatty acids in the liver.

> Nitrites, potent carcinogens, are formed during spray-drying, and a toxin called lysinoalanine is formed during alkaline processing. Numerous artificial flavorings, particularly MSG, are added to soy protein isolate and textured vegetable protein products to mask their 'beany' taste and to impart the flavor of meat.

> In 1996, researchers found women consuming soy protein isolate had increased incidences of epithelial hyperplasia, a condition that presages malignancies. A year later, dietary genistein was found to stimulate breast cells to enter the cell cycle—a discovery that led the study authors to conclude women should not consume soy products to prevent breast cancer.

> In vitro studies suggest that isoflavones in soy products inhibit synthesis of estradiol and other steroid hormones. Reproductive problems, infertility, thyroid disease and liver disease due to dietary intake of isoflavones have been observed in several species of animals.

> Scientists report infants fed soy formula, popular in the U.S., receive a huge amount of phytoestrogen compared to taking at least five birth control pills per day. Future patterns of sexual orientation may be influenced by the early hormonal environment. Learning disabilities, early puberty, and premature sexual development may

be linked to soy infant formula and soy products, later related to reproductive problems, infertility and breast cancer. Other problems of soy-based formulas reported by parents are: extreme emotional behavior, asthma, immune system problems, pituitary insufficiency, thyroid disorders and irritable bowel syndrome.

The following is other information from the Weston A. Price Foundation (www.westonaprice.org):

- Vitamin B12 analogs in soy are not absorbed and actually increase the body's requirement for B12.

- Soy foods increase the body's requirement for vitamin D.

- Soy foods contain high levels of aluminum, toxic to the nervous system and the kidneys.

If transitioning from cow milk, and still feeling the need for a replacement, it would be best to use rice milk, or even better, use live nut milk (such as almond milk), and avoid soy altogether.

Green leafy vegetables and small amounts of raw nuts and seeds provide sufficient quantities of minerals and vitamins as well as quality protein, without the problems of cooked beans—usually a big part of the vegan diet. I do recommend the quantities of nuts and seeds be limited from 1 to 4 ounces a day depending on the eater's size and degree of physical activity.

Ease of digestion is best, and raw food will make its way out of the body quickly. When my baby son was ill, my consumption of beans seemed to be a big part of the problem. When I ate beans during nursing, they caused him to have painful flatulence and mucus. Grains also contributed to these problems. The nutrients we need are made by eating plants in their most digestible form. Organic, ripe fruits and vegetables are digested with ease—the lighter you feel due to ease of digestion, the more energy you'll have.

After reading *Grain Damage* by Dr. Douglas Graham, I was clearly convinced grains had been a major culprit in my son's illness. A cooked vegan diet is morally responsible toward our animal friends and a step to reduce global warming. It's more healthful than diets containing growth hormones, antibiotics, and indigestible animal flesh, but it may still cause problems to our systems when consisting mainly of grains, beans and processed foods. *Grain Damage* is a must-read for anyone truly interested in achieving vibrant health and getting away from cooked grains permanently. Human beings didn't eat grains until as recently as 10,000 years ago with the beginning of agriculture. Their use became widespread 5,000 years ago. Grains are low in nutritional value and contain opiates which are addictive substances. They have little taste without the addition of salt and sauces. Although whole grains are certainly better than processed white grains, and can be used as the smaller percentage of a mostly raw food diet or in a transitional diet, I don't consider cooked or processed grains to be healthful. Those who do not wish to eat a totally raw food diet can still create a healthy alkaline/acid balance by keeping acid-forming foods such as whole grains to a smaller part of the diet.

Even whole grains, such as brown rice, are considered acid-forming, and white rice is still more acid-forming and toxic to the body than brown rice. Many reasons have been discovered to keep brown rice and other whole grains to a minimum percentage of the diet, if you are going to eat them. The following are some of the reasons: They cause mold and fungus; are acid-forming; are depleted of enzymes and minerals; they can become like glue in the body if they become a main food source; aren't water soluble; are processed by machinery; can be the cause of problems in the body such as Candida, chronic fatigue, parasites, gallstones, heart problems, and weight gain. They cannot be easily digested and assimilated. However, a vegan diet of fresh fruits, leafy greens and vegetables supplemented with cooked whole grains and lightly steamed vegetables can be a good dietary choice for those unable or unwilling to maintain a 100% raw vegan diet. This also provides a good transition, eating small amounts of these less harmful of the cooked foods in a predominantly raw diet.

Pasta and bread are two cooked starch addictions that are very difficult to give up. The reason for this is the chemical reaction to cooked starch in the body acts like a drug and has a sedative effect. I can recall many years ago eating a lot of cooked starches at dinner parties (potatoes, pasta, breads, etc.) and feeling extremely lethargic following the meal, sometimes having a difficult time getting up from the table. Some guests would fall asleep after eating this difficult-to-digest meal. How do you want to feel after you eat? Do you want to feel bloated and weighted down or do you desire to feel clear-headed and energetic? Does the way you eat coincide with the way you feel? Processed grains such as pasta, bread and chips can demineralize the bones. Minerals, such as calcium, cannot get properly absorbed into the bones on such a diet.

Complex carbohydrates will make you tired because of the digestive effort involved. They contain compounds which have a numbing effect similar to opium. Pasta, bread, potatoes and other complex carbohydrates require high temperatures to be broken down in order to be digested at all. Heating changes their molecular structure, and they ferment in the intestines. Alcohol and acetic acid are produced. A hyper or hypo thyroid condition can be the result of consuming heated complex carbohydrates. Over the years, the consumption of these complex carbohydrates can lead to many other health problems.

Not only do meat-eaters fall ill, vegetarians, vegans and raw foodists can also get sick. Many vegetarians and vegans consume too much starchy food (complex carbohydrates); processed starches are particularly problematic. The problems a raw foodist can develop are often due to poor food combining, improper acid/alkaline balance, lack of variety of foods and too much fat (such as are found in nuts and seeds). For more information on some of the dilemmas raw foodists can encounter, see the books *Your Natural Diet: Alive Raw Foods* by David Klein and T.C. Fry, *Raw Secrets* by Frederic Patenaude and other books in the Bibliography and Additional Resources.

When switching to a healthier raw food diet, a healing crisis often occurs. This healing crisis is necessary. Symptoms of a healing crisis can include: cold sores, mucus, rashes, bladder infections, diarrhea, fever, headache, running frequently to the bathroom, weakness, etc. In addition to consumption of toxic foods, we also inhale toxic chemicals into the body from paints, perfumes, cleaning detergents, lawn pesticides, and other pollutants. When I initially became a raw foodist in 1994, I developed a mouth filled with canker sores and a swollen tongue. This may have been my initial detoxification from a mostly cooked food diet, or it may have been a negative reaction to the significantly increased intake of acid-forming nuts and seeds in my diet during the transition to raw foods.

I believe the following "Thirty Prime Requisites of Glorious Health" by Dr. David Klein, from his book, *Your Natural Diet: Alive Raw Foods*, are absolutely essential for achieving optimal health. Couples planning for a beautiful, healthy and happy baby would do well to recognize and fulfill these concepts for themselves and their families:

1. Love of self
2. Healthy self image and esteem
3. Passionate love of all life
4. Awareness

5. Intention
6. Inner focus/listening
7. Abidance of the senses and intuition
8. True knowledge
9. Graceful, grateful, respectful, generous attitude
10. Organic, vegan, properly-combined alive raw food diet
11. Pure water
12. Pure air
13. Sunshine
14. Warm climate
15. Fitness and posture
16. Security and peace of mind
17. Rejuvenative rest and sleep
18. Heart-centered self nurturing
19. Sharing of love
20. Relaxation
21. Humor
22. Creative expression
23. Emotional flow and release
24. Rhythmic movement
25. Musical indulgence
26. Simple lifestyle
27. Communing with nature
28. Gardening
29. Service—Living your life's purpose
30. Engagement in self-improvement challenges

There are some people who can move from eating primarily cooked foods to eating fruit and leafy greens, and they do quite well. There are others who need to eat more greens while gradually adding fruit to the diet. I believe I experienced damage to my teeth from eating dried fruit, but also because even the fresh fruit I was eating was so detoxifying in a very acidic body. After years of medication, use of poisonous personal care products and abominable eating habits, my system was extremely acidic. The change to eating raw fruits, vegetables, nuts and seeds caused detoxification and oral acidity. I didn't want to continue eating cooked food because of its lifeless quality, but if I only knew then what I learned later, I would have eaten more greens initially and less fruit, listening to my body each step of the way. Each of us comes to the raw food lifestyle with a distinct individual history. We have to sift out the best information from books, experienced speakers, and those following similar paths in order to find our own unique way back to the natural diet. I personally have found, over time, fruit provides me with the most energy, and I also need to have plenty of fresh organic greens for the high mineral content. A close friend of mine became ill years ago. Her diet had consisted primarily of fruit, and sometimes she would eat melon for days. When she added a significant amount of green leafy vegetables and celery to her diet, she was able to heal. I also know of people who live in tropical climates who live largely on fruit and do well. Especially in the colder climates, we need significantly more greens because we don't get the amount of minerals we need from the imported fruit that never had the chance to ripen on the plant in the sun.

The food that makes up the American diet eventually causes premature death from infectious diseases, anemia, cancer, diabetes, mental illness, strokes, etc. Fire burns food, and destroys enzymes and nutrients.

It's very interesting to me that humans suffer from illnesses which animals in nature don't have. However, domestic animals develop diseases that are the same or similar to those of humans. We need to open our eyes and look at the world around us, and carefully observe how other animals raise their young. Living cells require raw nourishment with everything intact. If we are eating dead, toxic food, our lymph fluid is filled with poisons which will be stored in the cells. It makes sense, because our bodies are 72% water that we need to eat at least 70% water-rich foods if we want to be healthy. Most Americans eat only 5 to 10% water-rich fresh foods.

Our blood is meant to have a slightly alkaline pH, but cooked foods, with the exception of lightly steamed vegetables or vegetable broths, are acid-forming. Foods are either acid-forming (acidifying) or alkaline-forming (alkalizing) after they have been processed by the cells. Acid fruits, such as oranges, even though acidic, leave an alkaline ash once metabolized by the cells. When oranges are exposed to high temperatures, such as in Pasteurized orange juice, they lose their ability to form an alkaline ash, and remain acidic. We can only handle small amounts of acid-forming foods which acidify the body fluids. Dairy foods are high in sulfur and phosphorous which make them acid-forming. Dairy, grains (except millet), meat, refined sugars and nuts are high in the minerals which cause acidity. The body has to maintain a blood pH of about 7.3. When the body is stressed from too much acid-forming food, it resorts to leaching alkalizing elements such as calcium from the bones and teeth. To find out the pH of the saliva, pH paper can be used.

Fruit gives us the highest energy, the glucose we need to live active lives; and plenty of vegetables, especially greens, keep our blood at a healthfully alkaline pH. The most important nutrition for pregnancy exists in green leaves for their abundant minerals, and fresh fruit as the source for energy.

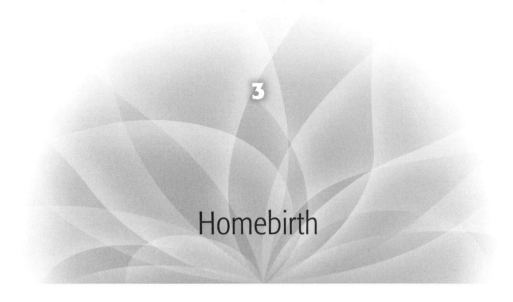

Homebirth

"Women of Earth, Take back your Birth."
LONNIE MORRIS, RN

*"One of the best ways to free a woman from institutional
constraints is to have a homebirth."*
ANONYMOUS

The parents should prepare for a homebirth. In the beginning of the twentieth century, hospital births were rare. If you decide to give birth at the hospital, you run a high risk of receiving medical intervention. Even midwives who assist in hospital births are more likely to revert to medical intervention than midwives who assist in homebirths. In your own home, you have control over what happens to mother and baby in the birth process and after. Your newborn does not have to be subjected to eye drops such as those containing dangerous silver nitrate. You will not be coaxed to use formula or sugar water. There will not be a vitamin K shot. The vitamin K shot is reportedly given to assist with clotting of the blood if a hemorrhage should occur. However, the development of leukemia from this shot can be a more likely result than a hemorrhage. There will be no pressure to circumcise and vaccinate when giving birth at home. No interference or pain for mother or baby! Circumcision and vaccination will be discussed in later chapters. Pregnancy and childbirth should be a healthy, easy, exciting time of life, but they're often considered as if they were diseases. The mother should be in wonderful, radiant health and should not require a doctor or medical intervention of any kind. A woman's body is created to give birth, and the natural birth at home is an empowerment for her.

In the article "Why Homebirth?," Jill Cohen says, "If intervention arose out of need to 'rescue' women from pain, results nevertheless show that under normal circumstances it is safer for mother and child to let the process of natural birth occur without medical intervention. Pain in childbirth is empowerment. Sure it may hurt, but the rewards women recognize on a cellular level drive them. When all is said and done, that empowerment paves the path to parenthood—the ultimate task at hand. A woman feels much more relaxed and safe in her own environment, whereas the hospital is unfamiliar and filled with strangers. Labors will often go on for longer periods in the unnatural surroundings of the hospital with its specific procedures and schedules because it keeps a woman from going into herself for the strength to give birth. When a birth happens at home, the birth most often just happens. But in the hospital, there will most often be some kind of intervention."

In her book *Gentle Birth Choices,* Barbara Harper RN, Director of Waterbirth International (www.waterbirth.org) points out, "In countries with the lowest mortality rates, midwifery care is an integral part of obstetrical care, and homebirth is commonly practiced. In the Netherlands, for example, homebirth and midwifery attended births for low risk populations are the norm. More than 70 percent of births are attended by midwives and nearly 40 percent take place at home. The infant mortality rate is 2.1 per 1,000 births. By comparison, in the United States, where the mortality rate is 10.8 per 1,000 births, only 2 to 3 percent of births occur out of the hospital with midwifery care."

Barbara Harper discusses the results of medical intervention:

> What price have we and our children paid for this supposedly advanced technology? Women who sought to liberate themselves from the more uncomfortable and sometimes lethal aspects of childbirth lost much in the process. Women and families must cope with children who have obvious birth-related injuries as a result of the use of forceps or drugs, or through mishandling of the labor. How do families rationalize the child whose abilities to love, trust, and learn may have been impaired by the drugs given to the mother during birth? How has the use of drugs altered women's perceptions of childbirth? What are the personal costs for women who experience intimidation, loss of freedom, humiliation, and even abuse while giving birth?
>
> Interventions in childbirth are usually administered by kind, well-intentioned hospital personnel for what they consider appropriate medical reasons. Unfortunately, those reasons do not alleviate the humiliation a woman feels when she is rendered helpless and attached

to monitors and IVs, preventing her from moving. It doesn't lessen her embarrassment when she is asked to remove her clothes and put on a hospital gown, or her helplessness when her loved ones are excluded and she labors alone. A woman's trust in her own body and her ability to birth normally is shattered by repeated vaginal examinations in order to assess her "progress" during labor. A mother's self-confidence wavers when her newborn is taken away to the nursery to be cared for by "medically superior" professionals.

In *Gentle Birth Choices*, Barbara Harper also points out the importance of mind-body response, listening to your body and listening to the baby:

> The concept of a vital energy force is shared by cultures throughout the world. Unconscious functions of the body, such as healing cancer or birthing a baby, can be strongly affected by thoughts and emotions that block the flow of this energy, or chi, through the body.
>
> Labor is extremely physical, but it is also emotional and spiritual in nature. Medical science is now discovering the body is made up of thoughts and emotions in addition to its physical components. Creating a harmonious womb environment requires the baby to be bathed in positive thoughts and healthy emotions.
>
> The object of being aware is not so much to be in control of your body or its emotions but to recognize and work with them. This allows you to take charge of your life. A woman who keeps herself from expressing or releasing emotions is storing them on a cellular level somewhere in the body. The hormonal shifts in a woman's body during pregnancy make her emotionally vulnerable. Many people view emotions as being either positive or negative, but expressing all emotions is healthy. The key to dealing with emotions during pregnancy and birth is to first recognize them and then to release the negative ones. Most women need a support person who can encourage them to express their feelings without judgment.
>
> For many years professionals have thought a baby's biology and behavior was determined only by the quality and number of genes he or she received in utero. Today, there is a growing awareness that what goes on in the womb from a hormonal and emotional perspective profoundly affects not only the life of this child, but actually influences future generations.

This connection does not end at birth; in fact, it becomes stronger because the infant now has the basis for his own emotional life. While perceiving his mother's mind-body state, an infant cannot communicate with words but uses his cries and body postures as cues to indicate what is going on inside of him and what he perceives in his environment.

A woman is able to release hormones easily during a homebirth which will help to reduce the pain of labor, but in a hospital environment the woman's insecurity may cause her to secrete adrenaline instead of the pain relieving hormones oxytocin and endorphins, resulting in her feeling more pain and slowing the labor process. The slowing of the woman's labor in the hospital often leads to intervention such as administration of drugs which can result in a Caesarean delivery.

It is important for a woman to move freely during labor. My first labor took 22 hours in length with a midwife in the birthing room of a hospital. Had I been permitted to move around more freely, and were able to birth in a kneeling or squatting position instead of a lying-down position, my labor would most likely have been significantly shorter. The lying-down position is inappropriate for delivery.

Barbara Harper emphasizes:

When lying on her back, the woman's enlarged uterus compresses the major blood vessels and diminishes the amount of oxygenated blood available to the placenta, possibly placing the fetus under distress. Additionally, the lithotomy position forces the woman to push against gravity during the actual birth. Rarely does a woman choose to lie down during labor or delivery because it is so painful. Most of womankind will give birth in the vertical position if there is no obstetrician or labor nurse around to make them lie down.

The two most widely chosen birthing postures throughout the world are kneeling and squatting. In cultures where women still control childbirth, women naturally squat, kneel, or lean against a support person in a semi-sitting position.

Birth is a rite of passage. It can be a positive life enhancing experience or a scarring traumatic experience. Very few medical doctors have ever experienced a normal birth, and they often find pathology where it doesn't exist. Drugs given at the hospital to induce labor make the mother's contractions longer and stronger and can place the unborn baby under significant stress, often leading to a Caesarean delivery. One of the biggest problems in the United States is that inadequate information is given to women about giving birth. People spend more time researching the purchase of a car or camera than childbirth options for their own child. Women in America are caused to be frightened of giving birth—often they're convinced they don't know how to do it, so the Caesarean Section delivery rate continues to rise. This trauma to both mother and baby can result in problems with bonding, such as difficulty in breastfeeding. It's time to give the power of giving birth back to the woman. Excellent films for parents and parents-to-be are: *Orgasmic Birth* (www.orgasmicbirth.com), *The Business of Being Born* (www.thebusinessofbeingborn.com), *Birth as We Know It* (www.birthasweknowit.com) and *Birth Without Violence* (www.newearthrecords.com).

What effect does the method of birthing have on our children's health? I've delivered or overseen about 10,000 births and wonder why I'm seeing so many healthy babies. I delivered very few babies who were brain damaged or later developed autism, learning disabilities, or other issues that plague our society today. For over 28 years, I delivered babies in a free standing birth center where interventions were not an option. When I reflect on the effects of those numbing drugs on the newborn, I wonder if the rise in autism is related to being born numb. Does the rising C-section rate have something to do with the rise in autism and other learning issues? These are questions that remain to be answered. Does taking charge of our children's development and health from the very beginning make a difference?
Lonnie C. Morris, CNM, ND

When deciding to have a homebirth, you are in control of your birth. The comfort of the surroundings provides the needed security for the woman to feel in charge. Having family and friends present, especially nurturing women, provides the needed support for the birth process. It is not possible to have family and friends present when giving birth in the hospital. Jingee and Storm Talifero's ebook on pregnancy and childbirth has the beautiful description of their unassisted homebirths in which Jingee tells how it created an even closer bond in her marital relationship with her husband. (www.thegardendiet.com)

Homebirth brings spiritual and personal empowerment, a significantly lower chance of interventions, superior safety and beautiful outcomes. Its time has come again; we need to embrace it.

4

Discovering the Truth about Circumcision: One Woman's Journey of Personal Transformation

"Many parents today realize that, if they had been given accurate information about circumcision, they would never have let anyone circumcise their baby. I am one of those parents, and that is why I do the work I do..."

MARILYN FAYRE MILOS, R.N., FOUNDER AND EXECUTIVE DIRECTOR OF NOCIRC

"The best reason to let a baby keep his foreskin intact is that it's almost a certainty, he will be glad you did."

JOHN A. ERICKSON

Just before I gave birth to my son, I read the chapter "Mutilation of Male Babies" in Dr. Herbert Shelton's book *Hygienic Care of Children*. I already knew I wouldn't allow a circumcision to be performed on my child, but I became extremely concerned for other baby boys while reading some of the details about the procedure. Later, I met my friend, Laurie Evans, who has done significant research on circumcision, and works to end this medical procedure in order to protect baby boys. She also supports Jewish parents who are questioning the religious ritual. I asked Laurie to write an article about circumcision for this book in order to explain rarely disclosed medical information and to share her inspiring and courageous personal story:

In 1984, an event occurred that changed my life. I was exhibiting at a health fair, to promote my work as an infant massage instructor. When I returned from a break, I noticed someone had left a pamphlet by Edward Wallerstein on the issue of circumcision. Since I am Jewish, I was disturbed by the information. How dare anyone challenge a religious tradition that has occurred for thousands of years? Jewish parents of newborn boys decide when and where, not *if*, the ritual Jewish circumcision will occur. In a sense, it was an odd reaction. I was teaching infant massage to foster peaceful beginnings, enhance non-verbal communication, and support parent-infant bonding. I was investigating nutrition, midwifery-assisted birth, and attachment parenting to prepare myself before I became a parent. Why was my reaction to circumcision so visceral? I soon learned this response is very typical and one of the reasons, every year, over one million newborn boys are routinely circumcised in hospitals in the United States, even though 80 to 85% of the men in the world are intact.

I could have thrown the pamphlet away. In 1984, at age 31, I was a French and Spanish teacher as well as a massage therapist, and had studied anatomy and physiology. I was reading many childbirth education books and attending workshops. No one had ever explained or even mentioned circumcision, so it is not surprising that I knew nothing about the issue—I had not even thought about it. Why? More importantly, why had Edward Wallerstein, a Jew, written a brochure on the topic, a brochure people were distributing? Despite my discomfort, I made a conscious choice to explore the topic further.

> "The worst foreskin problem most intact males ever have is that someone thinks they have a problem."
>
> JOHN A. ERICKSON

Before I proceed, I would like to ask you to reflect, how often have you heard anyone speak about the issue of circumcision? Do you discuss it with friends, relatives, and colleagues? If not, is there a reason? Have you attended a *bris*? How have the parents and other participants reacted? What about the baby? Have you seen photos or a video of the surgery? Have you seen a newborn's penis immediately after a circumcision? What have you read about circumcision and where? If you are a parent, what information did you have before your child was born? Would you know where to get accurate up-to-date information?

This chapter will take you on the journey which led to my personal transformation. Although my story is written from a Jewish perspective, the topic is of utmost importance for everyone, since most circumcisions in America are done routinely in the hospital for supposed medical reasons. I have included the information I learned about the function and care of the foreskin, explained where you can find support should you need it, and provided resources to enable you to answer any medical, legal, ethical, or religious questions you may have.

In 1985, I co-presented on infant massage at the international Pre- & Perinatal Psychology and Health Congress. There, I attended a rebirthing workshop by Stanislav Grof. To my surprise, two men were rebirthing their circumcision. At the time, I did not fully understand how significant this was, but I have always remembered the incident. This confirmed what I had learned from watching babies in the infant massage classes. Babies' bodies remember, even if they are in the pre-verbal state at the time of an experience.

Whenever I attended a conference or class, I would ask the presenter about the issue of circumcision. I found it surprising that most people, even those who were open to homebirths, would avoid the issue. It was very frustrating that so few people had any useful information to share. At the Whole Life Expo, I enrolled in a workshop by Dr. Robert Mendelsohn, the beloved pediatrician, and author of *How to Raise a Healthy Child...In Spite of Your Doctor.* When I questioned Dr. Mendelsohn about the topic of circumcision, I was pleasantly surprised by his response.

Dr. Mendelsohn was an Orthodox Jew; yet, he spoke candidly about the harm of circumcision and shared with us what he had written about it. "If performed for other than religious reasons, it is a useless, unnecessary, and potentially dangerous procedure."..."If your doctor suggests circumcision for your baby boy, ask him why he wants to expose the poor kid to the pain, the possibility of infection and hemorrhage, and the risk of death from surgery that has no medical justification." Dr. Mendelsohn was not yet ready to abandon circumcision for religious reasons, but he was honest enough not to mix his religious beliefs with the medical issue—a rare quality for many doctors, even today. Finally, I had found some accurate information regarding this medical practice. However, I still felt I needed support from Jewish parents, so my quest continued.

In 1985, I became pregnant for the first time. I was lucky our childbirth educator showed us slides and discussed the issue of circumcision. I still did not understand how the foreskin worked, but I knew babies do feel pain, and I wouldn't want to hurt my child. There was one huge obstacle; my husband vehemently opposed my view, feeling if we were to have a son, as a Jewish male, he would have to be circumcised.

Now what? Soon thereafter, I unexpectedly met my childbirth educator and she told me she was going to attend a meeting at the United Nations to protest female genital mutilation, which is practiced in regions of Africa. I did not even know this custom existed. My reaction was visceral, instinctive, and automatic; in a split second, I realized I would not want that done to me or a daughter. And, I knew I could never allow that for a son either. But, how was I going to find the courage to stand up to my family and my religion?

The continued discussions with my husband were intense. I regret I did not know then, something I have learned since that time. When circumcised men are insistent their sons be circumcised or are resistant to discuss the issue, it is helpful to empathize with them about what they lost and the harm that was done to them. They need immense compassion because it is difficult for them to consciously think about their own painful experience. It can be helpful to say, "I wish I could have been an ally for you and your parents when they were making their decision." Sometimes when men hear this, they switch from *thinking* about their son's possible circumcision to *feeling* and *remembering* their own. Luckily, our first born was a girl. Time was on my side.

When our daughter was six months old, I was invited to my first *bris*, ritual Jewish circumcision. I shared some information with the parents, but since I didn't have a son, I was not a convincing or strong advocate. I did not want to attend, but I had been at the homebirth and, reluctantly, I agreed. I remember being sick to my stomach. I wanted to grab the baby and run. I felt like an accomplice. I wanted to scream "How dare you!" I do not say this to blame because we are all victims of the culture, but I couldn't understand how the baby's relatives could comply with a tradition that required a newborn's penis get cut by a knife, watch, do nothing, and call this a welcoming ceremony. The baby's pain and my own silence sickened and tormented me. I began to write anonymous letters to *Mothering* magazine.

Finally, in the summer of 1987, I found what I had been looking for. *Mothering* magazine published an article about the *bris shalom*, covenant of peace, a welcoming ceremony, which includes the prayers and omits the cutting. It was a relief to learn there were other Jews questioning this issue and opting for an alternative bris. However, in the article, the mother and father were in agreement. Luckily, the article gave contact information for Natalie Bivas, the director of the Alternative Bris Resource Center.

A few years later, I was invited to another bris, for a child whose homebirth I had also attended. This time, it was harder to go. I stayed in another room; still, once again, my feelings were deeply agonizing. This time, I vowed, in order to be true to myself, I would never attend another bris.

In 1989, I was pregnant again. The discussions with my husband began all over again and continued to be frustrating and unproductive; we were at an impasse even at the time of our son's birth. At this time, I called the Alternative Bris Resource Group. Natalie Bivas shared her story with me.

She was a Conservative Jew who belonged to a synagogue. Though she still practiced the religion, she was willing to change what she thought was a hurtful custom. Most importantly, she explained that due to her prolonged insistence, her husband had finally agreed with her. This was a turning point for me; I was inspired by Natalie's courage to follow her conscience and stand up to the expectations of her religion and family members.

> "Routine circumcision is not a medical issue or a social issue. It is a sexual issue and a human rights issue."
>
> FREDERICK HODGES

Natalie offered me tremendous support. However, I was still troubled, as I was unsure if my son would be upset with me for making him different, so Natalie gave me the phone number of an intact Jewish man. He assured me he was proud to be a Jew and grateful to be intact. It was the first time I had spoken to an intact Jewish man; our conversation helped to alleviate some of my fears. I still needed reassurance from more Jewish parents who had had this experience, so Natalie provided me with the phone numbers of other Jewish parents who had chosen an alternative bris. During a phone conversation, one of these parents asked me, "What if the person who opposes you changes his mind or dies?" Another asked, "Is our religion in our heart and souls or our son's genitals? And why must Jewish boys be cut to be Jewish? Why are women considered Jewish without surgical alteration?" After my long quest, I finally had the support of Jewish parents. At this time, I knew that after arranging a gentle homebirth, I would never be able to explain to my son why I had not protected him, since now I *was* informed. Although it hurt me to realize how much pain this was causing my husband, I knew in my heart I would never forgive myself if I allowed my son to be cut.

Ultimately, our son was left intact. This decision took every ounce of courage and emotional strength I had, but I followed my conscience, felt proud, and never had regrets. Some relatives were angry and avoided visiting for months. In time, because family relations were important to me, healing occurred, and the subject was dropped—temporarily.

During a tai chi class, a woman told me she was concerned because her seven-year-old intact son's foreskin had not yet retracted. I knew little about this. I had heard about the National Organization of Circumcision Information Resource Centers (NOCIRC), and I phoned to see if someone could offer information. Marilyn Milos, the founder and executive director, provided phone time and printed materials, as she still does today. During our conversation, she told me there were several other Jews offering support and information.

Equally important, I finally learned detailed information about the anatomy and physiology of the foreskin as well as the care of the intact penis.

The foreskin has protective and sexual functions, and is not just 'a little piece of skin'. The skin that is removed grows to become about 12 to 15 square inches, which includes the inner mucosa and the outer foreskin layer. This is about one-third to one-half of the outer skin of the penis. The glans, head of the penis, is meant to be a moist internal organ like the eye. No one would think of rubbing his or her eye without using the eyelid. The foreskin has tens of thousands of nerves and provides a gliding mechanism which enhances the sexual pleasure of both the male and his partner. I finally understood how this mechanism functions when I saw the graphics at http://www.circumstitions.com/Works.html. At birth, the foreskin is attached to the glans, like the fingernail is attached to the nail bed. This protects the glans from feces and abrasion during the diapering years. It also means the foreskin must be forcibly torn from the glans before it can be surgically removed.

Circumcision causes both physical and psychological harm. All foreskin sensitivity is lost. The glans becomes dry and keratinized because it is no longer a moist internal organ. Many circumcised males also suffer from tight, painful erections, curvature of the penis during erection, and skin tags or bridges. As with any surgery, there is risk of hemorrhage, infection, as well as complications from anesthesia. Very often, anesthesia is not used, therefore, one can imagine the pain involved in this procedure. Sometimes a second surgery is recommended to repair a botched circumcision. However, this causes additional trauma and loss of more erogenous tissue. Surgical mistakes have included loss of the glans or the entire penis. Although rare, deaths do occur.

Ron Goldman explored the psychological aspects of the issue in *Circumcision: The Hidden Trauma, How an American Cultural Practice Affects Infants and Ultimately Us All*. Dr. Goldman helps readers to focus on the long-term impact of circumcision and how it affects men's self-esteem, sexuality, and relationships. He shares insightful information on the hurtful effects of circumcision on babies, mothers, and adult men. During the surgery, the baby's cortisol, stress level hormone, increases. After their circumcision, babies who were cheerful can become fussy and inconsolable for days or even weeks. Every baby is in pain after the surgery; this can negatively affect breastfeeding. Often, when mothers see their baby's raw wound, they deeply regret allowing their sons to be circumcised. This remorse can last a lifetime. Dr. Goldman reports some men become enraged when they consciously realize they have been circumcised, especially if they understand the function of the foreskin.

Some men admitted they were hesitant to discuss their thoughts and feelings about circumcision because people dismissed their concerns.

Dr. Goldman raises many poignant questions. What is the impact of having pain inflicted on the genitals, an erogenous area that is supposed to provide pleasure? What does an infant learn about trust when his parents have not protected him when he was most vulnerable? How does a man cope when he realizes just what was done to him? How does a woman feel when her strongest desire to protect her son has been overridden by a patriarchal custom? Is the high incidence of impotence in middle-aged men a result of circumcision? How does the removal of so much erogenous tissue impact a couple's sexual relationship? How is a marriage impacted when partners vehemently disagree about their son's circumcision? How does this impact the way men feel about women and their capacity for intimacy?

Dr. Goldman explains one reason circumcision continues is some adults do not realize or accept that babies are fully capable of feeling pain and remembering. For this reason, these adults are willing to do to infants what they would not want done to themselves. Once educated, however, they can become empathetic with the child and choose to protect him from an unnecessary, harmful surgery.

It is especially important for parents to be informed about proper intact care since most American healthcare professionals are not educated about the structures, functions, development, and care of the foreskin. Forcibly retracting the foreskin before it is ready can cause pain, bleeding, infection, and adhesions. Therefore, do not permit any healthcare professional to attempt to retract your son's foreskin and be vigilant about this. Healthcare professionals have been known to suddenly retract a boy's foreskin, even after being told not to. When you diaper or bathe your baby, a gentle wiping of the outside of the penis is all that is necessary. Anyone who changes your son's diaper, such as grandparents, should be given this information. The foreskin is usually retractable by the time the boy has completed puberty, although the foreskin of some boys may retract when they are as young as three years old. The child should be the one to retract his own foreskin *after* it has separated from the glans.

There are several organizations that can offer assistance if a doctor ever recommends circumcision for an older child, if you have a question about intact care, or any other medical, legal, ethical, or religious concerns. They can provide pamphlets, websites, books, videos, referrals to foreskin friendly doctors, and can connect you with local *intactivists*, volunteers who are

> *"The foreskin protects the glans throughout life."*
>
> AMERICAN ACADEMY OF PEDIATRICS

dedicated to informing people about the benefits of genital integrity.

The *National Organization of Circumcision Information Resource Centers* (NOCIRC) has the most comprehensive and multidisciplinary information on the benefits of being intact as well as the care of the intact penis. NOCIRC has over one hundred centers in fifteen countries, hosts biennial international symposia and publishes the symposium proceedings.

NOCIRC refers parents to knowledgeable professionals for any question. It has resources for parents of many denominations, i.e. Jewish, Muslim, Christian, and Catholic parents, as well as parents who are planning to adopt.

Doctors Opposing Circumcision (D.O.C.) educates medical professionals about the anatomy and physiology of intact genitalia as well as the bioethics and conscientious objection of circumcision. One of D.O.C.'s goals is to have this information included in medical textbooks. D.O.C. can suggest nonsurgical alternatives when a circumcision is erroneously recommended for an older boy.

Nurses for the Rights of the Child is an organization of conscientious objector nurses who refuse to participate in the circumcision of babies. These nurses educate their colleagues, doctors, and midwives as well as parents.

Attorneys for the Rights of the Child (ARC) is an international network of attorneys. ARC encourages professionals in various fields, including medical ethics, psychology and children's rights, to incorporate genital integrity awareness into their work. In addition, ARC assists in legal cases when a baby is circumcised without the consent of his parents or when there is a complication or death due to a circumcision.

Jewish Associates of the Circumcision Resource Center and *NOCIRC* offer information and support to Jewish parents. They can put expectant parents in touch with other Jewish couples who have left their sons intact. They can also supply a variety of texts for an alternative bris, a *bris shalom,* or covenant of peace.

You may wonder when, why, and how circumcision evolved from an ancient religious ritual or puberty rite to a common, accepted medical practice in the United States. It began in the mid-1800s during the Victorian era in an attempt to curb or prevent masturbation. At that time, people thought masturbation would cause blindness, epilepsy, and a myriad of other diseases. But why has it continued in the United States when no national medical organization recommends routine circumcision and most countries have stopped the practice or never started it?

Circumcision persists in the United States for several reasons. Although human rights organizations have made tremendous strides in educational outreach for more than twenty years, cultural resistance in medical associations and in the press has kept many people still unaware of the efforts of these organizations. Every few decades, doctors devise new medical myths, such as, "it's cleaner," or, "circumcision prevents urinary tract infections." These are rarely challenged. Parents are usually not told the long-term harm. Some physicians want to perpetuate the practice, so the avoidance is done intentionally. In 2005, two decades after my search began, many childbirth classes and medical books still do not include this topic, and those that do, are often confusing or in favor of the surgery. Thus, the current medical myths get perpetuated.

Earlier in this chapter, I asked, why the silence? The topic of circumcision brings discomfort to many people. Men do not want to reflect upon the pain, trauma, and loss they have suffered. Women may not want to be reminded that they allowed it for their sons. Doctors and midwives find it uncomfortable to recognize or admit they have caused harm to newborns. Nurses routinely prepare babies for their circumcisions. Inwardly they may question the procedure, yet they remain silent out of fear of upsetting parents and/or losing their jobs.

Despite this silence, progress has been made. When parents learn the truth, they will usually opt against circumcision. In the past twenty years, the annual circumcision rate in this country has dropped from 85-95% to 55%, evidence that educational outreach is making a difference. Still, every 26 seconds in America, a baby boy is circumcised, 1.1 million boys a year—proof there is more to be done.

What will enable the circumcision rate to decrease further? It is essential to break the silence and taboo. Accurate information on the harm of circumcision and the functions of the foreskin must be disseminated to parents and health professionals. Photos and videos should be included. It would be useful for people to discuss the issue with friends, relatives, and colleagues. More parents need to have the courage to leave their sons intact and to tell expectant parents about their decision. More doctors must refuse to perform circumcisions.

This issue has changed my life. In 1997, when I couldn't prevent my relative's bris, I was distraught. In order to heal my sorrow with a positive action, a colleague encouraged me to start a NOCIRC chapter; I agreed. I also decided, when people ask me what I do, I would break the taboo and let them know I am the director of the NOCIRC NY Hudson Valley chapter. This has made for some interesting conversations. My outreach work includes exhibiting at health and baby fairs as well as medical conferences. Whenever I have the opportunity, I speak publicly and write articles. Through this work, I have met many courageous, compassionate people. It brings me joy to work with them to ensure that children are seen, heard, and believed.

In our family, my husband, children, and I refuse to attend a bris—even for a relative. Both my children have accompanied me to NOCIRC conferences and educate their peers on this issue. My husband is supportive of my outreach work. Most importantly, my son is grateful he is intact.

Personally, I was transformed from being quiet and obedient to courageous and outspoken. Once that shift occurred, I was less influenced by fear and the status quo; it was easier to follow my heart and my conscience with trust and love.

It is time for routine infant circumcision to end in the United States. If more people join our efforts, our generation has the ability to end this practice in our lifetime. While some people fear this change, others are joyful to be working towards a cultural shift that will ensure the bodily integrity of our precious newborns.

Laurie Evans, M.A., is the Director of NOCIRC NY Hudson Valley. She is a contributor to *Questioning Circumcision: a Jewish Perspective* by Dr. Ron Goldman, and author of "Counseling Couples in Disagreement about Circumcision: A Jewish Perspective" printed in the *Journal of Prenatal and Perinatal Psychology and Health,* (17) 1, Fall 2002, pp.85-94. Ms. Evans has been interviewed on radio and television. Her daughter graduated from SUNY New Paltz. Both her children were born at home and were homeschooled.

Karen Ranzi's comment:

I attended a showing of *Cut*, a documentary film available as a DVD, by Eliyahu Ungar-Sargon, raised an Orthodox Jew. The film examines the subject of male circumcision from a religious, scientific and ethical perspective. Using cutting-edge research, in addition to interview footage of rabbis, philosophers, and scientists, *Cut* challenges viewers to confront their biases by asking difficult questions about this age-old practice. It's a powerful film, important for all parents to see before making a decision about circumcision.

Genital Integrity Websites and Organizations

Intact America www.intactamerica.org

Educational aids and handouts for parents and birth care providers (comprehensive) www.coloradonocirc.org

Myths and Facts www.coloradonocirc.org/myths.php, www.coloradonocirc.org/files/handouts/HIV_Talking_Points.pdf, www.coloradonocirc.org/hiv.php

Doctors Opposing Circumcision (Medical school curriculum and ethics) www.doctorsopposingcircumcision.org

National Organization of Circumcision Information Resource Centers www.nocirc.org (Pamphlets for professionals and parents in English and Spanish–support on medical, legal, and ethical issues)

Nurses for the Rights of the Child (Education and conscientious objection) http://nurses.cirp.org

Attorneys for the Rights of the Child www.arclaw.org

Circumcision Information and Resource Pages (Reference library) www.cirp.org

International Coalition for Genital Integrity www.icgi.org

National Organization of Restoring Men www.norm.org

Jewish Associates of the Circumcision Resource Center www.circumcision.org

Catholics Opposing Circumcision www.catholicsopposingcircumcision.org

Christians for Wholeness www.Acts15.org

Students for Genital Integrity www.studentsforgenitalintegrity.org

Intersex Society of North America www.isna.org and www.accordalliance.org

Religious Info for Jews, Muslims, and Catholics, and Counseling Couples in Disagreement (Click religious then click Jewish) www.notjustskin.org

Female Genital Integrity www.forwarduk.org.uk

Hypospadias Resources www.isna.org/search/node/hypospadias

Videos and Photos on the Internet

Film: *Cut: Slicing through the Myths of Circumcision* www.cutthefilm.com Director: Eliyahu Ungar-Sargon

Video Clip of Gomco Clamp and Plastibell Methods http://circumcisionquotes.com/video.html

Video (19 minutes detailed description of function of the foreskin) www.doctorsopposingcircumcision.org

Anatomy of the Penis, Mechanics of Intercourse http://www.cirp.org/pages/anat

How the Foreskin Works—Animation http://www.circumstitions.com/Works.html

Photos: Circumcision Tools and Procedure http://www.intact.ca/vidintro.htm

Books:

Denniston, G., F. M. Hodges, and M. F. Milos, (Eds.). *Male and Female Circumcision: Medical, Legal, and Ethical Considerations in Pediatric Practice.* New York, NY: Kluwer Academic/Plenum Publishers, 1999.

Fleiss, P. M. and F. M. Hodges. *What Your Doctor May Not Tell You about Circumcision: Untold Facts on America's Most Widely Performed—and Most Unnecessary—Surgery.* New York, NY: Warner Books, 2002.

Glick, Leonard. *Marked in York Flesh: Circumcision from Ancient Judea to Modern America.* New York: Oxford University Press, 2005.

Goldman, R. *Circumcision: The Hidden Trauma—How an American Cultural Practice Affects Infants and Ultimately Us All.* Boston, MA: Vanguard Publications, 1997.

Goldman, R. *Questioning Circumcision: A Jewish Perspective.* Boston, MA: Vanguard Publications, 1997.

Ritter, T. J. and G. C. Denniston. *Doctors Re-examine Circumcision.* Seattle: Third Millennium Publishing Co., 2002.

Whitfield, H. (Ed.) British Journal of Urology International, 83, Circumcision Supplement 1, 1999.

Videos:

Dillon, L. (Director), and T. Hammond (Producer). *Whose Body, Whose Rights?* San Francisco, CA: Dillon Wood Productions, 1995.

Ellsworth, B. *The Nurses of St. Vincents: Saying "No" to Circumcision.* New York, NY: Fireball Films, 1994.

Markuze, K. (Producer and Director). *The 8th Day: Examining Circumcision.* (www. BirthingTheFuture.com), 2002.

Nurses for the Rights of the Child. **Facing Circumcision: Eight Physicians Tell Their Stories**. Santa Fe, NM: Nurses for the Rights of the Child, 1998.

Schonfeld, V. (Director). *It's a Boy!* New York, NY: Filmmakers Library, 1996.

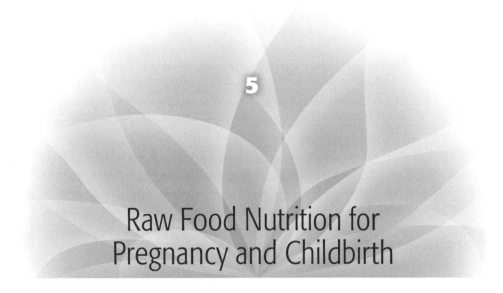

5

Raw Food Nutrition for Pregnancy and Childbirth

"Beauty and vitality are gifts from nature for those who live by her laws"
LEONARDO DA VINCI

Women who have eaten healthfully prior to pregnancy have the opportunity for a much easier time becoming pregnant, and have a greater likelihood of experiencing a vibrantly healthy pregnancy as well as a longer life expectancy and healthier babies.

Diets high in fat, protein and processed foods may cause an increase of the hormone estrogen, and are related to the early onset of menstruation which has been correlated with a greater risk of breast cancer later on. Both animal fat and plant fat (such as vegetable oils) increase estrogen and cause free radicals in the body which can trigger the initiation of cancer. Lack of exercise and a sedentary lifestyle also contribute to early onset of menstruation. Poor diet and lifestyle can affect a woman's ability to become pregnant, maintain a full-term healthy pregnancy and experience a natural childbirth, as well as affecting her own life expectancy and that of her children. The substances that make up such a poor diet end up becoming the mother's tissues and then become the baby's. The child you create is formed from the food you have eaten during pregnancy and lactation, and later, the food he or she continues to eat.

John Robbins, author of *Diet for a New America* and *The Food Revolution,* states, "Tests done at several major universities have found that nearly 25% of today's college students are sterile. This is a terrifying trend. Only thirty-five years ago, the sterility rate was less than one-half of one percent."

According to Dr. William J. Pizzi and June E. Barnhart of the Department of Psychology, Northeastern Illinois University, in *Neurobehavioral Toxicology* Vol. 2:1-4, "MSG (Monosodium Glutamate), a common flavor enhancer added to foods, was found to cause infertility problems in test animals. Male rats fed MSG before mating had less than a 50% success rate (5 of 13 animals), whereas male rats not fed MSG had over a 92% success rate (12 of 13 animals). MSG is found in ACCENT, flavored potato chips, Doritos, Cheetos, meat seasonings, many packaged soups, Bragg Liquid Aminos and other products."

According to *Health Facts*, Vol. 19 (176), January, 1994, "Infertility treatments are a $1 billion dollar a year industry."

Many women who have experienced difficulty becoming pregnant may have a greater chance to become pregnant after adopting a healthy vegan raw food lifestyle. Studies have reported the higher the woman's iron intake, the lower the risk of infertility. Plant-based iron, as contained in many raw plant foods, provides adequate iron intake during pregnancy. Dark leafy greens, particularly spinach, are excellent sources of iron. Raw pumpkin seeds and watermelon are also noted sources of iron.

I know women who have experienced severe PMS symptoms (premenstrual syndrome), and were able to completely recover after having switched to raw foods. I was definitely one of these women so happy not to experience any more severe cramps, bloating and depression during that time of the month.

Studies have reported the early development of breasts is linked with breast cancer. Many girls now develop breasts and pubic hair as early as age 8 or 9, and there are many girls who begin menstruating as young as age 9 to 12. This is most often influenced by a diet high in animal protein, including meat, dairy, poultry, fish and eggs.

Dr. John McDougall discusses the startling sexual changes occurring in very young children, observed in early breast development, pubic hair and earlier onset of menses:

> As a result of this accelerated rate of development, girls are entering puberty at younger and younger ages. Scientists have calculated that every ten years, the age at which girls experience puberty drops two to six months.
>
> This is happening in developed countries throughout the world. In Norway, the age of menarche, or the first menses, has dropped steadily during the past 160 years. In 1830, girls experienced their

first period—and thus were capable of bearing children—at the age of 17.2 years. In 1950, girls began menstruating at the age of 13.2 years. Similar changes have been seen in other western European countries during the same period.

In the United States, girls started their first periods at age 14 years in 1900; by 1960 they were menstruating by an average age of 12.7.

In Japan, in 1875 girls became women at 16.5 years of age. In 1950, they started their first periods at age 15.2. By 1960, the age of menarche was 13.9; by 1970, it fell to 12.5.

With the steady adoption of the Western diet since World War II, Japanese girls now experience sexual maturity at the same age as American girls.

Interestingly, the oldest onset of sexual maturity was observed among native women of Papua New Guinea in the 1960s, who did not get their periods until sometime between 18 and 19 years of age. These native people ate largely vegetarian foods, with only very small amounts of animal foods. Needless to say, the diet was exceedingly low in fat and cholesterol, but rich in fiber and plant nutrients.

For those interested in eating healthfully on a raw plant diet, the information in this book and those in the bibliography and recommended books will help in creating the best diet possible for mother, baby and child.

The mother should create a clean internal environment for her unborn child even before becoming pregnant. The human body will not suddenly heal from drugs and/or a toxic diet. Rather, it takes a period of time, different for each individual, to detoxify the body. To make a dramatic change toward exclusively raw vegan foods during pregnancy could start a huge detoxification. If the diet is changed, it would need to be done gradually over a period of months. A large amount of toxins suddenly released into the system could have a negative effect on the fetus, so it's important to detoxify slowly, especially if changing to 100% raw foods during pregnancy. Some women have been successful at gradually transitioning during a period of two to three months, but it would be more advisable to make this dietary change prior to pregnancy. A change to 60 to 70 percent raw vegan foods during pregnancy is encouraged, with the remaining 30 to 40 percent being the least harmful of cooked foods—steamed vegetables. This diet will still be quite healthful and easier on mother and baby. Mother can then move to totally raw foods after the birth of the baby when detoxification will have less, and eventually, no effect on the baby.

Individual histories are important. A woman with a recent history of drug, tobacco, caffeine or alcohol abuse should not think of becoming pregnant unless she has been transitioning to healthful vegan foods and is drug, tobacco, caffeine and alcohol free for at least one year prior to pregnancy.

In his book *Disease-Proof Your Child: Feed Your Child Right*, Dr. Joel Fuhrman lists the things known to be the most risky for you and your unborn children:

- Caffeine

- Nicotine, including secondhand smoke

- Alcohol

- Medications, both over-the-counter and prescription drugs

- Herbs and high-dose supplements, vitamin A

- Fish, mollusks and shellfish, sushi (raw fish)

- Hot tubs and saunas

- Radiation

- Household cleaners, paint thinners

- Cat litter (because of an infectious disease called toxoplasmosis caused by a parasite found in cat feces)

- Raw milk and cheese

- Soft cheeses and blue-veined cheeses such as feta, Roquefort, and Brie

- Artificial colors, nitrates, and MSG

- Deli meats, luncheon meats, hot dogs, and undercooked meats

Smoking and high cholesterol increase the risk for Arteriosclerosis. Arteriosclerosis is a major contributor to two leading causes of death in the modern world: stroke and heart disease.

Dr. Fred Bisci, Ph.D. in nutrition, author of *Your Healthy Journey: Discovering Your Body's Full Potential*, and raw foodist since the mid 1960s, emphasizes in his lectures, "What you don't eat is more important than what you do eat." With his patients, he finds for each toxic item left out of the diet, there is a "reciprocal degree of improvement." He believes a diet for children should consist of at least 80% raw plant foods with the remaining 20% of food intake consisting of cooked whole plant foods. For better digestion and healing, he emphasizes the importance of waiting at least four hours after the last meal of the day before going to sleep (www.fredbisci4health.com).

Most of the difficulties of pregnancy are caused by poor health. Women who gain 30 to 40 pounds or more, and eat mostly cooked foods, animal flesh and other animal products, particularly dairy, a lot of beans, wheat and other glutinous grains may have problems during pregnancy and childbirth. A diet laden with fat, cholesterol, too much protein and excessive calories can cause these problems. Animal products are high in protein, but quite deficient in vitamins and minerals. Some of the problems that can be the result of an unhealthy diet during pregnancy include shortness of breath, bloating, cramps, difficulty walking, difficulty sleeping, body swelling, constipation, morning sickness, fatigue and backaches, strong cravings, and worse problems such as gestational diabetes and preeclampsia. Symptoms of preeclampsia include high blood pressure, edema, and protein in the urine, which may be related to consumption of animal products. It is very rarely seen in vegan women. Preeclampsia, or toxemia, seems to be highly linked to improper diet.

The above problems during pregnancy, as well as excess weight gain, can result in long and difficult labors which may require medical intervention. Malposition of the fetus may also be an outcome of these problems. Excess weight gain can lead to a fat, bloated newborn.

Dr. John McDougall, author of *The McDougall Program for Women* (www.drmcdougall.com), provides the following important information on weight gain during pregnancy:

> Only thirty-seven years ago a Joint Expert Group of the Food and Agriculture Organization of the World Health Organization pronounced, "Nutrition is of no great importance in pregnancy." Today, of course, we know differently. However, even to this day, experts in prenatal and infant nutrition disagree widely on such fundamental matters as how much weight a woman should gain and what her requirements are for energy, protein, and micronutrients. This confusion among the experts, not surprisingly, explains why so many women are bewildered about what to eat during pregnancy.
>
> Gaining excess weight during pregnancy is a bad idea with many negative consequences. One of the most common responses to this confusion is for a woman to eat lots of high-fat animal foods in the hope she will get all she needs to produce a healthy baby. Unfortunately, such a diet often makes both mother and baby too big to produce a normal delivery. Thus, an increasing number of women require Caesarean

sections. Fully one-fourth of pregnant women require surgical removal of their babies. In developed countries throughout the West, pregnant women usually gain between 22 and 35 pounds. Compare that to the 14 pounds pregnant women gain on average in many traditional cultures and undeveloped countries. Many of these places, it should be pointed out, have lower infant mortality rates than we do in the U.S., and much lower Caesarean section rates. (The U.S. Caesarean section rate is the third highest in the world.).

Let's consider the effect of this weight gain on the mother. The more weight you gain during pregnancy, the more likely you will retain that weight afterwards. On average, women who gain less than 25 pounds during pregnancy are, six months after giving birth, about 2.6 pounds lighter than their prepregnancy weight. On the other hand, women who on average gained 36 pounds or more are 11 pounds heavier than their prepregnancy weight, six months after delivery.

Dr. McDougall points out gestational diabetes and preeclampsia are often the result of excess weight during pregnancy.

During my second pregnancy, I listened to inaccurate information about diet and weight gain from my midwives, and gained 35 pounds. I believe, as a result, I encountered serious problems during childbirth, as my son was too large for me at 8 pounds, 14 ounces and presented with shoulder distosia, where his head was already out but his shoulders were too large and difficult to deliver, requiring me to have an episiotomy. Babies that are too big can be injured during birth.

Due to my excessive weight gain, my son was bloated for quite some time after birth. During my pregnancy with my daughter, I gained only about 20 pounds. My daughter was easier to birth as she weighed only slightly over 6 pounds. As I have been observing women on raw food diets experiencing pregnancies, I've noted the weight gain is often in the range of 15 to 25 pounds, and the baby is easier to deliver in the 6 to 7 pound range.

Excessive weight gain during pregnancy is often the result of overeating. Since a pregnant woman already has to eliminate the fetal waste products in addition to her own, it would not be wise to overeat on protein, especially animal protein. A pregnant woman requires only slightly more food than she would require under ordinary circumstances. Assuming the mother is eating whole natural foods, all or mostly uncooked, she will easily obtain the additional protein she needs by increasing her overall food consumption only slightly.

In the March/April 1997 McDougall newsletter, vegan advocate, John McDougall, M.D., writes about the "Energy Required to Grow a Healthy Baby":

> Many pregnant women are on medications for diabetes and high blood pressure.
>
> One-fourth of these women end up with surgical removal of the baby. The dairy and meat is usually the source of the trouble. Since the 1960s most doctors have encouraged their patients to eat, and not to worry about extra weight gain. Mother and baby too often become too big, carrying an increased risk of death and need for Caesarean Sections. With unrestricted weight gain for the mothers, babies these days are weighing in at 10 to 12 pounds- a size often too big to comfortably fit through the mother's pelvis. Big babies are harder to deliver and as a result, injury and death are more likely.
>
> In some parts of the world, such as the Philippines and rural Africa, pregnant women do not eat more food, instead gaining the extra calories by increased body efficiency.
>
> These women take in no more, and often fewer calories, than prior to pregnancy. Their foods are primarily nutrient-dense vegetable foods which will easily provide the raw materials to grow a healthy baby.

Dr. Timothy Trader, Ph.D., N.D. believes weight gain during pregnancy is all about consumption of the proper foods. He looks more at the woman's energy than weight on the scale. He asks, "'Are you eating too little or too much' in relation to how much energy you have and how you are feeling. The body is an excellent regulator if provided with the proper nutrition. We need to keep in mind the baby will grow much bigger in the first six months after birth than when in the womb."

There are proteins in everything that grows as long as it's not refined. Bananas contain about 5% complete protein. Lettuces are 34% protein. Mangos and bananas contain all 8 essential amino acids. If some of our foods are deficient in certain amino acids, this will be compensated by their abundance in other foods. We should eat the food to which we are naturally adapted. Protein is required for the development of the human baby, but the protein consumed should be of the highest quality. Green leafy vegetables and smaller amounts of nuts and seeds provide this high level of nutrients. Sprouts are an excellent source of protein. A pregnant and lactating mother can get all the protein she needs eating raw vegan foods.

Eating meat floods the body with protein waste products. The kidneys then need to eliminate these acidic wastes, requiring calcium as a buffer in the process. Calcium is continually lost in the urinary waste, and may result in osteoporosis or bone loss. Vegetable protein is much more easily absorbed into the bloodstream without the loss of calcium from eating animal protein. There are many protein-rich food sources among fruits and especially green leafy vegetables and sprouts that supply the pregnant woman with all the protein necessary at this time.

Nuts and seeds are rich in fat, and there should only be a slight increase in their overall consumption. Many raw foodists already overeat on nuts and seeds, so it might not be necessary to deliberately eat more of them. Nuts, except for almonds, are acid-forming, and an excess could cause health problems, including decalcification of bones and teeth.

Too much protein places a great stress upon the liver and kidneys. Dr. McDougall explains in his book *The McDougall Plan*, "It's extremely hard for anyone to become protein deficient. Unless you gave up eating altogether, I don't see how you'd ever manage it. Virtually all unrefined foods are loaded with proteins. The unfortunate reality is that most Americans consume enormously excessive quantities of unnecessary proteins, which must be excreted through the kidneys, harming them and the rest of the body." Dr. McDougall points out in his book, "The results of prolonged consumption of excess protein can cause kidney stones and also osteoporosis (as a result of the calcium imbalance which occurs due to excess protein)."

According to "Sources of Protein in the Diet" from www.Krispin.com/protein.html, nuts and seeds contain 2-3 grams of protein per tablespoon, fruit contains 1 gram per fruit, and vegetables contain 1-3 grams per 4 ounces.

The following list, from *Nutritive Value of American Foods in Common Units*, U.S.D.A. Agriculture Handbook No. 456, shows the percentage of calories from protein in raw plant foods:

Fruit	Vegetables	Nuts and Seeds
Cucumber 24%	Spinach 49%	Pumpkin seeds 21%
Tomato 18%	Watercress 46%	Sunflower seeds 17%
Honeydew 16%	Kale 45%	Walnuts 13%
Watermelon 8%	Chinese cabbage 34%	Pistachios 13%
Raspberries 8%	Parsley 34%	Almonds 12%
Cherries 8%	Lettuce 34%	Pine nuts 8%
Orange 8%	Peas (green) 30%	Pecans 5%

Papaya 6%   Dandelion greens 24%   Coconut milk 5%
Avocado 5%   Cabbage 22%   Coconut meat 4%
Banana 5%   Celery 21%

To add to this list, hempseeds contain 22% calories from protein, and flaxseeds contain 17%.

As can be observed in the above chart, raw plant foods provide significant amounts of protein. Notice that green vegetables contain the most protein of all the above plant foods. People are always surprised when I tell them the amounts of protein in green veggies.

Dr. Douglas Graham, author of *The 80/10/10 Diet* and other raw food nutrition books, points out: "Protein consumption should be a function of total calories consumed, not a number to strive for in terms of grams per day. As total calorie intake goes up, so does protein intake, at a rate of a maximum of 10% of calories consumed. I would imagine most pregnant and nursing moms will find their total food intake will rise, gradually, to a peak of almost 1000 extra calories per day when nursing, which, depending upon food choices, will represent anywhere from about 14 to 25 extra grams of protein per day."

This makes great sense since most women's appetites naturally heighten when nursing to create a good milk supply and to meet the increased energy demands. I ate significantly more food when nursing. Women I have observed throughout pregnancy and nursing have often talked about the natural heightening in appetite when lactation began. This is the time when extra ounces of nuts, seeds or avocados may be most desired by the lactating mother.

Dr. Graham recommends:

A maximum of 10% of total calories consumed come from protein. If one is consuming 2000 calories per day that would equal a maximum of 50 grams daily. If, as typically happens during pregnancy and nursing, as well as during extended periods of great degrees of physical activities, total calorie consumption rises, protein consumption should and will rise accordingly, based on my percentage suggestion. Therefore, an athlete consuming 6K calories per day would be consuming close to 150 grams of protein per day.

Dr. Joel Fuhrman writes in *Eat to Live*:

> When your caloric needs are met [by eating whole foods], your protein needs are met automatically. Focus on eating healthy natural foods; forget about trying to get enough protein. Your protein needs increase in direct proportion to the increased caloric demands and your increased appetite. Guess what? You automatically get enough. The same is true during pregnancy. When you meet your caloric needs with an assortment of natural plant foods, you will receive the right amount of protein—not too much, not too little.

You certainly don't need to eat all the amino acids at one meal for "complete protein." Fresh fruits and vegetables contain all the amino acids to make complete protein. Cooked protein foods require large secretions of stomach acid, but the human stomach doesn't produce much stomach acid. The lower protein raw food diet results in freedom from stomach acid secretions, resulting in more energy and a lighter disposition.

On the website, http://nov55.com/hea/food.html, Gary Novak, biologist and moral philosopher, presents the following:

> New research shows the critical nature of glycosides (sugar complexes) in physiology and immunity. Glycosides are found in the structural components of cell walls. They give cells an identity. This allows cells to communicate with each other, and it allows the immune system to distinguish self from foreign. These molecules are complex and difficult to synthesize. They are normally abundant in raw food but easily damaged by cooking. The damage to these molecules by cooking could explain why raw foods have such marvelous effects upon physiology. Evolution did not account for cooking because it is such a recent practice.

Dr. Gabriel Cousens has explained in one of his lectures:

> Forty three thousand children die each day because of beef consumption. Sixty million people die each year. While Guatemala sends thousands of pounds of cattle to the United States, 75% of its children suffer from malnutrition. Veganism creates longevity. The high protein diet of meat eaters causes osteoporosis. Breast cancer is four times greater in meat eating women. Pythagoras used live foods

to treat poor digestion. He used apples to produce enzymes, resulting in improved digestion.

In the book *Nutrition and Physical Degeneration*, Weston Price wrote about fourteen primitive tribes who developed abnormalities after adopting the Western diet of processed and refined foods. The resulting nutritional deficiencies caused crowded teeth, narrowed facial structure, and birth defects.

The suggested dietary during pregnancy is fruit, vegetables, nuts and seeds.

Other living creatures are not ill because they don't eat cooked and processed foods. Only human beings and their pets have degenerative disease, due to the foods they eat. Humans continue to eat even when sick, whereas a wild animal would cease to eat for a week if not well.

Professor Rozalind Graham of Great Britain said, "Animals in their wild habitat know by instinct how to live, and what to eat and drink. They know how to fast by natural instinct when they get hurt or sick. Naturally, animals are led to eat what is good for them. But man eats and drinks anything and everything—consuming the most indigestible concoctions, washing it down with poisonous slops, and then wonders why he is sick and does not live to be a centenarian."

I found in my own journey toward a healthy raw food lifestyle that I have felt best when staying totally 100% raw, eating simply of fresh fruit, greens and vegetables with smaller amounts of soaked nuts and seeds. I haven't felt as well when eating dehydrated foods, prepared live foods from the health food store, supposedly all raw (but often not), soy sauces and unsoaked nuts and seeds. When trying to create imitations of cooked foods, I often began to crave cooked foods again, until I went back to eating simple fresh produce and got back on track. I do not recommend emphasizing nuts and seeds as I did for many years. I also do not advocate eating dried fruit, and especially the poor combination of dried fruit with nuts and seeds other than on exceptional occasions as in a live dessert recipe for the holidays. I do highly recommend a balanced and varied diet of fruits and vegetables, with plenty of "green" leafy vegetables, accompanied by small amounts of nuts, seeds or avocados. Have a green smoothie, raw green soup or blended salad every day! Be sure to chew these blended foods for best digestion. One of the mistakes raw foodists often make is not consuming enough green leafy vegetables. When an abundance of these mineral rich greens become part of the diet, cravings for cooked food will noticeably diminish. Victoria

Boutenko, in her book, *Green for Life,* focuses on the importance of eating delicious green smoothies.

Fiber in fruits, vegetables, nuts and seeds is fundamental for health. An essential nutrient entirely missing from animal foods, including dairy, fiber lowers bad cholesterol, raises good cholesterol, contributes to heart health, keeps the bowels toned and healthy, and helps distribute oxygen to the brain. Thanks to all the above benefits, eating fiber prevents cancer.

On a raw food diet, one receives all of the nutrients of the plant. One feels lighter and more energetic.

It is essential to eat organic, ripe fruit. Fruit is easy to digest, and especially necessary during pregnancy. Fruits are predigested by their enzymes in the ripening process so they pass through the stomach and into the intestines very quickly. Fruit is a precursor to serotonin in the body. It is imperative to a baby's nerve and brain development and especially important during pregnancy.

Many people question the nutrients we can get from fruits and vegetables because of the poor quality of the soil. Most of the fruits come from trees with deep roots that are not affected by the top soil. However, much of the fruit is sprayed with pesticides, even some of the organic fruit that is imported, and this can eventually cause us harm. In addition, fruit is often picked unripe and then does not ripen properly the way it would have had it been left to ripen naturally on the plant. The goal is to purchase local organic food, and to consider the enormous benefits of having your own organic garden or farm. Working toward sustainability is the best way to know you are eating 100% organic produce.

According to Dr. Douglas Graham, "Over 90% of all disease is food-related." He asks, "Does your mouth water in an orchard of ripe fruit or in a pasture of cows?" He goes on to say, "People are sicker than you give them credit for. Death is often the first symptom of heart disease."

The pregnant and nursing mother needs to eat whole, ripe, organically grown foods that are not poisoned by additives and pesticides. These poisons will get through to the placenta and can affect the blood and tissues of the growing embryo and fetus. The placental barrier cannot stop harmful chemicals from getting through. If such substances are ingested during the embryonic period, they can cause birth defects and have other serious consequences in the process of normal development.

In their article "Nutrition Hints," Betty Kamen, Ph.D., and Dr. Michael Rosenbaum, M.D. discuss the following contaminated foods: Foods with the most pesticides include apples, bell peppers, celery, cherries, grapes, nectarines, peaches, pears, potatoes, red raspberries, spinach, and strawberries, and so, if possible, should be purchased only if organic. You can lower your pesticide intake by 90 percent by avoiding those top twelve most contaminated fruits and veggies. Nectarines have the highest percentage of pesticides among fruits, and celery the highest likelihood of multiple pesticides on a single vegetable. Avocados have the lowest chance of contamination. Washing may reduce some pesticides, but when these foods were tested, they had all been thoroughly washed.

Other studies ranked Mexican cantaloupes, apricots, green beans, cucumbers, and Chilean grapes among the highest in pesticides of fruits and vegetables.

Many pesticides are taken up internally in the plant. Pesticides cause adverse effects from cancer to nervous system damage to reproductive problems. Many pesticides mimic estrogen and become endocrine disruptors that affect hormone balance and have been associated with breast and prostrate cancer, deformities of the reproductive organs, fertility problems, altered fetal and child development, learning disorders and more. Of course children are more vulnerable to the damaging effects of pesticides than adults. There was a 21.5% increase in childhood cancers from 1950 to 1986, a period during which production and use of pesticides skyrocketed. A more recent study showed children who live in homes where lawn chemicals are regularly used have a 6.5 times higher risk of developing leukemia. Other studies relate use of pesticides to a higher rate of brain cancer among children. An analysis of the major baby food brands found samples of the most commonly used foods contained 16 different pesticides. Conventional farming contributes toxins to the air, water and earth. Because we know pesticides contaminate many fruits and vegetables, you should always choose organic if possible.

In an article titled "New Studies Back Benefits of Organic Diet", by the Inter Press Service, on Saturday, March 4, 2006, Toronto, Canada, Stephen Leahy reveals the following crucial information:

> Organic foods protect children from the toxins in pesticides, while foods grown using modern, intensive agricultural techniques contain fewer nutrients and minerals than they did 60 years ago.
>
> A U.S. research team from Emory University in Atlanta analyzed urine samples from children ages three to eleven who ate only organic

foods and found they contained virtually no metabolites of two common pesticides, malathion and chlorpyrifos.

However, once the children returned to eating conventionally grown foods, concentrations of these pesticide metabolites quickly climbed as high as 263 parts per billion, says the study published February 21, 2006.

Organic fruits and vegetables had significantly higher levels of cancer-fighting antioxidants, according to a 2003 study in the Journal of Agricultural and Food Chemistry.

A 2001 report by Britain's Soil Association looked at 400 nutritional research studies and came to similar conclusions: foods grown organically had more minerals and vitamins.

In Epidemiology, March 2001, Eric Bell, Ph.D. of the University of North Carolina, School of Public Health, stated, "Miscarriage rates were higher when living near agriculture. Mothers who lived near crops where certain pesticides were sprayed faced a 40 to 120 percent greater risk of miscarriage due to birth defects."

In July 2009, scientific research has implicated pesticides, which affect the nervous system, as a causative factor for Alzheimer's and Parkinson's. What better reason could there be to choose organic foods?

It is important to eat locally grown produce as much as possible. It would be best to eat locally grown organic produce from your own garden or a local organic farmer, such as from CSA (Community Supported Agriculture). Since we should really live in an environment where we can have local organic produce year-round, moving to a tropical place where we can grow our own food would be ideal. If living in colder climates, most of our natural food needs to come from long distances where organically grown produce is still available during the winter months. Although organic produce is certainly preferable, when it is unavailable in some cases, conventional raw produce is still less harmful than cooked. However, do avoid the top 12 most heavily sprayed fruits and vegetables, listed in this chapter.

As a pregnant or lactating mother, the focus should be on "organic," and "locally grown" as much as possible. Wild edibles in unsprayed areas provide excellent nutrients for those who forage for food.

As of 2009, most of the organic produce taken over by large distributors gets irradiated. Consequently, it's important to support local organic farmers or local farmers who use organic methods (although uncertified), who *do not* irradiate their produce. One way you can investigate if organic produce has been irradiated is to slice an apple and leave it exposed to air for 10 minutes. If the slices have not "rusted," this apple most likely was irradiated.

In a talk I had with author Victoria Boutenko, she expressed the following information on the importance of eating organic produce: "If you eat organically grown plants, you're consuming insects or their eggs, and they're totally inseparable. Conventional produce, with all the pesticides, no longer contains insects—no bee would go to a conventionally grown plant. You will never find a worm inside a conventionally grown apple. Those who eat all organic produce usually don't have problems with B12 deficiency due to the insects or their eggs in the produce. This is called conscious veganism."

The pregnant and lactating woman can begin the day with high water content foods, such as very juicy fruits: melons, grapefruits, oranges or just water, as the body is still detoxifying during the early morning hours. Some pregnant women do well with green juices or with green leaves blended with fruits to make delicious green smoothies.

The body detoxifies each night during sleep which continues into the morning, unless heavy foods are eaten. Because ripe fruit is predigested, by eating only watery fruits, water or nothing at all in the early morning, the detoxification can continue. My daughter has often liked green juices sweetened with half an apple or a single carrot in the morning (3 leaves of kale, half a cucumber, 2 stalks of celery, 3-4 leaves of Romaine lettuce and a quarter to half an apple or a small carrot). Or we frequently enjoy a morning green smoothie using the variety of recipes from the books *Green for Life* or *Quantum Eating*.

Our brains require glucose which is provided by fruit. Fruit enzymes become available only when the fruit is ripe. For example, for optimum digestion, a banana needs to be ripe with small brown dots. In nature, the ripe banana on the plant would not have any dots, but would be bright yellow inside and out. A more important indication of ripeness is the absence of green at both ends of the banana. In the false "forced ripening" process, the ends still remain green which to the knowledgeable consumer means the banana is not really ripe. Fruit kept in the refrigerator cannot ripen properly. Eat celery and/or lettuce with sweet fruits such as bananas or papayas to balance the fruit sugars with minerals. Be sure to brush teeth at least twice a day, and especially before bedtime. Floss at least twice a day to keep teeth free of food particles and to prevent the buildup of plaque near the gums.

Although cruciferous vegetables—broccoli, kale, cauliflower, cabbage, and collards are easier to chew after cooking, heating changes their molecular structure and causes toxic chemicals to be formed. I eat these vegetables raw by chopping them finely or by using a blender for easier assimilation, such as in a soup I make with kale in the Vita-mix, a large high-powered blender. Any blender would work well also. All of the vegetables are well-blended, and mixed with other easily digestible vegetables. Frederic Patenaude's book, *Instant Raw Sensations*, has quick, well-combined soup and smoothie recipes as well as blended salads. In Victoria Boutenko's book, *Green for Life*, she explains green smoothies are an excellent way to obtain the benefits of green vegetables with their abundance of minerals in a very digestible form. The combination of fruit and green leafy vegetables into a green smoothie provides the energy we need from the fruit along with the minerals and alkalinity from the green leafy vegetables, and includes the fiber we need. Raw smoothies are predigested and high in enzymes. They are quick to prepare and require little time to eat if you should happen to be a busy person. Although these smoothies are wonderful for their easy assimilation, because they've been blended, they require less chewing. It's still important to eat solid fruits and vegetables to provide proper chewing exercise required for correct jaw development.

The best greens for your salad are the dark green lettuces, young dandelion and other wild edible greens, baby greens, spinach, kale, and sprouts such as sunflower greens, broccoli sprouts, clover sprouts, buckwheat greens, etc. The two popular varieties of kale are curly kale and Lacinato kale. I find the Lacinato kale (often called dinosaur kale) is more tender and great in a salad or used as a wrap for a veggie roll. It has a sweeter, more delicate taste than the curly kale. Kale is reportedly rich in immune boosting vitamins C, E, B1, B2 and B6, iron, phosphorous, magnesium, calcium, potassium, fiber, omega-3 fatty acids and protein. Dandelion is also a most nutritious leafy green. It is full of vitamins A, C, and K, iron and calcium. It has been known to prevent vision problems, fight infections, create bone strength and assist in nerve function. Healers have used it to help with digestion, decrease swelling and treat conditions such as jaundice, acne and eczema. Baby spinach has less oxalic acid than mature spinach. All dark greens add plenty of alkaline minerals and are great in salads, green smoothies, raw soups or juices.

We'd do best to eat at least 80% alkaline-forming foods, and not more than 20% of acid-forming foods. Fresh fruits, green leaves and vegetables are alkaline-forming in the body. Nuts, except for almonds, can be acid-forming. Our blood is meant to have an alkaline pH, and when the body becomes overloaded with acid-forming foods from eating cooked and processed foods, grains, animal products or an excess of nuts, it struggles to return to an alkaline pH (refer to *Alkalize or Die* by Theodore A. Baroody or *The pH Miracle* by Robert O.Young, Ph.D.). As mentioned previously, twenty-five percent of all college freshmen are said to be infertile. This is not surprising when one considers the typical acid-forming foods eaten by today's college students.

In a study by Francis M. Pottenger, Jr. M.D., along with Alvin Ford, a ten year investigation beginning in 1932 involving 900 cats, revealed cats fed with exclusively cooked food could no longer reproduce after the third generation. Cats fed with raw food had no difficulty birthing and nursing in any generation.

Roger Haeske (www.HowToGoRaw.com) has researched which of the raw foods have the highest alkalizing mineral content. In an article titled "Maybe Popeye Was Right," he presents the following information on alkaline minerals in plant foods:

> The major alkaline minerals are calcium, magnesium, sodium and potassium. Any raw foods that are high in those minerals will be alkaline-forming. It is very important to keep the body properly mineralized and at the same time functioning at the proper blood pH level of about 7.4.
>
> Eating cooked food will acidify the blood. Eating too much fat will have the same effect because fat interferes with the body's ability to deliver oxygen to the cells. Also, nuts and seeds tend to be higher in the acid-forming minerals: chlorine, phosphorous and sulfur. A high protein diet will also overly acidify the blood.
>
> It is also possible to be too alkaline. The key here is the proper balance.
>
> A mistake I've noticed many raw foodists make is not eating enough mineral rich, leafy green vegetables. This is vital to their success. When you consume a high quantity of mineral rich foods, you'll notice your cravings for cooked foods will diminish dramatically.

Roger analyzed raw food for its alkaline mineral content, and found spinach was high not just in minerals but in virtually every major beneficial nutrient. "Maybe that is why Popeye was so strong when he ate his spinach!" Roger provides an analysis of the alkaline minerals in 25-calorie servings of celery, spinach, kale, Romaine lettuce, banana, orange, cucumber, okra, zucchini, tomato and avocado. Measuring by calories is the most accurate way to compare food nutrient levels. Many more calories are consumed when eating fruit compared to green leafy vegetables. For example, six bananas contain 2,921 mg of potassium, while 10 ounces of raw spinach yield 1,585 mg of potassium.

Roger did his research at the following website:

http://www.nal.usda.gov/fnic/foodcomp/search/
Each food below represents a 25 calorie serving.

Celery
Calcium: 62.0 mg. Magnesium: 17.0 mg. Potassium: 403 mg. Sodium: 124.0 mg.

Spinach
Calcium: 109 mg. Magnesium: 87.0 mg. Potassium: 614 mg. Sodium: 87.0 mg.

Kale
Calcium: 68.0 mg. Magnesium: 17.0 mg. Potassium: 224 mg. Sodium: 22.0 mg.

Romaine Lettuce
Calcium: 48.0 mg. Magnesium: 20.0 mg. Potassium: 358.0 mg. Sodium: 12.0 mg.

Banana
Calcium: 1.0 mg. Magnesium: 8.0 mg. Potassium: 100 mg. Sodium: 0.0 mg.

Roger points out:

Food	Calcium mg	Magnesium mg	Potassium mg	Sodium mg
Celery	62	17	403	124
Spinach	109	87	614	87
Kale	68	17	224	22
Romaine Lettuce	48	20	358	12
Banana	1	8	100	0
Orange	21	5	96	0
Cucumber w/peel	26	21	243	3
Okra	65	46	242	6
Zucchini	23	26	406	16
Tomato	14	15	332	7
Avocado	2	4	76	1

All of these green vegetables are alkaline-forming foods, but spinach is the overall best. Spinach also has a better than perfect amino acid score of 119. It's high in dietary fiber and its sodium is of course in the organic form, which our bodies utilize naturally. It's the inorganic sodium which is toxic to us and every cell in the body. Spinach is also very high in vitamins A, C, E, K, B6, thiamin, riboflavin, niacin and folate, as well as the minerals iron, zinc, copper and manganese. Per calorie, spinach has over six times more potassium than bananas. Some people are concerned they'll leach calcium by eating spinach, but this is unlikely to be a problem for most people.

Dr. Gabriel Cousens makes a point about oxalic acid in his book *Conscious Eating*:

> In one extensive study on children put on a high-spinach diet and other high-oxalate foods, no evidence of any alteration of calcium, vitamin D, or phosphorous metabolism was found. It is possible, however, if a person has a low calcium intake or poor calcium metabolism, a high-oxalate diet could cause a calcium deficiency.

Roger describes the difference between eating cooked and raw spinach: "It is believed the oxalic acid will not bind with the calcium when the spinach is raw, so eat as much spinach as you want as long as it is raw." Roger provides the following easy to assimilate, nutritious green smoothie:

Banana, Blueberry and Spinach Smoothie

3 ounces water—Add more or less depending on how thick or thin you want your smoothie to be.
2 bananas
4 ounces of fresh or frozen blueberries
3 or more ounces of raw spinach

[To avoid the controversy over the high oxalic acid content in spinach, I recommend using primarily baby spinach leaves which are far lower in oxalic acid content.]

Salt added to food will dehydrate the body. Any dehydrated food will reduce the percentage of energy we have. Table salt should be avoided as it tends to raise blood pressure. It puts excessive pressure on the tiny capillaries of the eyes. Salt can contribute to a loss of calcium in the urine. We can get natural sodium instead quite easily from organic fruits and vegetables such as organic tomatoes, leafy greens and celery. Sea vegetables can be included in the diet, as they provide organic minerals and quality protein. Dr. Brian Clement, Director of Hippocrates Health Institute, believes sea vegetables and sprouts, according to his testing, are the most important of foods. I enjoy dulse in my salads. Whole dulse can be soaked to rid it of most of the salt, and then added to salads.

According to Dr. Timothy Trader, seaweed contains high levels of sodium chloride, mercury, PCBs and other chemicals. He says, "Sodium chloride causes the arteries to tighten, thus raising the blood pressure. After completely removing salt from the diet for two months, the blood pressure will return to normal."

Pregnancy is often looked at as a disease, and childbirth as a surgical operation. I have observed many healthy women who were eating raw vegan foods during pregnancy, and not only were they more radiant than ever, they never experienced all the problems that often come with pregnancy. If one does exhibit the symptom of morning sickness, it's a sign of detoxification, and light juicy fruits or green juices for a day will usually provide relief. As morning sickness is a sign of the body's need for detoxification, it may be best for mother to abstain from solid foods to detoxify properly. Pregnant women need not worry fasting may harm the fetus. In the book *The Live Food Factor* by Susan Schenk, Dr. Tosca Haag states, "A pregnant woman in reasonably good health can safely fast for three to five days without any harm to the fetus."

In the March/April 1996 issue of Health Science Magazine, an article describes a woman's change to a healthful vegan diet and its positive effects on her childbirth. She had read the popular nutrition bestseller *Fit for Life* by Harvey and Marilyn Diamond. After suffering from allergies for many years, she decided it was time to try diet and lifestyle changes. She became a full vegan, and when she became pregnant, she desired to pay even closer attention to what she was eating. She spoke with Dr. Joel Fuhrman, M.D. of Flemington, N.J. about how best to eat during pregnancy. He said to eat a variety of leafy greens and two salads a day, in addition to fruit, including bananas each day. She followed his recommendations and believed she had a very easy delivery because of it. She had a wonderful pregnancy with no problems—no blood sugar problems, no bloating, no backaches, no cramps, none of the things that are supposedly normal during pregnancy. She experienced a very short labor, only four and a half hours from when her water broke until her daughter was born. Her midwife was envious because the delivery of her own first child lasted 25 hours. At 13 months, the vegan's daughter began chewing on solid foods such as strawberries, watermelon, and cucumbers but still nursed for 95% of her diet. The baby was "very happy and very rarely got fussy."

Our ideal diet consists of easily digestible raw plant foods: fruits, vegetables, nuts and seeds. The results of the raw food diet are superior. Fruits and vegetables provide an abundance of all the necessary macro and micro nutrients, including protein. It is important to include a variety of colors in your intake of fruits and vegetables. Phytochemicals are compounds found in plant foods that have beneficial effects on our bodies. Each plant food has its own specific phytochemicals. The different colors provide all we need in order to get all the nutrients. Green and orange colors are easy to find. The red, purple and blue pigments can be included when we eat berries. However, stay away from conventionally grown berries because they're loaded with pesticides. Raspberries and strawberries are on the most contaminated foods list, so it's important to buy only organic berries. Cooking berries has a negative effect on their antioxidant activity, so it's important to eat them fresh.

To learn more about the beneficial nutrients of individual fresh fruits and vegetables, read *The Healing Power of Nature Foods: 50 Revitalizing Super Foods and Lifestyle Choices to Promote Vibrant Health* by Susan Smith Jones.

Professor Rozalind Graham explains: "When eating, there are four vital questions you should ask yourself: 1. Would I find this food in my natural environment (a tropical/subtropical forest)? 2. Would I find this food presented in exactly this form? 3. Could I obtain this food without protection or weaponry? 4. Would I choose to make a meal of this food in and of itself? If you can answer "yes" to all four of these questions, then this food is appropriate to our human digestion."

Successful long-term raw foodists strive to follow a diet high in alkaline minerals. Over time, many raw foodists cannot thrive on commercially grown fruits, vegetables, nuts and seeds, which are chemically treated, genetically engineered and irradiated. As much as possible, it's important to eat organic, wild and native foods containing high alkaline minerals and trace elements. Gardening and foraging for wild native foods that grow in your area in season would be extremely beneficial. Any commercially grown produce is going to contain some degree of chemicals used in pesticides and fertilizers. In August 2003, the EPA reported high levels of rocket fuel were found in lettuce grown in areas using the Colorado River for irrigation. The perchlorate levels in the lettuce were more than 30 times the accepted EPA standards. Perchlorates are well-known endocrine disrupters. They can cause brain damage in babies. It is best for your family to have your own garden and to buy organic local lettuce grown by farmers in the area you live when available.

When eating nuts and seeds, it's important to remember they combine best with green leafy non-starchy vegetables. For optimum digestion after eating nuts and seeds, it's best to wait for a minimum of 4 to 5 hours before eating again. If a piece of fruit should be eaten before the nuts and/or seeds can be digested, the result will be fermentation.

Mixing fruits and vegetables will create alcohol in the stomach. However, celery, cucumbers, and lettuces can be mixed with fruit. Predominantly starchy foods do not digest optimally with foods high in protein when combined at the same meal. Sprouts, rich in protein and starch, are digestible. David Klein, publisher of Vibrance Magazine, has an excellent food combining chart available for purchase at www.livingnutrition.com.

A study done at the University of Stockholm, Sweden in 2002 demonstrated the toxic effect of high cooking temperatures. For example, potatoes when cooked at high temperatures in trans fat become the potent cancer-causing plastic compound called acrylamide, as in French fries. Most commercial chips are high in trans fats, cooked in polyunsaturated oils like canola, soybean, safflower, corn and other seed and nut oils which produce large quantities of free radicals in the body. Dr. Joseph Mercola states, "These oils can cause aging, clotting, inflammation, weight gain and cancer." He says, "One French fry is worse for your health than one cigarette." In "New Research Supports the Link Between Cooking and Cancer" (www.mercola. com), "the study reports fried, oven-baked and deep-fried potato and cereal products contain high levels of acrylamide. Researchers at Stockholm University summarized evidence of acrylamide's presence in foods and performed a detailed analysis of acrylamide during heating. Carbohydrate-rich foods had high levels of acrylamide, with potato chips and French fries at the top of the list. Any item containing potatoes produced significant acrylamide upon being heated in microwaves or conventional ovens. The study also found greater amounts of acrylamide are formed as foods are heated to higher temperatures. Boiling at 100 degrees Celsius appears to be the only safe cooking method. In potato-based foods, even cooking at a moderate temperature of 120 degrees Celsius began the process of acrylamide formation." Dr. Mercola expressed, "I am sure there are many more surprises produced in these foods that seriously damage health and lead to the development of chronic degenerative disease. 90% of the money Americans spend on food goes toward processed foods."

In press release/51 of June 27, 2002, the World Health Organization (WHO) disclosed: "Acrylamide is a chemical used in the manufacture of plastics. It was first discovered to be present in certain foods cooked at high temperatures as the result of work announced in Sweden in April 2002. It is a known carcinogen and causes nerve damage. Foods in which acrylamide develops when cooked at above 120 degrees Celsius include potato chips, French fries, bread and processed cereals."

In her article, "Turning Up the Heat on Acrylamide," in the FDA Consumer Magazine (U.S. Food and Drug Administration), January—February 2003, Linda Bren explains: "Acrylamide was not found in uncooked or boiled food—studies indicate that it appears to form during certain high-temperature (greater than 250° F) cooking processes, such as frying and baking, and that levels of acrylamide increase with heating time. Home-cooked foods, as well as pre-cooked, packaged and processed foods, have been found to contain acrylamide. Based on high-dose experiments in animals, acrylamide is classified as a potential human carcinogen, as well as a genotoxicant, a substance that can mutate and damage genetic material."

The high temperatures used to cook French fries, bread, crackers and biscuits, chips, cereal and even pasta can cause the formation of this carcinogenic substance, acrylamide. The formation of acrylamide should give you much reason not to eat these things, especially during pregnancy and lactation. When hearing of such reports, it makes even more sense to follow the diet that was given to us by the Creator, and utilize Nature's laws, which will bring us directly to unheated fruits, vegetables, nuts and seeds.

Popcorn, potato chips and crackers not only contain unhealthful amounts of salt, but they are processed at high temperatures causing chemical reactions that produce the toxic plastic acrylamide in the food. The acrylamide stiffens the food and gives it that crunchy feeling. If you want "crunchy," eat celery or an apple.

In their book, *Prescriptions for a Healthy House*, Paula Baker-Laporte, Erica Elliot and John Banta state: "The act of cooking generates significant amounts of indoor air pollution in the form of vapors and airborne particulate matter such as grease. In addition, food particles left on burners are incinerated and release combustion by-products."

Dr. Herbert Shelton wrote, "The sufferings of mothers during pregnancy and delivery are consequences of the wrong ways of life. The inability of women to breast-feed their babies is also a result of the wrong mode of living. The processed and refined foods of the American diet fail to supply the materials needed for the proper development and growth of the embryo and fetus, and after the birth, for the production of an abundant supply of wholesome milk."

Before continuing on nutrition, it's very important to point out the emotional outlook of the mother during pregnancy. Many mothers have told me their children took on the mood they had during pregnancy. It's crucial for the mother to have a happy outlook and a serene view of life. Relaxation and a feeling of contentment, combined with pleasurable and supportive relationships are as important as nutrition. Babies are very much in tune with their surroundings, and will take in any negative energy in their environments and be affected by it. I often felt my son as an infant was like an emotional radar system. He seemed always to be able to detect any upsets or negative energy I was feeling. To raise happy and secure children, it's important to be a relaxed, self-confident positive parent.

It may be necessary to disassociate with some family and friends who don't understand and accept your lifestyle choices for the protection of your child. For this reason, it's so crucial to be sure that prior to conception both spouses are in agreement as to their beliefs on raising healthy and happy children.

Mother's comfort and degree of rest and relaxation are so important to her mood during pregnancy and her ability to have an easy childbirth. Lying down comfortably to receive the best sleep possible during the later months of pregnancy can sometimes be challenging. Sleeping on your back is not recommended because of restricted blood flow to the fetus, and sleeping on your stomach may no longer be comfortable. I found that sleeping on my side with pillows between my legs was most helpful to providing the necessary comfort during the later months of pregnancy. A warm bath, gentle yoga, meditation, and/or a massage from your partner prior to bedtime can create the relaxation of body and mind during this important time in the life of mother and baby.

Women have told me when they sang frequently or were musically engaged during pregnancy, often playing instruments and singing, their babies became musically oriented.

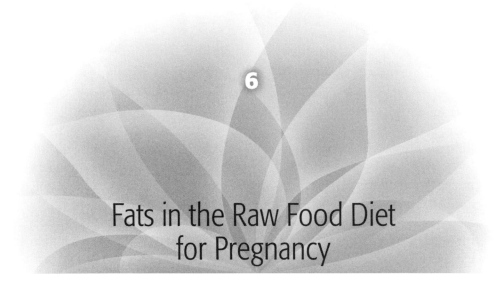

Fats in the Raw Food Diet
for Pregnancy

"The rest of the world lives to eat, while I eat to live."

SOCRATES

The diet of most Americans contains 35% or more calories from fat. A raw food diet high in fruits and vegetables with the addition of a small daily serving of half an avocado or a small whole avocado, or a handful of soaked nuts or seeds, should constitute a healthful amount of fat without going overboard. However, many raw foodists adhere to an unhealthful diet consisting of as much as 65% of their calories from fat. This type of raw food diet, which was my diet for many years, is extremely detrimental to one's health. In my early raw food days, I was quite misinformed, believing all raw foods were equal. When I began the raw food journey, I ate way too many nuts and avocados, foods with high percentages of fat. When traveling, nuts and dried fruits were the main staple—big mistake! Some nuts and seeds can be helpful while traveling in order to stay raw, but continuing to eat large amounts of these fatty foods for an extended period is not advisable. The intense oral detoxification I thought I was having when transitioning to raw foods may have been a negative reaction to the abundance of acid-forming nuts in my new diet. The oral symptoms of a swollen tongue and canker sores may have been related to the change from a cooked vegan diet to an even more acid-forming diet by eating great quantities of nuts and seeds. During my first few years on raw vegan foods, even showering every day made little difference in getting rid of my strong underarm odor which was the result of having eaten an unnecessarily large amount of nuts and seeds. At the time, I thought the body odor was due to detoxification, but when I significantly reduced the amount of fats in my

69

diet, the odor disappeared immediately. According to Dr. Timothy Trader, "We get plenty of fats from our plants. Overeating fat and protein causes disease. Fats from nuts, seeds and avocados are hard to digest. It takes a great deal of energy for the body to convert fat into sugar, overburdening the body. Nuts are 80 to 90 percent fat. This high fat content blocks nutrients to the cells, including oxygen, and calcium is lost in the process. A high fat diet also inhibits the intrinsic factor which supports the absorption of vitamin B12, thereby causing a B12 deficiency."

The research of vegan Ph.D., Dr. T. Colin Campbell, and M.D.s, Dr. John McDougall, Dr. Joel Fuhrman, Dr. Neal Barnard, Dr. Michael Greger and others, supports the low fat vegan diet.

When sweet fruit and fat are eaten together, the result is fermentation. The addition of fat causes the digestion to work harder. Fruit should be eaten alone or with compatible vegetables such as lettuces, celery or cucumber. Many raw foodists create a hazardous diet which can result in many problems by frequently combining sweet fruits and fats. The cakes and pies in raw food dessert menus often consist of this combination, which should only be an occasional treat (nuts and seeds with fresh and dried fruit) for a party or celebration.

When asked about omega 3 fatty acids, and getting enough of it during pregnancy, Dr. Trader responded, "We get some from fruit and some from vegetables. It appears the human body is able to make fatty acids omega 6 and omega 9 on its own, and we need them in much lower amounts than most Americans are taking in with animal products and oils. Most Americans have an imbalance of too much omega 6 compared with too little omega 3. We know we only need to consume omega 3s." A pregnant woman eating fruits, lots of greens and half a large avocado, or a whole small avocado, or a handful of raw nuts a day will be getting what she needs, as long as she's eating enough fruits and vegetables. These are suggested guidelines. The avocado needs to be eaten on separate days from nuts and seeds. Leafy green vegetables are reported to be high in omega 3 fatty acids. Nuts instead of an avocado a few times a week would be sufficient. EPA (eicosapentaenoic acid) and DHA (docosahexaenoic acid) can be made in the body from the omega 3 fatty acids through fruits and vegetables and a small portion of avocado or nuts and seeds to be sufficient. If a mother is eating great quantities of nuts and seeds, then it would be harder for her to deliver oxygen and nutrients to the baby because the blood would contain too much fat. Eating foods with high fat percentages for breakfast, lunch and dinner would be too much fat in the diet.

Dr. Trader pointed out a segment in the well-known film documentary *Diet for a New America* by John Robbins, which showed the blood of a man who had consumed a meal high in animal fat. The blood was filled with sludge, moving sluggishly. Animal fats are more dangerous for human beings due to their high levels of saturated fat—solid at body temperature. Nevertheless, Dr. Trader stresses: "Fat is fat, whether it be of animal or plant origin. If the blood is low in fat, then it will deliver the nutrients to baby more readily and efficiently. In addition, most nuts are heat-treated while others are chemically treated. It's difficult to find nuts that are sun-dried. At 110° Fahrenheit, the fat starts to break down. The high temperature causes the fat to decay. It becomes carcinogenic and unusable because high temperatures change the structure of fats. A healthful raw food diet should consist of lots of fruits and vegetables. Sweet fruits and leafy green vegetables contain fat. Without consuming foods with high percentages of fat such as nuts, seeds and avocados, you could still get 5 to 10% of your total calories from fat. Our closest animal relative, the bonobo chimpanzee, eats about 1% of his diet from fatty foods. Everyone needs differing numbers of calories depending on body size, type, and degree of activity. We need to eat fruit and greens until satisfied. The stomach releases a hormone to the hypothalamus in the brain that 'we've had enough.'"

Rich sources of omega 3 fatty acids are purslane, flaxseeds and hempseeds. Nuts can replace the avocado several times a week (such as a nut and veggie dressing or some nut or seed paté with a big salad, instead of the avocado). Two ounces of nuts or seeds in a day or 1 to 2 tablespoons of raw nut butter would be sufficient for a person of average weight and physical activity. Soaking of nuts and seeds overnight is imperative to release enzyme inhibitors, which keep them from sprouting. Soaking nuts and seeds in purified water makes them more easily digestible. All nuts benefit from soaking which replaces the water that was in the nuts at harvest, before they were dried for market.

Dr. Brazos Minshew, who writes for the Trivita Weekly Wellness Newsletter, provided the following information on English walnuts, under Small Snacks with Powerhouse Fats, March 8, 2008:

> English walnuts—It takes about 100 calories of energy for me to walk a mile, and about 130 calories to run one mile. A one-ounce serving of English walnuts (about 7 pieces) provides 180 calories of energy—that's enough fat energy for me to walk nearly two miles or to run 1 1/4 miles! Plus, walnuts are very high in omega-3 fats.

As you can see, a small number of nuts go a long way.

An over-abundance of fat congests the liver. Too many avocados, nuts and seeds can congest the liver with fat, causing diabetes. Fruits and vegetables move easily and quickly through the stomach, but these high fat foods take longer to digest (four or more hours) and provide less energy. We need some, but most people eat too much fat on the raw food diet.

Dr. Ruza Bogdanovich, author of *The Cure is in the Cause*, explains: "I eat nuts in the wintertime cracked from the shell. The calories from nuts are more needed in the winter. By eating nuts whole and raw, you become satisfied. By the time you crack three to four nuts, you feel full. But in the summertime when it is warm, you don't need to eat nuts. Nuts roasted with flavor enhancers don't have nutritional value. After eating them, the body isn't satisfied because it didn't get what it needed. You can eat a whole bowlful and still not feel full. The excess protein and fat from too many nuts and seeds can cause hair loss, as the hair follicle can't handle the extra protein and grease. The kinds of nuts you eat should depend on the part of the world where you live—coconuts in Hawaii and macadamias in New Zealand."

Dr. Douglas Graham recommends 10% of total calories as the maximum for fat intake, as an average. He points out: "There can be specific times during pregnancy when eating a bit more fat can work to the mother's advantage, as other foods just don't seem to satisfy. There is room for flexibility here, but as an overall average, I still recommend a maximum of 10% of calories come from fat."

Dr. Gabriel Cousens, in his book *Conscious Eating* recommends that no more than 20% of the total calories come from fat.

In the film, *Eating,* (www.RaveDiet.com), Caldwell Esselstyn, M.D., formerly with the Cleveland Clinic Foundation and conductor of the longest and most successful heart disease reversal program ever, stated, "A 30% fat diet causes heart disease."

I've often been asked about eating olives. I eat them only on occasion and in small quantities because of their high salt and fat content. If you purchase dried or cured olives, soak them for three days, changing the water twice daily to rid them of much of the salt. I sometimes use olives to enhance the flavor of delicious raw food preparations for holidays or parties.

A woman needs to be observant of how she feels and how much weight she is gaining during pregnancy. As a woman follows her intuition on the raw food path, she will be naturally able to listen to her body, and will have a built-in protection through eating for herself and her growing child.

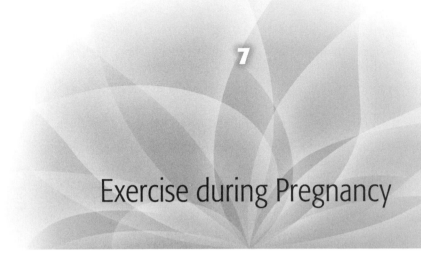

Exercise during Pregnancy

"Physical activity is more than a necessity; it is the law of life. It generates health and strength for mind and body. Without it—stagnation, deterioration, and finally death, ensue."

CELIA HOROWITZ

"It is exercise alone that supports the spirits, and keeps the mind in vigor."

MARCUS TULLIUS CICERO

I did a great deal of walking and hiking throughout both of my pregnancies. During the second pregnancy, I also rebounded up until the time I felt uncomfortable toward the end of my final trimester. Rebounding, or jumping on a mini trampoline, is a wonderful form of exercise. It gets all the organs of the body working, is an aid to digestion, is a complete cardiovascular workout, and is great for the lymphatic system, which continuously cleans the body of waste material. It would be extremely beneficial to jump for a half hour a day, but even as little as ten minutes a day is good. In an article titled, "The Bounce That Counts – Rebounding" in Options Magazine, August 2002, my husband and I were interviewed about the benefits of rebounding:

> The rebounder, a mini trampoline, has a round mat suspended on heavy-duty springs in the center of a round metal frame. Its legs can be collapsed and in some versions rebounders can be used for group workouts at gyms as well as by individuals who purchase them to use at home.

Dr. Harvey Diamond, internationally known author, teacher and health consultant, perhaps best recognized for his *Fit for Life* series of books, has written, the body's lymph system is its "defense system," a network of "fluid, organs, nodes and nodules, ducts, glands and vessels that continuously and aggressively cleans the system of waste matter." He endorses rebounding as an extremely easy exercise in which all that's basically required is "a slight up-and-down bounce, which subjects the body to a change in velocity and direction twice with each jump... As little as five or six minutes a day can be of immeasurable value."

Once Karen Ranzi stepped onto the rebounder with a headache, and by the end of her session the headache was gone. She finds the exercise helps her think more clearly as "it gets things moving," and she recommends its use to the members of a group she leads in Manhattan called "Accent on Wellness." The organization is involved with a change of lifestyle towards a more natural style of living.

Her husband Harvey, a sports enthusiast, also uses their re-bounder. He likes the continuous motion of jumping on a flexible surface as opposed to a hard one, and he finds the exercise has helped him gain greater speed on the tennis court. It has aided in his general conditioning and has also built up his stamina.

Anna-Inez Matus, who lives in Pine Grove, Pennsylvania, uses her rebounder every day, preferably outdoors in the sunshine. An educator who teaches others "how to achieve optimal health naturally, according to the principles of Life Science," Matus listens to music which reflects her mood as she exercises. She adds: "Rebounding increases my capacity for breathing, keeps my body well oxygenated, is a complete cardio workout in twenty minutes, flushes out my lymphatic system, and it helps the body to build good, healthy bone mass so I won't get osteoporosis."

Toward the end of pregnancy, if jumping on the rebounder becomes un-comfortable, some women might prefer to take advantage of the flexibility of the rebounder's springs to bounce lightly up and down without the feet leaving the mat. Although this is a lower activity level, there will still be a beneficial increase of lymphatic movement.

It is crucial to have an exercise program throughout pregnancy. Deep squats are important to develop the thigh muscles, sit-ups to develop the abdominal muscles, leg lifts, at least 50 Kegal exercises a day, calisthenics, and regular aerobic exercise (walking, jogging, biking, swimming, rebounding, dancing, whatever is fun and you enjoy!). I recommend reading the book *SPARK: The Revolutionary New Science of Exercise and the Brain* by John J. Ratey, M.D. which reports the important connection between aerobic exercise and lifting mood, beating stress, fighting memory loss, sharpening intellect and functioning at one's best by elevating the heart rate and breaking a sweat. The book reveals how aerobic exercise physically remodels our brains for peak performance, demonstrating the mind-body connection. In review of the book, "Startling research proves exercise is truly our best defense against everything from depression to A.D.D. to addiction to aggression to menopause to Alzheimer's. SPARK is the first book to explore comprehensively the connection between exercise and the brain."

Use of weights and resistance exercises for upper body strengthening is also extremely beneficial. Yoga is an excellent means of toning, stretching and relaxation during pregnancy and beyond. The internal organs are strengthened and toned by the additional flow of blood brought to them by the various yogic postures. The raw food lifestyle and yoga compliment eachother—both enhance energy and rejuvenation and offer composure to the mind and serenity to the spirit. Yogic postures, deep relaxation and meditation are beneficial at all times of life to bring our spirituality to light, revealing our inner energy. It's also important to breathe deeply each day.

Many people in our society consider pregnancy a time not to be physical, a time to double the food intake and live a sedentary lifestyle. The absence of physical exercise during these nine months can result in pain and problems in birthing. A moderate exercise program throughout pregnancy contributes to a radiant pregnancy and childbirth.

8

The B12 Question: How to Obtain It for You and Your Children

"In the nonindustrialized world, where bacterial contamination commonly brought traces of B12 to foods, B12 deficiency is largely prevented. However, modern hygiene has eliminated this source, just as indoor living has largely eliminated sunlight, nature's source of vitamin D."

WWW.VEGSOC.ORG

There has been intense discussion about the B12 issue, particularly in the past decade. Some leaders in the raw food arena have changed their views, recommending supplementation because of the dangers involved with low B12 levels. However, the information is inconclusive, and I have tried here to present views for and against supplementation, and other related issues that can directly affect B12 levels. Adequate B12 levels during pregnancy and lactation are important because the mother is supplying both herself and her baby with this vital nutrient.

In an article titled, "Vitamin B12: Are You Getting It?," Jack Norris explains, "For success in moving society away from a reliance on using animals for food by way of adopting vegan diets, it is of great importance for vegans to have optimal health." He says many vegans go back to eating animal products, and thinks:

It is possible some of the people who go back are feeling the effects of reduced B12 status. Most vegans do not think a lack of B12 could have caused someone to feel bad because they've been told humans need very little B12, and the body stores it for many years.

77

Norris reports the early signs of B12 deficiency according to Crane et al from the 1994 Journal of Nutritional Medicine:

> Early manifestations are unusual fatigue, faulty digestion (no appetite or nausea), and loss of menstruation. Other symptoms are nervousness, numbness, and tingling of the hands and feet, mild depression, striking behavioral changes, paranoia, hyperactive reflexes, fever of unknown origin, frequent upper respiratory infections, impotence, impaired memory, infertility, sore tongue, and diarrhea. Because they can be irreversible in some cases, neurological symptoms are the biggest problem in B12 deficiency.

This article is directed to vegans, and is a crucial read when deciding about B12 supplementation. The original version with full citations of this detailed article (2000) can be found on the web at http://www.veganoutreach.org or ordered from Vegan Outreach at 211 Indian Drive, Pittsburgh, PA 15238. Phone: (412) 968-0268. It can also be found at www.veganhealth.org/b12/.

Many vegan doctors now feel it is safer to supplement B12 or to have blood tests done regularly than to take the risk of eventually getting B12 deficiency symptoms. Homocysteine levels can rise if the body does not contain adequate B12 stores.

Dr. John McDougall writes:

> The actual risk of experiencing a B12 deficiency is extremely small, since it is stored for years. However, B12 deficiency has been reported in infants born to mothers who have been long time vegans and to macrobiotic mothers who have avoided all animal foods for many years. No significant neurological disorders or symptoms were reported in either case. However, to avoid any risks, pure vegetarian women who are pregnant or breast-feeding must add a non-animal source of B12, such as a vitamin supplement, to their daily diet (approximately 5 micrograms/day).

For many years, I did not supplement my 100% raw food diet with B12 vitamins. Instead, I did not wash all of my organic and biodynamic produce, hoping the traces of soil would create the necessary B12 for my system to assimilate. I did not supplement during my second pregnancy, my blood work was normal, and I had no symptoms of a deficiency. On a subsequent visit to Dr. Joel Fuhrman for blood work, a low B12 level was revealed. I decided to use a B12 supplement twice a week.

Dr. Gabriel Cousens (www.treeoflife.nu), researcher and a leader in the vegan and live-foods movement, reports the following information from his book *Spiritual Nutrition:* "The research conclusion is that it is a reasonably safe bet that about 80% of the vegan and live-food population, over time runs the risk of B12 deficiency...An even higher percentage of newborns run this risk." Dr. Cousens explains that vegan foods which were thought to contain human-active B12, such as spirulina and sea vegetables, are B12 analogs which are not useful, and can lead to deficiency. He recommends supplementation with an actual B12 human-active supplement which "allows us to be totally success-ful, vegan, live-fooders." The Tree of Life Rejuvenation Center in Patagonia, Arizona sells an activated B12 sublingual supplement in the form of hydroxo-cobalamin. It contains no GMOs, preservatives or MSG.

Dr. Fred Bisci, New York raw vegan nutritionist of 45 years, says many raw vegans who don't supplement B12 end up with long-term deficiencies.

A Tufts University study on B12 stated: "Anyone over 50 should take B12 supplements because after 40, many people are not able to absorb B12 through their digestive tracts. B12 is known to be essential for blood forma-tion, neurological function, a healthy heart, energy and optimism." Another report from the Netherlands researched blood levels of Vitamin B12 and bone mineral density. The result was osteoporosis occurred more often in those with marginal or deficient B12 levels. Therefore, the study revealed B12 may be important for bone density as well.

There are also some who think it is possible that since man has been eating meat for hundreds of generations that our bodies may have adapted to a greater level of vitamin B12, and therefore continued supplementation may be necessary when adopting a vegan diet.

Jingee, the mother of five children raised on living foods, writes: "Supplements are far inferior to foods. Hippocrates said to 'make food your medicine.'" She feels all the nutrients you need can be found in fresh fruits and vegetables, including vitamin B12. Jingee reports the findings of Joel Robbins, M.D., N.D., D.C., Ph.D., author of *Eating for Health and Wellness:* "B12 is found in alfalfa leaves, bananas, comfrey leaves, Concord grapes and raisins, ginseng, hops, mustard greens, plums and prunes, sprouts, sunflower seeds and wheat-grass." She also points out celery is a nerve-cell re-builder, and if you include enough celery or celery juice in your diet, then you will not end up with nerve damage. It is also a good source of sodium and alkaline salts. Vitamin B12 is also present on the surfaces of wild plants. Jingee's husband, Storm, has been a raw foodist for over 30 years without supplementation.

A high-quality supplement can be beneficial for someone who cannot get fresh organic produce year-round or eat wild, native plants. If choosing not to supplement during pregnancy, a urine sample and blood analysis should be taken to check B12 levels before and during pregnancy.

Rhio, author of *Hooked on Raw*, believes B12 becomes available in food through the action of bacteria that grows on or is present in food. She explains: "Since a family of yeasts and bacteria is what causes food to ferment, B12 would be present in fermented foods, as well as the other foods mentioned by Jingee. B12 as well as other vitamins of the B complex family are produced in a well functioning intestine." Rhio also sites Dr. Robert O. Young from his book *Sick and Tired? Reclaim Your Inner Terrain*. He expresses: "As long as you have plenty of friendly bacteria (probiotics), Vitamin B12 is synthesized." Rhio feels if we eat seaweeds and pollen as well as fermented foods, there can be bacterial action which creates B12. Rhio and Jingee add that 40% of Americans are deficient in B12, and only 10% of Americans are vegetarian, so many other people have B12 deficiencies. Additionally, most of the B12 in food is destroyed by cooking, just as other vitamins and minerals are destroyed. Rhio points out, "Catalytic converters for car emissions and industrial pollution also deplete our B12."

Other experts in the raw health field suggest alternative options instead of vitamin supplementation, such as use of chlorella or E3Live. Further views on chlorella will follow.

The following article is by Dr. Vivian V. Vetrano, well-known doctor of Natural Hygiene, who worked with Dr. Herbert Shelton, author of numerous Natural Hygiene books. Dr. Vetrano is a respected leader in the raw vegan community. Her articles have appeared frequently in Living Nutrition Magazine:

Rethinking and Clarifying the B12 Issue
by Dr. Vivian V. Vetrano (http://vetrano.cjb.net)

There is no such thing as a deficiency of vitamin B12, even in 100% raw vegans. They do not have to eat dirt, animal products, or take pills to secure coenzymes of B12. Bacteria in the intestinal tract make it for us, and the metabolically usable and necessary forms of coenzyme B12 are contained in unprocessed, fresh natural plant foods, particularly in nuts and seeds. The real problem in so-called B12 deficiency is a failure of digestion and absorption of foods, rather than a deficiency of the vitamin itself.

Vitamin B12 coenzymes are found in nuts and seeds as well as in many common greens, fruits, and many vegetables. If we ate 100 grams of green beans, beets, carrots, and peas we would have half of our so-called daily minimum requirement of Vitamin B12 coenzymes, provided that our digestion and absorption are normal. From Rodale's *The Complete Book of Vitamins*, page 236 we find the following clarification: "As you know, the B complex of vitamins is called a 'complex' because, instead of being one vitamin, it has turned out to be a large number of related vitamins, which appear generally in the same foods."

A little publicized source of active Vitamin B12 coenzymes is from bacteria in the mouth, around the teeth, in the nasopharynx, around the tonsils and in the tonsilar crypts, in the folds at the base of the tongue, and in the upper bronchial tree. This source alone will supply sufficient quantities of Vitamin B12 coenzymes for the very small requirement of total vegetarians, especially considering their needs for this vitamin are not as great as for those on conventional diets.

I have studied this issue thoroughly, and have learned biochemists, neutraceutical scientists, and many writers mistakenly use the term Vitamin B12 for cyanocobalamin, which is not usable by the body but is included in all vitamin B12 supplements. When speaking of Vitamin B12 they are referring to the semisynthetic Vitamin B12 (cyanocobalamin), initially contaminated with poisonous cyanide during its chemical extraction from animal tissues. Carbon columns are used during the extraction process and the carbon combines with nitrogen from the medium forming the poisonous cyanocobalamin, that scientists insist on calling Vitamin B12. The original method used to extract Vitamin B12 from its sources included heating the medium in a weak acid, the addition of cyanide ion, and exposure to light. In this process the coenzymes were converted to cyanocobalamin, yet this was overlooked. (*Review of Physiological Chemistry*, Harper, Harold A., Lange Medical Publications, New York, 1977, page 181. Also refer to *Cobalamin: Biochemistry and Pathophysiology*, Wiley. N. and F. Sicuteri, New York, 1972.) Moreover, in the manufacture of vitamin supplements, cyanide is added to the medium because the carbon and nitrogen are needed to form large molecules as are found in vitamins; and, additionally, they need it to extract the B12 from fermentation liquors and liver homogenates. Carbon is needed in great quantities when making vitamins or any other manufactured vitamin or substance that mimics the natural vitamin normally containing a lot of carbon.

The two Vitamin B12 coenzymes known to be metabolically active in mammalian tissues are 5-deoxyadenosylcobalamin and methylcobalamin (methyl-B12). When extracted in light, these two coenzymes undergo photolysis and are destroyed. Natural B12 is found solely in plants and animals, and that is the only form that can be called "coenzyme B12."

If an animal or individual is given cyanocobalamin, the body removes the cyanide because it is not usable as a coenzyme and it is toxic. Then the cobalt of the former cyanocobalamin can combine with other nontoxic substances and actually form Vitamin B12 coenzymes that are usable by the body. These normally existing Vitamin B12 coenzymes are labile and break down easily unless inside living tissue. Potassium in the body can react with the cyanide found in cyanocobalamin—the "Vitamin B12"—and form toxic potassium cyanide (KCN). Potassium cyanide is a poisonous compound used as a fumigant. This is one reason why the body jettisons the "Vitamin B12" (i.e., cyanocobalamin) injections so rapidly. Within 24 hours most (about 90%) of the cyanocobalamin in supplements has been eliminated.

The names of cobalamins formed by the body or in a laboratory are: 1. hydroxocobalamin if it combines with a hydroxyl ion (OH), and 2. aquocobalamin, when it combines with water. Cobalamin also combines with anions such as nitrite, a form of nitrogen, chloride, and sulfur. These are not usable by the body. The two active coenzymes that can be formed after stripping off the cyanide are 5-deoxyadenosylcobalamin, or adenosylcobalamin for short, and methylcobalamin. The problem is the cyanide is toxic and makes many people sicker than they were before taking the supplement. Cyanocobalamin is in [most] every vitamin B12 supplement known because it is stable and less costly to manufacture. But it is not usable in the body. If the body has sufficient energy, it may be able to offload the cyanide and benefit from the useful component. Mainly, what people experience after taking cyanocobalamin supplements is stimulation. The toxic effect of the cyanide triggers a rush of energy as the body works hard to excrete the poison, and this fools people into believing the supplement has "worked" to heal them. Meanwhile, if their blood tests show an increase in B12, it mainly reflects the amount of the cyanocobalamin in the bloodstream. The usable forms are carried into the cells and can't be discovered by testing the blood as is the current practice. Blood tests are often inaccurate and, as previously stated, in the case of cyanocobalamin supplementation and B12 injections, about 90 % of it has been eliminated from the body in 24 hours.

Looking at it Hygienically, no Vitamin B12 therapy can cause a recovery from any so-called deficiency disease. It may only hide the symptoms and cannot promote health. When people report their apparent B12 deficiency symptoms have been relieved by cyanocobalamin supplementation, they are mistaken. They are not getting usable Vitamin B12 coenzymes, and their bodies are forced to convert the cyanide form into the active forms, methylcobalamin, and adenosylcobalamin. This extra function stimulates but wastes nerve energy, and they are actually getting worse, not better. They have not addressed the cause of their troubles.

In summary, vegans and raw fooders all have sufficient amounts of co-enzyme B12 in their diets and from that produced in their bodies. The most common basic cause of a natural cobalamin deficiency is a failure to digest, absorb and utilize the various cobalamins from food and from the intestinal tract as in the case of gastritis or gastroenteritis. The cause of malabsorption is commonly a gastrointestinal disorder and this was known by pathologists way back in the 1800s. In this case, one's lifestyle must be assessed and brought into unison with the needs of the living organism. Furthermore, absorption of the natural B12 coenzymes can take place in the mouth, throat, esophagus, bronchial tubes and even in the upper small intestines, as well as all along the intestinal tract. This does not involve the complex enzyme mechanism for absorption (intrinsic factor) in the small intestine as required by cyanocobalamin. The coenzymes are absorbed by diffusion through mucous membranes.

The following article was written by Dr. Rick Dina:

B12 Testing The gold standard test for Vitamin B12 is known as Methyl Malonic Acid (MMA), as it is the best functional indicator of B12 status in the body. B12 is involved in breaking down MMA, therefore the MMA level of the blood and urine should be low. When levels of MMA are high, that means the B12 in your body is not working effectively, no matter what your actual blood B12 level shows. For example, someone can show adequate levels of B12, but could still have high MMA. This could mean the B12 detected was potentially B12 analogs, and therefore was not performing the functions B12 is designed to do. I performed a long series of B12 experiments on myself a few years back, in which I consumed spirulina to see if my B12 status changed. Before and after I consumed 2 heaping tablespoons of spirulina daily for three months, I had both my serum (blood) B12 and MMA levels measured. My lab data prior to consuming spirulina revealed my B12 was low, and my MMA was elevated. The lab report at the end of the three months indicated my serum B12 level went way up, but my serum MMA did not change. This experiment suggests spirulina is not a reliable source of

B12. There is a plethora of peer-reviewed scientific research supporting the outcome of my personal experiment.

In addition to the serum MMA test described previously, MMA can also be tested in the urine. The urine test is considered to be the most accurate, especially in people with compromised kidney function.

Serum homocysteine can also be an indicator of B12 status, but is not as reliable as the MMA test. Homocysteine will be elevated with B12 deficiency, but inadequate levels of B6 or folic acid will also cause elevated homocysteine. Therefore, homocysteine is not the most accurate test for B12 status, unless you are absolutely certain your B6 and folic acid levels are normal. MMA is elevated only as a result of B12 deficiency.

B12 Physiology / Deficiency The two active forms of B12 are *methyl*cobalamin and *5-deoxy-adenosyl*cobalamin. *Methyl*cobalamin is the active form utilized by the body, and *5-deoxy-adenosyl*cobalamin is the liver storage form. Another form, *Cyano*cobalamin, is the most stable form of vitamin B12, which is why it is the form found in most B12 supplements. *Cyano*cobalamin is not directly utilized by the human body, so a biochemical process in the liver removes the cyanide molecule from cobalamin and adds a methyl group to the cobalamin forming *methyl*cobalamin.

One of the main sources of the methyl groups that combine with cobalamin to create methylcobalamin comes from N-Methyl-Tetrahydrofolate, which is a fancy word for the inactive form of folic acid. When N-Methyl-Tetrahydrofolate gets "de-methylated" by cobalamin, it changes to the active form of folic acid. This active form of folic acid performs many important functions, one of which is an essential role in the replication of DNA. This is the basis of how B12 deficiency can lead to a certain type of anemia known as macrocytic anemia. Our red blood cells have a faster turnover rate than most other cells in the body. An average red blood cell lives about 120 days. If the DNA responsible for the formation of our red blood cells is unable to replicate properly, the result will be not enough red blood cells to carry oxygen to the rest of the cells.

Symptoms of this may manifest as weakness, fatigue, lightheadedness, shortness of breath upon exertion, a pale appearance, bleeding gums or a sore red tongue, a rapid heartbeat or chest pain, a loss of taste and appetite, or intermittent diarrhea or constipation. Often times the symptoms occur gradually over many years, or are very mild; therefore we may not even notice them or may just attribute them to the aging process in general. Sometimes these symptoms are not even noticed at all, especially in those who consume large quantities of folic acid from their diet, which is often times the case with whole food vegans and raw foodists.

If this situation persists over a longer period of time, damage to the nervous system can result, as nerve cells cannot replicate fast enough to keep pace with the normal rate of cell turnover. These symptoms can include numbness or tingling in the fingers or toes, poor balance and coordination, impaired thinking, depression, a decreased ability to sense vibration, ringing in the ears, tremors or dementia. If caught early enough, these symptoms can sometimes be reversed, but if this continues long enough, most experts have found some of the neurological deficits are indeed irreversible. This is no situation to gamble with, no matter what philosophy you subscribe to.

When cobalamin takes the methyl group from inactive folic acid, thus activating it, the methyl group is then transferred to the amino acid homocycsteine, which converts homocysteine into methionine. Homocysteine is well known to create inflammation that damages blood vessels. Methionine on the other hand does not damage blood vessels, and is a precursor to serotonin, an important brain neurotransmitter involved in proper brain function, responsible for the creation of the moods of happiness. We can see then by this mechanism that inadequate B12 causes increased levels of homocysteine, which therefore increases our risk for vascular disease and can simultaneously contribute to a general failure to feel good via low levels of serotonin. If we don't convert homocysteine to methionine, which is the precursor to serotonin, we don't make enough serotonin. Our bodies will then have to rely more heavily on our diets to get enough methionine to make serotonin. Additionally, inadequate amounts of methionine caused by a B12 deficiency decreases the availability of another substance made from methionine, s-adenosylmethionine, also known as SAM. SAM is required for the maintenance of the myelin sheath layer that covers nerves and helps the nerve cells conduct electrical impulses. This is another mechanism by which B12 deficiency can contribute to the neurological symptoms mentioned in the preceding paragraph.

Now that we understand a little more about how cobalamin transfers methyl groups from one place to another, we can see how it takes a methyl group off of methyl-malonic acid (MMA), thus lowering its levels.

In summary, B12 is involved in activating folic acid, lowering homocysteine, and making serotonin and SAM. This in turn keeps our red blood cells, blood vessels and nerve cells functioning properly, keeps oxygen flowing to all of our cells, and keeps us in a good mood.

Let's now go back to *cyano*cobalamin breaking down to cyanide and cobalamin. Some will argue this form of B12 is toxic because of the cyanide. In a nutshell (quite literally), there are many common foods such as almonds and stone fruits (i.e. apricots, peaches, plums, nectarines, etc.) that contain cyanide in larger amounts than we would consume in a B12 supplement. The minute amount of cyanide found naturally in these food sources is easily detoxified by the liver. Our bodies have no problem dealing with this small amount, so let's not take things out of perspective. The ramifications of long-term B12 deficiency are much more devastating than the miniscule amounts of cyanide from B12 supplements. For those who are still concerned, B12 supplements are also available in the *methyl*cobalamin form.

The most common reason for a B12 deficiency is gastric atrophy. In fact, up to 15% of the elderly population suffers from this, despite adequate dietary B12 intake from animal products. With gastric atrophy, cells that line the stomach known as parietal cells do not work properly, possibly resulting from many years of unhealthful dietary practices. Parietal cells produce hydrochloric acid (HCl) as well as another substance known as intrinsic factor. We need strong enough concentrations of HCl to break B12 off of food in order for it to be absorbed. Additionally, intrinsic factor combines with B12 and is involved with the absorption of B12 at the end of the small intestine, called the distal (or terminal) ileum. Without intrinsic factor, B12 absorption is very poor, and without enough HCl, B12 cannot be liberated from food to be utilized.

There are other reasons for B12 deficiency as well, including parasites, malabsorption, liver and kidney disease, and lack of dietary intake. This last reason is sometimes unfortunately the case for long-term vegans. Clinicians are now realizing B12 deficiency in this population is much more prevalent than we previously thought. This includes raw food vegans as well. Just because there are reasons for B12 deficiency other than lack of dietary intake does not mean we can ignore this as a potentially major health concern.

We need very small amounts of B12, and the liver can store many years and sometimes even decades worth of B12. Just because one has been a vegan for many years and still feels great does not necessarily mean his B12 status is optimal. Many people on an unhealthy traditional American diet claim to feel "just fine" right before they drop dead of a heart attack. We cannot feel high cholesterol, high blood pressure, arterial damage, cancer development, etc. as they are occurring, but the consequences of these will certainly be felt later on. The same is true with B12 deficiency.

Elevated MMA and homocysteine will show up well before any major B12 deficiency problems such as the neurological or anemic conditions mentioned above. I share the view of the great majority of vegan oriented clinicians in recommending either B12 supplementation or annual MMA testing to be sure your B12 status is optimal.

B12 Sources The traditional view is that B12 is found only in animal products, and not at all in any plant foods. As I mentioned earlier, I found spirulina did not improve my B12 status, despite consuming 2 heaping tablespoons per day for three months on three separate occasions. At the beginning and end of each of the three trials I tested my B12, MMA, and homocysteine to determine any change in my B12 status. Before I began these experiments, after 12 years as a mostly raw vegan, my B12 was low, and MMA and homocysteine were both elevated. At the time, I felt great and did not have anemia or any neurological problems. I had been reading the debates about vegan sources of B12 for years and did not know whom to believe. I decided to take this opportunity to see for myself what worked and what did not. For several years prior to finding out about my poor B12 status, I consumed very large quantities of dulse, a sea vegetable purported to contain human active B12. I also occasionally ate small amounts of miso, which is also supposed to have B12 formed in the fermentation process. I didn't always rinse my vegetables in the hopes some B12 manufactured by bacteria in the soil would be attached to the vegetables. I also assumed bacteria in my intestines, gums, nasopharynx, etc. was producing all the B12 I needed. After I found these assumptions to be wrong, I was not willing to allow any philosophy or dogma to put my long-term health in jeopardy.

After I determined spirulina was unsuccessful in improving my B12 status, I began consuming a product called Vitamineral Green, a whole food raw vegan product containing a large variety of algaes, grasses, green vegetables, and natural soil organisms. The bottom line is, I was able to improve my vitamin B12 status—my B12 levels went up, serum homocysteine decreased, and urinary and serum MMA went down—from consuming Vitamineral Green. I was very happy I was able to do so without taking a supplement.

At this time, I strongly suspect the chlorella in Vitamineral Green contained human active B12, which led to the improvement of my lab values. There is some recent peer-reviewed research that supports this assumption. For example, a recent Finnish study looked at the B12 status of long-term raw food vegans. They found the majority of the people in the study to have inadequate levels of B12, except for those who consumed chlorella on a regular basis. Other studies that have looked at different foods directly have shown chlorella to be a reliable source of human active Vitamin B12.

In an ideal world, all of our food producing plants would be grown in healthy soil that contains bacteria producing B12. The plants could then absorb and fix the B12 in their tissues, so the B12 would be bioavailable to those who consume them. In today's civilized world, this is rarely the case. If you have been a vegan for several years, even if you consume chlorella or a product containing it, I would still strongly recommend that you have your B12 status tested via urinary MMA. This will give you the information you need to make an informed decision on this critical health issue. I would be very interested in knowing the lab results of any long-term vegans. Feel free to contact me through my website for any suggestions or support you may require.

I hope you found this information to be eye-opening and useful in your pursuit of optimal health.

Rick Dina, D.C.
www.rawfoodeducation.com

References

Coppen A, Bolander-Gouaille C, Treatment of depression: time to consider folic acid and vitamin B12, J Psychopharmacol. 2005 Jan;19(1):59-65.

Groff, James L. and Gropper, Sareen S, Advanced Nutrition and Human Metabolism, Belmont, CA: Wadsworth/Thompson Learning, 2000: p. 302

Rauma AL, et al, Vitamin B12 status of long-term adherents of a strict uncooked vegan diet ("living food diet") is compromised, Journal of Nutrition. 1995 Oct;125(10):2511-5,

Watanabe F, et al, Characterization and bioavailability of vitamin B12-compounds from edible algae, Journal of Nutritional Science and Vitaminology (Tokyo). 2002 Oct;48(5):325-31

Dr. Gina Shaw of the UK expresses her opinion on the B12 supplementation issue:

In the vegan movement, there is so much hype about the B12 issue that for people to ignore the classic signs and symptoms and not to recognize them would be pretty unbelievable.

Muscle fatigue, paranoia, depression, tingling in the extremities, burning in the extremities, irritability, insomnia, etc. I noticed it when I had it and felt much better after fasting (so have clients, and their clinical results and improvement prove their recovery). Supplementing without cause is in my opinion unnecessary. If the symptoms or signs are there, fair enough, do what you feel is right on a personal level, but I personally would recommend clients fast to overcome the CAUSE (providing the CAUSE isn't a dietary issue), not deal with the symptoms (if you're not absorbing there could be a whole range of other problems besides vitamin B12). I know people who have been supplementing for years and still seem to have overt signs of B12 deficiency. These people would rather die than fast and, in my opinion, the problem is they are refusing to look at the CAUSE, which will not go away. From my studies, chlorella like other algaes contains B12 analogs which may well show up as B12 in serum tests, but aren't actually bio-available and so could skew the test results leading to a false positive reading. Also, MMA tests are not 100% reliable indicators of a B12 deficiency as genetic defects, kidney failure, low blood volume, dysbiosis, pregnancy and hypothyroidism (the latter which, in my experience, many clients seem to be suffering with these days) will cause a high MMA reading (although know it is probably one of the most reliable tests, especially the urine one).

Although it is clear to the client and me that after fasting the client is very much rejuvenated and healed on many levels, the only documented case I have with clinical results is as follows: A male client who presented with overt B12 deficiency symptoms. His clinical serum level was 141pc/mol. Post fast his B12 serum level was 415pc/mol. At last contact, the client is doing well on high raw food diet, with renewed energy levels. I recently fasted a male client with a cancer diagnosis who had severe neurological problems as indicated by iris analysis. His nervous system was very inflamed but upon the last iris examination, his nervous system is almost completely healed. I suspected he had some quite serious B12 problems too as he had low HCl levels and some neurological symptoms were reported.

Dr. Shaw's experience with B12 is as follows:

In December 2004, I experienced overt B12 deficiency symptoms including muscle fatigue, tingling and numbness in extremities, insomnia, memory problems, stress, fatigue, etc. after a very stressful year. I was diagnosed with B12 deficiency through serum level testing. My level was very low, at 99pc/mol. I fasted and experienced much healing including neurological healing. I felt much better afterwards but about a month later I started to experience symptoms again. It wasn't a good time to fast again as I had only just started to regain my weight since I had lost a lot of weight after the fast. I thought I'd experiment with some vegan supplements recommended by someone who felt they had lessened symptoms. I actually tried for several weeks but none of the symptoms improved. I realized I had to fast again—and did for just three days on water—and felt much better and have not had problems since. Certainly, the latter fast was an issue of malabsorption, but the first fast probably had to be done because of stress and that my diet had become quite limited due to poor quality of fruits in the UK at that time, and because I wasn't taking in sufficient nuts/protein. It is important to take Dr Vetrano's advice and include sufficient raw nuts/seeds and other B12-rich foods in our diet and a variety of organic leafy green vegetables.

http://www.vibrancy.homestead.com/pageone.html

[A sufficient amount of nuts and seeds in the diet should not mean overeating on these high fat foods. The detrimental effects of over consumption of nuts and seeds have been elaborated upon in the section on *Fats in the Raw Food Diet for Pregnancy and Lactation*.]

The following beliefs are expressed by Dr. Timothy Trader:

You ask, "What did people ever do two or three thousand years ago before B12 supplements were ever invented? How did the human race ever survive?"

When people talk about food being cleaned of its bacteria, they are not so much talking about the washing of the food (although that can contribute), but about the sterilizing of the soil in which the food is grown. B12 was not discovered until 1948. By then, modern agriculture, with its chemical fertilizers and pesticides, had been practiced for about half a decade. B12 is actually the waste matter of bacteria. They excrete it into the soil, and the animals (including us) who eat plants grown in that soil thus ingest B12. If you totally devitalize the soil of all its microbial life, as conventional farmers have been doing for 60 years now, you can rest assured there is no bacteria excrement. In contrast, plant foods grown in composted, highly bioactive organic soils have been shown to uptake B12 into their structure (in other words, the B12 is not only in the soil but in the plant itself). I have heard this from permaculture farmer and scientist David Blume (www.permaculture.com), as well as from Dr. T. Colin Campbell, Cornell professor of nutritional biochemistry. On page 232 of *The China Study,* a 1994 study published in the journal "Plant and Soil" by a man named Mozafar, Campbell cites, "Research has convincingly shown: plants grown in healthy soil that has a good concentration of vitamin B12 will readily absorb this nutrient."

Thus, Nature put the B12 and all other nutrients we need in our foods. Unnatural farming practices have made this nutrient unavailable to the masses. And unnatural dietary and lifestyle practices have made sure we do not absorb and properly utilize this nutrient even if we do ingest it. Many factors, including eating animal foods, impair our absorption of B12. At the same time, carnivorous animals concentrate B12 within their tissues. Thus, meat/dairy/egg-eating humans experience a compensating over consumption of B12 that masks the subclinical pancreatic and other damage caused by eating those same foods. Eventually, as described at http:/www.lifesave.org/ VitaminB12.htm, (part 2) the subtle but ultimate occurrence, over time, of animal tissue triggered B12 absorption breakdown may well be simply deemed, written off, or accepted as part of "normal aging!"

Don Weaver of Earth Health Regeneration in California, author of *To Love and Regenerate the Earth*, and co-author of *The Survival of Civilization* (http: www.remineralize.org) points out:

The soil must have all the minerals including the cobalt for the cobalamin molecule(s) if we expect B12 and much else to be microbially synthesized. As my late publishing partner John Hamaker once wrote, "The legitimate purpose of agriculture is to feed the soil microorganisms," and he meant their complete natural diet including the full spectrum of rock-borne soil elements. To explore the topic of remineralizing the soil and thus our inner microflora and ourselves, read about this topic at www.remineralize.org. I think it would be wise to never forget the connections of soil health and personal-planetary health when we consider any sub-field such as one of the 100+ essential and inter-related nutrients.

Dr. Ruza Bogdanovich, author of *The Cure is in the Cause*, explains:

Statistics are only tools, not facts. We are all a bit different. The test numbers are always changing to accommodate pharmaceutical companies and doctors so they can prescribe. What is normal and what is not, and according to whom? When people are on an all raw vegan organic varied diet, many things will look different and tests will not show the same results. How do you feel should be the question. I have found many of my patients have problems because they live complicated lives, do not have a garden, worry too much about unnecessary things and hold grudges toward their brothers and sisters. That alone depletes the body of very important nutrients and brings the immune system down.

9

Digestion and Assimilation of Nutrients during Pregnancy and After

"Nature is the best physician."

HIPPOCRATES

Some doctors and nutritionists believe certain nutrients in vegetables become more available through cooking, and that heating vegetables even improves their digestion and assimilation. An example of this regards the lycopene in tomatoes, said to be better absorbed from cooked tomatoes. Classically, according to the teachings of Natural Hygiene, cooked tomatoes are to be avoided because heating prevents the tomato acids from turning alkaline, whereas the acids in raw tomatoes turn alkaline as soon as they touch the lips. Once tomatoes are cooked, the acids become fixed and remain acidic.

Most people cook their food at high temperatures. Once heated, food becomes limp and lifeless-looking. If you put fire to your hand, it would be burnt or even totally destroyed. It makes sense this is the same thing that happens with food, making it poor or devoid in nutrients and difficult to digest. In all of my years of cooking food, I don't remember being careful to heat food at the very lowest temperatures to preserve nutrients. Even the lowest temperatures on stoves are not low enough to preserve most nutrients.

If food is not chewed sufficiently, there will be digestive difficulty. It has been written in a number of books (such as *The Power Eating Program* by Lino Stanchich) that chewing is of utmost importance to digestion and assimilation of nutrients. One of the most important classes taught at the Ann Wigmore Institute in Puerto Rico focuses on proper chewing. Upon entering the mouth, the digestion of food begins, and it then needs to be thoroughly chewed into a mushy, liquid-like consistency prior to swallowing. This is further described later. Fruit smoothies, green smoothies, blended salads and raw soups further enhance digestion because these foods are pre-chewed through blending.

93

Nevertheless, liquefied foods should be further chewed to help release enzymes. Examples of green smoothies are in the kid-tested recipe section and the chapter on Raw Pregnancy. Also see Victoria Boutenko's valuable book, *Green for Life*, which describes in detail how green smoothies can improve health.

Good food combining is also important. The fewer combinations of food eaten at one time, the easier it will be for the food to be digested. When only a single food is eaten at a given time, a mono meal, digestion functions best. When creating a salad, no more than 3 to 4 ingredients should be used because each food requires a different time period and type of digestion. Meals need to be easy on the system and uncomplicated.

David Klein, health educator, author, and publisher of "Vibrance" Magazine, sells a Food Combining Chart (www.livingnutrition.com) that I've displayed on my refrigerator and referred to often over the years. It is especially important to have a food combining chart when first learning proper food combining. At a time when baby is placing pressure on mother's internal organs, more easily digestible well-combined meals will be most beneficial.

I've often been told that digesting fresh fruits and vegetables is difficult. First of all, fruit must be eaten only when completely ripe to be properly digested. I've also frequently observed when food combining is properly followed, the digestion significantly improves, even if there is still some cooked food in the diet. For example, over time, eating grains with fruit (such as cereals and fruit, bread and fruit, etc.), results in poor digestion. Some people have said they can't eat fruit, and even vegetables, because they don't digest them properly, resulting in gas and other problems. Almost always when I recommend eating fruit by itself (or just with lettuce and celery) or vegetables alone (or combined with some nuts, seeds or an avocado), and not to combine fruit with complex starches or fat, the digestion improves.

Heavy meals are often followed by dessert containing fruit. I was recently at a gathering where the meal was chicken, rice, beans, pasta, salad and various cooked vegetable dishes. Following dinner, a big bowl of fruit was the dessert. Fruit doesn't need to stay in the stomach to be digested. Rather, it needs to go directly to the intestines, but this can't happen when the rest of the complex meal of fats, proteins and starches is already in the stomach. Putrefaction and fermentation are often the results of such combinations.

On page 95, see the Food Combining Chart by David Klein, Ph.D. for best combinations of raw fruits, vegetables, nuts and seeds.

If mother were to embrace a healthful raw food lifestyle with an awareness of food combining during pregnancy, there would often be reduced or no morning sickness. There would be a slight weight increase, and childbirth would be quicker and smoother.

Food Combining Chart

DO NOT EAT FRUIT WITH ANY OTHER FOOD EXCEPT GREEN NON-STARCHY VEGETABLES

ACID FRUIT		SUB-ACID FRUIT		SWEET FRUIT	MELON	
Blackberries	Pineapple	Apple	Kiwi	Bananas	Cantaloupe	Honey Dew
Grapefruit	Raspberries	Apricot	Mango	Dates	Casaba	Persian
Lemon	Strawberries	Blueberries	Nectarine	Dried Fruit	Crane	Sharlyn
Lime	Tangerines	Cherimoya	Papaya	Thompson &	Crenshaw	Watermelon
Orange	Tomatoes [1]	Cherries	Peach	Muscat Grapes	[Eat with no other fruit]	
[Eat before other fruits]		Fresh Fig	Pear	Persimmon		
		Grapes	Plums	Raisins		

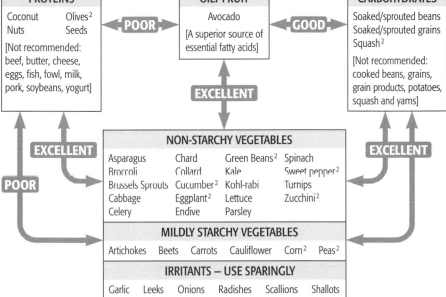

PROTEINS		OILY FRUIT	CARBOHYDRATES
Coconut	Olives [2]	Avocado	Soaked/sprouted beans
Nuts	Seeds	[A superior source of essential fatty acids]	Soaked/sprouted grains
[Not recommended: beef, butter, cheese, eggs, fish, fowl, milk, pork, soybeans, yogurt]			Squash [2]
			[Not recommended: cooked beans, grains, grain products, potatoes, squash and yams]

POOR — POOR — GOOD — EXCELLENT — EXCELLENT — EXCELLENT — POOR

NON-STARCHY VEGETABLES

Asparagus	Chard	Green Beans [2]	Spinach
Broccoli	Collard	Kale	Sweet pepper [2]
Brussels Sprouts	Cucumber [2]	Kohl-rabi	Turnips
Cabbage	Eggplant [2]	Lettuce	Zucchini [2]
Celery	Endive	Parsley	

MILDLY STARCHY VEGETABLES

Artichokes   Beets   Carrots   Cauliflower   Corn [2]   Peas [2]

IRRITANTS — USE SPARINGLY

Garlic   Leeks   Onions   Radishes   Scallions   Shallots

[1] Tomatoes only combine with non-starchy vegetables, seeds, nuts, olives, avocados, cucumbers and sweet peppers.
[2] Botanically classified as a fruit, but its bio-chemical composition places it in a non-fruit food combining category.

Source: David Klein, Ph.D., Colitis & Crohn's Health Recovery Center, http://www.colitis-crohns.com

10

Breastfeeding Is the Best Choice
for Mother and Baby

*"A baby nursing at a mother's breast... is an undeniable affirmation
of our rootedness in nature."*

DAVID SUZUKI

Human breast milk is made for the human baby to digest. Women's breasts were made to produce milk for their babies. Human milk is perfect for the human baby's digestive system, just as cow milk is perfect for the calf, and goat milk is perfect for the kid goat's digestion. When animals suckle the milk of their own species, more energy is available for development of the offspring's body and brain. Vegetarian animals provide an adequate supply of milk for their young. The horse, camel, bison, cow, rhinoceros, elephant, giraffe and gorilla are exclusively raw foodists, and as all raw vegetarians, provide plentiful amounts of milk.

My father told me he encouraged my mother to breastfeed me. She breastfed me for two weeks, but then her doctor discouraged her, and she discontinued. My father emphasized this was one of the most important things I could give my children, and I listened to him very carefully, nursing my own children for years until they decided to wean. My children never had pacifiers or blankets to suck on, because in addition to milk, their mother's nipples provided them with security, relaxation and bonding.

There is a long list of benefits that come with providing baby with the most natural milk which the Creator so miraculously created. The presence of strontium 90, a heavy radioactive material from nuclear fallout, is reportedly more concentrated in bottled formulas and animal milks than in human milk. According to Dave Rietz, past webmaster of www.notmilk.com, "Most cow milk has measurable quantities of herbicides, pesticides, dioxins (up to 200 times the safe levels), up to 52 powerful antibiotics (perhaps 53, with LS-50), blood, pus, feces, bacteria and viruses. (Cow milk can have traces of anything the cow ate…including such things as radioactive fallout from nuclear testing…the strontium-90 problem so widespread in the Fifties)." (www.rense.com/general26/milk.htm)

Beth Montgomery, author of *Transitioning to Health: A Step by Step Guide for You and Your Child*, examined lacto-free formula. She found it is "98% corn syrup and oil, which is sugar and oil. It consists of less than 2% vitamins and minerals which are not in a natural form. They are synthetic, and sprayed into the powder—and the doctors don't prescribe vitamin and mineral supplements for babies under one year old."

Breast milk enhances baby's immune system and protects against infection. Dr. John McDougall points out the risk of influenza and spinal meningitis for bottle-fed babies is as much as sixteen times greater than the risk for breastfed babies.

The breastfeeding benefit to mothers includes a reduced risk of premenopausal breast cancer and release of stress-relieving hormones.

Gabriel Cousens, M.D., in his book *Rainbow Green Live–Food Cuisine*, claims infant formula is inappropriate nutrition for infants: "The formulas do not contain the GLA (gamma-linolenic acid) and DHA (decosahexaenoic acid) which are so important. Breast milk is perfectly formulated for maximum neurological growth." "DHA is the essential long-chain omega-3 fatty acid needed for brain development and the fatty acid found in highest concentration in the brain. A deficiency of DHA is associated with post-partum depression in women and lower IQ in DHA-deficient babies."

Hygeia Halfmoon, author of *Primal Mothering in a Modern World*, in an article in the 1997 Fall-Winter "Living Nutrition Magazine," expresses she produced an optimum milk supply for her three children as a raw vegan for more than 11 years. She says, "The nutritional composition of mother's milk is nearly identical to that of fruit, and that explains why our children thrive so well on fruit as a transition food when they are nursing less and less. Many mothers are concerned that without dairy products in their diet they won't have adequate protein and calcium in their milk supply, but all fruits contain predigested proteins that are quickly assimilated. Just one orange gives you more calcium than a glass of cow milk because calcium from cow milk is poorly assimilated."

Calcium cannot be absorbed in the presence of high protein content, and the protein content of cow milk is significantly greater than that of human

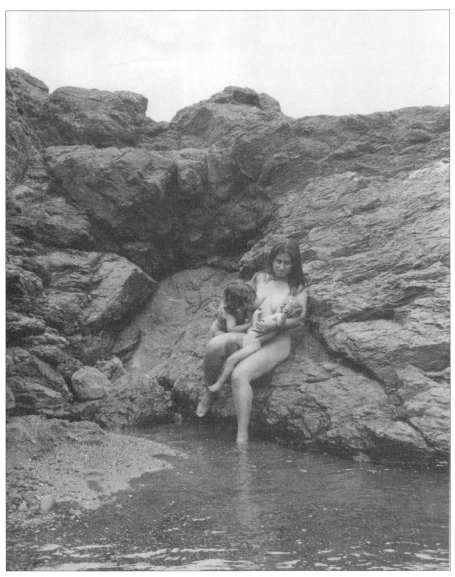

Beautiful loving mother, Yemaya Kimmel, nursing her two babes.

milk. Nature meant for it to be used for calves so they could grow into a large 2000 pound animal—the cow.

In terms of total calories, mother's milk is about 6% protein. Babies double in size in six months consuming nothing but mother's milk. Fruit contains a similar percentage of protein, and vegetables and nuts have even more protein.

Cow milk is reportedly about 15% protein. We know a cow grows much more rapidly than a human, and grows to be much bigger. This is why the calf has a significantly greater protein requirement.

Tests have shown breastfed babies develop about 90% of bone growth expected at nine months, whereas bottle-fed babies only have 50% of their bone growth by that time. In the article "Breastfeeding in Early Life and Bone Mass in Prepubertal Children: A Longitudinal Study," by G. Jones, M. Riley and T. Dwyer, the aim was to determine whether breastfeeding in early life is associated with bone mass in 330 8-year old male and female children from Southern Tasmania. Breastfeeding intention and habit were assessed in both 1988 and 1996. The results demonstrated breastfed children had higher bone mineral density at the femoral, neck, lumbar spine and total body compared with those who were bottle-fed.

Mother's uterus normally contracts more rapidly when breastfeeding her baby. Baby needs less burping from a breastfeeding mom because he or she won't swallow as much air. When nursing, a woman has more time and lower costs because she will not be making frequent purchases of formula. Psychological tests have shown breastfed children are better adjusted. They are held very near to mother in her arms. Baby hears mother's breathing and heartbeat as in the womb, and mom relaxes and gets to know her baby. The frequent feedings breastfed babies require will assure babies get the nourishment and the attention they need from their mothers. Mothers who breastfeed have a significantly lower risk of breast cancer later in life as do the young who receive their milk, as reported by numerous studies.

Because human milk proteins are digested more quickly and efficiently than formula proteins, breastfed babies begin to get hungry more quickly than formula-fed babies. Well-meaning advisors had recommended I nurse my infants every three hours, emphasizing the importance of keeping baby on a strict schedule. When I very briefly attempted these strictly timed intervals, it caused tremendous stress to my baby and me, and I found the baby could not nurse properly or relax under this pressured situation. Mother needs to recognize that baby knows when nutrition or comfort is needed—nursing on demand must be the only choice.

It takes much more energy to digest formula than the little energy required to digest human breast milk. If the stools of formula-fed infants are big and bulky, it's because excess protein that cannot be assimilated will come out in the stool. On the contrary, breastfed infants are able to absorb all of the protein in mother's milk.

Another surprising benefit to breastfeeding: My children's bowel movements did not have the awful smell typical of bottle-fed babies' excrement. And breastfed babies have even better smelling feces when their mothers are living the raw foods lifestyle. Even our raw fed dogs' bowel movements were easy to clean up because of their lack of foul odor.

I teach a class called "Creating Healthy Children." Sometimes, an adoptive mother gets upset when I talk about the many benefits of breastfeeding. Lactation consultants can help the adoptive mother get a flow of milk. There is also the practice of infant massage, which can facilitate wonderful bonding behavior between mother and baby. A book I recommend is *Infant Massage: A Handbook for Loving Parents*, 3rd Edition, by Vilmala Schneider McClure, Bantam Books. Another option for adoptive parents is breast milk banks which have sprouted up in different places around the country. In his article, "Donating Mother's Milk: The Gift of Life," Charles Downey writes, "According to Sony Riviera, M.D., president of the Mother's Milk Bank and medical director of Newborn Nurseries at St. David's Medical Center in Austin, Texas, 'Human milk is incredibly complex. Science is discovering more nutrients, immunities, essential fats and proteins that can only be found in human milk. The July 1999 issue of the British Medical Journal reported a study in which German children nourished exclusively with breast milk during the first three to five months of life were less likely to suffer from obesity when they reached school age than those raised on other foods. Human breast milk is also used to help heal babies with infectious diseases, severe diarrhea and pneumonia. Children with renal failure, cardiac problems and burns may also benefit from mother's milk.'" Most of these problems would never have arisen in the first place had the mothers been nourished on raw plant foods and nursed their babies.

The milk obtained from milk banks is pasteurized to kill bacteria. Pasteurization destroys the enzymes, but it is still preferable to formulas. Milk banks attempt to match the donors with the ages of the receiving baby since the composition of breast milk changes as baby grows. There are eleven breast milk banks across North America. It might be difficult to obtain the milk since there is a great shortage, and ill children would most likely have priority in receiving this milk. Other countries are more progressive. Brazil has 300 breast milk banks. A higher quality option is to find a local wet nurse and pay for milk that is not pasteurized. A woman should be willing to undergo a health screening before being paid for her milk. There are facilities in Europe where mothers can donate or sell their milk to those who cannot breastfeed. A website exists through which mothers donate breast milk to babies who would otherwise go without it: www.milkshare.birthingforlife.com.

A small percentage of mothers fail to have sufficient milk and/or can't find a wet nurse. In this dire situation, if mother's milk is not available either through nursing, a wet nurse, or a milk bank, a last resort would be to use raw organic goat milk. Some studies suggest that specific proteins known to cause allergic reactions may be present in cow milk in significant quantities yet largely absent in goat milk, allowing it to be better tolerated by humans. Raw organic goat milk may be preferable to giving formula to baby. Goat milk is sometimes used as a replacement for cow milk-based infant formulas, but unfortunately, goat milk is lacking in several nutrients necessary for growing infants. According to www.kellymom.com, "Feeding goat milk before 6 months or regular feeding between 6 and 12 months is not recommended." Mother's milk contains everything the baby needs and will always remain the best choice. Some mothers just don't want to nurse their children—an unfortunate circumstance for mother and child.

Use of medications and an unnatural diet can negatively affect mother's milk supply. Alcohol and caffeine can be responsible for infertility, miscarriages, and may also negatively affect mother's milk supply.

When I changed to a raw food diet and natural lifestyle, my milk supply became so much more abundant. I felt I could have fed many more babies.

Mammals that take the longest to mature also have the longest breastfeeding periods. Since humans take longer to mature than any other mammal, their nursing phase needs to be longer than that of any other mammal, ranging from three to five years and longer. Women who nurse for at least two years are providing breast cancer prevention for themselves as well as future immunity for their young. I nursed my daughter for four and a half years and my son for almost six years. The earlier nursing years provided nutrition and emotional bonding, and as the years progressed, and their nutritional needs were filled by eating solid foods, nursing became less frequent albeit always available for emotional needs. The child should decide when to wean, not the mother. I always instinctively felt my children were protected by the long-term nursing. The perfect amounts of fat and protein and the many vitamins and minerals (many probably still unknown) and the excellent bonding it provides are the key to forming strong, healthy children. And a mother eating 100% raw, or mainly raw foods, will be giving her fortunate child the gift of abundant health.

The components in human milk can never be duplicated. When bottled formula was being developed, there was a formula lacking in Vitamin B6. No one knew B6 was present in human milk. Many babies had convulsions and died. There are many nutrients not yet identified in mother's milk. Until we realize the Creator made only mother's milk to be consumed in the child's early life, we will see all kinds of deficiencies deriving from the early feeding of food or formula. A mother who is experiencing difficulty in nursing her baby should contact a lactation consultant from La Leche League. La Leche League can be reached at 800-LA-LECHE. Nursing is extremely important for the nutrients as well as for the emotional bonding. La Leche League can also be contacted at www.lalecheleague.org. To get support for nursing as a first-time mother, I had attended monthly La Leche League meetings in my area. I recommend these meetings to all parents for the support given for long-term breastfeeding. Women who need help with breastfeeding, especially parents of multiple babies, premature babies and adoptive parents, should seek the help of a board certified lactation consultant or La Leche League.

In his book, *Spontaneous Creation: 101 Reasons Not to Have Your Baby in a Hospital*, Volume 1 (www.spontaneouscreation.org), Jock Doubleday cites the following studies linking breastfeeding with intelligence and higher IQ:

"Many studies demonstrate the superiority of breastfeeding to bottle-feeding in relation to infant and child intelligence. Studies consistently show breastfed children have higher IQs and perform better academically than formula-fed children. One study, published in *Pediatrics* in January 1998, followed more than 1,000 children over an 18 year period. The authors concluded: 'There were small but consistent tendencies for increasing duration of breastfeeding to be associated with increased IQ, increased performance on standardized tests, higher teacher ratings of classroom performance, and better high school achievement.' Another study found, after controlling for family, social, and economic variables, early breastfeeding was associated with better picture intelligence at eight years of age, and better scores in mathematics and better sentence completion at 15 years of age.

No need to take just two studies' word for it. Studies published in 1982, 1988, 1994, and 1996 also concluded breastfeeding enhances cognitive development in preschool children. Studies published in 1978, 1982, 1984, 1992, 1993, and 1994 concluded breastfeeding enhances cognitive development of children in their early school years. (The 1993 study above tested both preschool and school-age children.) Researchers found breastfed children scored higher on both the Bayley and McCarthy scales, and the longer infants breastfed the higher were their intelligence scores. A March 2003 study published in *Acta Paediatrica* found that full-term infants who are born smaller than normal scored an average of 11 points higher on I.Q. tests if they were breastfed exclusively."

Although the protein content of human breast milk is relatively low, the types of amino acids that form these proteins are crucial. One of these amino acids, taurine, is abundant in human milk. Studies have shown taurine is important in the development of the brain and the eyes.

Breast milk is the only food baby should receive during much of the first year of life. It contains the important fat and protein that cannot ever be replaced by other foods or formulas. Even loving, well-meaning parents cannot use raw vegan foods to replace breast milk. Many infants are unable to properly digest almond milk or avocados at so young an age, and may not increase in weight because of their inability to absorb these fats and proteins. These infants risk malnourishment. Many children are allergic to nuts, specifically because they were introduced too early in life. Many years ago, I attended a class on healthy foods for the young child in which recipes were given for almond milk, and it was stated this alternative milk could replace mother's milk completely if the mother were absolutely unable to nurse. I believe this to be totally untrue. Almond milk and avocados are high in fats that are more difficult to digest than those in breast milk. It would be best not to introduce them until at least the second year, and to wait even longer before feeding whole nuts and seeds. Although some success has been reported with almond milk in Germany when babies were found to be allergic to cow milk, I strongly feel mothers have got to find a way to feed their babies with mother's milk—if not their own, from another mother.

The 6% protein content of mother's milk is perfect for the infant's digestion. I nursed my son exclusively until toward the end of his first year of life, giving him no other nutrients, and he had no problem with calories and adequate weight gain. Later, when I transitioned to a raw food diet, I was amazed at how my milk supply dramatically increased. I also drank a lot of water. The combination of the increased amounts of water and the water-rich diet while still lactating made for a plentiful supply of mother's milk.

After the weaning stage, there is no need for any kind of milk. The advertisements focusing on the benefits of animal milk are only for commercial gain since the dairy industry makes a huge profit from the sale of milk. Dairy products actually rob us of our calcium. Studies point to dairy as a cause of SIDS (Sudden Infant Death Syndrome).

Matthew Grace, author of *A Way Out: Dis-ease Deception and the Truth about Health*, points out the women of the Bantu tribe don't drink milk, and they have 7 to 9 babies all with strong teeth and bones.

Milk from another mammal, especially cow milk, may cause asthma, mucus, colds, allergies, ear infections and even worse problems down the road. Robert Cohen, scientist and author of *Milk: The Deadly Poison* and *Milk: A–Z*, provides documented illnesses that can occur as an outcome of dairy consumption, including breast cancer, Crohn's disease, diabetes, heart disease, iron deficiency, osteoporosis, rheumatoid arthritis, sudden infant death syndrome, tuberculosis, uterine cancer, vitamin D-deficiency, and many others.

I sometimes presented the following situation to my children so they would fully understand why we don't eat animals or animal products:

"If you were driving past a farm and were hungry and saw a cow grazing in the pasture with a nearby orchard of apple trees, would you run to suck the cow's udders, or would you pick an apple from the apple tree?" Which one do you think was my children's choice?

MILK BENEFITS ONLY THE YOUNG OF THE SPECIES FOR WHICH IT WAS INTENDED.

Many baby food manufacturers proclaim the importance of getting baby to eat solids as early as possible when in reality this is detrimental to baby's growth and development. Women who nurse their babies long-term are often ridiculed or made to feel they're doing something inappropriate. I recall well-meaning neighbors telling me it was wrong to nurse my two year old son, and there was plenty of food for him to eat instead. My son needed to nurse for a long time, perhaps because of the insecurity he felt by being separated from me when he was hospitalized, but also because many children require a lengthier bonding time. It's normal for a child to nurse exclusively for two years, and to begin solid foods when ready. And as solid foods are introduced, nursing continues to provide valuable nutrients and plays an important part in the development of the emotional bond between mother and child. At the end of the first year of life, only if the infant is ready, fruit can be introduced with continued breastfeeding. Fruit is sweet, similar to breast milk, and will be warmly accepted when the child develops some teeth for chewing and shows the desire to eat.

In the December 2007 issue of Pear Magazine (http://www.PearMagazine. com): "According to new research, breastfed babies typically won't have to be deceived into eating fruits and veggies like recent popular cookbooks encourage. Instead, if their mom regularly eats fruits and vegetables, the baby will acquire a taste for healthy foods. Flavors from the mother's diet are transmitted through amniotic fluid and mother's milk. So, a baby learns to like a food's taste when the mother eats that food on a regular basis."

In the article "The Weaning of Babies" for Living Nutrition Magazine, Volume 18, Professor Rozalind Graham states the implications of premature weaning: "Weaning an infant prematurely can result in a multitude of serious and potentially life-long health problems such as obesity, dyspepsia, leaky gut syndrome and consequent auto-immune problems, such as rheumatoid arthritis. Psychological problems, such as insecurity, can also result from premature weaning."

Professor Graham's daughter, Faychesca, received the majority of her nutrients directly from her mother's milk at 21 months of age. At that age, she ate three meals a day, and sometimes four, but they were quite small: one banana, or half a mango, or several small tomatoes and a piece of pineapple. At this age, approaching two years, about 80% of her food intake is still coming from mother's breast milk. Rozalind Graham, a well-nourished mother living on healthy raw vegan foods, provides her child with superior nutrients and long-term emotional bonding necessary for self-assurance and esteem.

Even when my children had begun to walk, talk and eat solid food, they still sometimes wanted to nurse when we were out in public. Since the public frowned on a mother nursing her toddlers, not to mention four and five year olds, I felt the atmosphere of general disapproval. Our solution was a secret code we called, "Come mommy!" Whenever either of my children wanted to nurse in public, he or she would say, "Come mommy!" People would think they just wanted to be picked up and held. This worked well for us in that I knew when they wanted me to create a private space for nursing, away from people who wouldn't understand their need.

11

Attachment Parenting, Skin-to-Skin, and the Family Bed

Attachment parenting, a phrase coined by pediatrician William Sears, is a parenting philosophy based on the principles of the attachment theory in developmental psychology. According to attachment theory, a strong emotional bond with parents during childhood, also known as a secure attachment, is a precursor of secure, empathic relationships in adulthood.

WIKIPEDIA DEFINITION

One reason I'm so passionate about disseminating this valuable information on raw food nutrition and attachment parenting is that earlier, I hadn't understood how to follow my mothering instincts. I've learned from my mistakes, and I would like to help other parents benefit from this information. Had I been properly educated in how to return to my true maternal instincts, I would have understood my children's needs for attachment parenting and skin-to-skin contact. It took time to learn this beautiful way of parenting that instills a sense of security and trust in children. When my children were babies, none of our friends were practicing this style of parenting, but starting with my visits to La Leche League meetings, reading *The Continuum Concept* by Jean Liedloff, and later with my attendance at a Continuum and Attachment Parenting group, led by Sandy Rzetelny, I saw the loving approach of attachment parenting made more and more sense as the best way to raise secure and happy children. Because my wonderful father had told me for years how important it was for children to be nursed, I was sure this was something I wanted to give them long-term. And during the breastfeeding years, there was a lot of skin-to-skin contact without my realizing just how beneficial it was.

A healthy child nursing, and later eating raw foods, must also be given the focused love and attention that is crucial for positive self-esteem and emotional development. The two work hand-in-hand. The infant and young child should not be brought into this world to adhere to the needs of the adult. Our responsibility as parents is to keep our children close to us and held by us until it is their choice to be more independent. Baby should be carried constantly in contact with mother's skin, inside her clothing, during the first year. Babies held mostly against mother's body feel safe and very much loved, a feeling that, like breastfeeding, is a continuation of life in the womb. A close friend of mine, a postpartum doula and lactation consultant, practiced skin-to-skin contact and long-term nursing—two important aspects of attachment parenting, with her third child. The results were an extremely happy, independent, self-confident child at a very young age (described in the article by Carole Blane, "Carrying Your Baby and Skin-to-Skin Contact," which appears later in this chapter).

Many women feel insecure about carrying their babies skin-to-skin because of outside pressures to put the baby down. When traveling in Mexico, I met a young Czech woman who was so beautifully carrying her baby skin-to-skin inside gorgeous, colorful light Mexican clothing. I told her how wonderful this was for her and her baby, for the baby's security, trust and brain development. She expressed to me how happy and relieved she was to hear that information since so many others had told her the baby would be more comfortable in a stroller. I assured her the baby needs to be close to her, warmed by her skin and close to her heart. Professor Rozalind Graham, in a November 2005 talk, explained the human infant fears being attacked and eaten by an aggressor and therefore needs to be held constantly by the mother. When the baby enters our world, he/she does not know or understand its surroundings and wholly depends upon its mother for survival.

The family bed is also essential for the baby and the growing child. When my children were born, I tried to put each of them into a crib by nursing them to sleep first, but as soon as they experienced the crib, they rebelled against staying in that empty, lonely and confining space. The infant neither knows nor understands the world around him or her and needs always to be close to the mother's body. I attempted to place my babies in the crib right next to my own bed, but they would wake up and I took them in with me because I could not bear to hear them cry. Had I taken my children in bed with us from the start, everyone's sleep would have been much easier as the baby feels more secure next to and touching the parents. Everyone usually receives more sleep in the family bed. Many babies wake frequently to nurse, and it's easier for mother if she can nurse while lying in bed. Many women have told me nursing during the night doesn't wake anyone in the family bed.

When I finally understood attachment parenting, I was able to follow my children's needs and I slept next to them as they grew. My husband, a sensitive sleeper, needed to get up early in the morning, so I slept with the children. However, many families are able to work out arrangements with king-size beds, or mattresses and futons lined up on the floor, so everyone, including father, gets enough sleep. One of the many benefits of the family bed is that it helps fathers who are away from home all day to establish close bonds with their babies. My daughter, Gabriela, desired her own space earlier, but she continued to come in and sleep with her brother Marco and me whenever she wanted. She still remembers sleeping with us frequently until she was about nine, and even after that time if she was emotionally upset and needed our comfort, as when our dog died. Marco shared the family bed for twelve years. In the middle of his twelfth year, he told me he needed more space and didn't want me to sleep next to him any more. I cried because my baby was growing up, and the time goes more quickly than one can imagine.

If you want to have time with your husband at night and believe the child should be placed in a crib down the hall to scream-it-out alone until falling asleep, please study the benefits of intuitive parenting and the emotional needs of children by reading the recommended books. As far as the marital relationship, the mother and father will need to be creative in finding their time together, such as when the child is napping, or when the children are fast asleep at night. I recommend reading *The Continuum Concept* by Jean Liedloff, *The Attachment Parenting Book* by Dr. William Sears and *The Family Bed* by Tine Thevenin. Leaders of La Leche League meetings can also help parents to understand the importance of sleeping with their children.

Throughout the growing years and beyond, your child will benefit from parents who keep a close eye to his or her needs, relying on their intuition in creating a happy and healthy person. Many years ago when Marco was almost five and Gabriela was seven and a half, I became part of a continuum or attachment parenting group. It was led by a warm, nurturing psychotherapist and mother, Sandy Rzetelny, who taught me a lot about following my children's needs. The mothers who made up this group were more devoted to their children than any mothers I'd ever met. They practiced long-term nursing and carried their children until the age when the child signaled or asked to be put down. Marco was in kindergarten at the time I started attending this group. When I would go to get him at school, he would run to me and jump into my arms. At age five, he still very much needed to be carried, and so I followed his lead and carried him everywhere. Other mothers who saw us at the school frequently reprimanded me on how inappropriate it was for me to carry a big five year old boy around. Some even expressed they thought I had separation problems. I knew I was following my intuition as far as my mothering to my child, and I finally felt comfortable in paying no attention to the remarks of others. I carried him as much as he desired, which was frequently, for about 1 1/2 years. He stayed home from school whenever he wanted, and the following year he chose not to continue into first grade.

As Gabriela and Marco grew, we knew our neighbors viewed us as "different" since we're vegetarians and eventually homeschooled, but they didn't know I was preparing live vegan foods and nursing the children for many years. Being different teaches you to think "outside the box" in many situations. The people around us can put a lot of pressure on us to follow more conventional behavior, going along with what the masses are doing. Your extended family, friends, acquaintances and perhaps even your spouse may not agree with your lifestyle. They may scare you into thinking your raw food diet will hurt you and your children, that long-term nursing is unacceptable in our "modern" civilized world, and sleeping next to and holding your baby all day will spoil him or her. You as parents need to take a step back from what is considered "normal" in society, and meditate on your own beliefs and intuitions about the values that will best serve your child and your family. There is no need to argue and defend yourself to others. Inner peace and confidence will give you strength to live in the midst of others who are in disagreement with your style of parenting and choice of diet. I always dreamed about how wonderful it would have been to live in a raw food community that supported a continuum attachment parenting approach to raising a family. I dreamed my children could happily eat whatever the other children were eating, and that they could nurse as a young child without hearing negative remarks.

At the time when some people were still telling me I was too attached to my son, I read a book called *The Courage to Raise Good Men* by Olga Silverstein. I learned so clearly that my intuitions as a mother were important and that I should listen to them and keep my little boy close to me, whereas so many mothers force early separation between themselves and their sons.

I highly recommend the loving and compassionate parenting book, *Whatever Happened to Mother?—A Primer for Those Who Care about Children* by James Kimmel. This is a short, easy-to-read book of tremendous value—an absolute must-read for all prospective parents. Some of the questions answered in this book are: "Are our conventional infant care and child rearing practices detrimental to children? Why has bottle-feeding replaced nursing as the major method for feeding infants? Why has the abuse of children been tolerated through centuries of civilization? Why do we believe if we nurture children, it will spoil them? Why do so many mothers no longer mother?" James Kimmel shows great concern for the mother-baby relationship in today's world when he says:

> Lots of mothers put earning money, taking care of the house and their husbands, and having time for themselves before being there for their baby. This doesn't mean the mothers of today don't like their babies or don't think they are important. What it does mean is that, in our world, we don't believe it's important for a mother to always be there for her baby. Obviously our government doesn't consider it very important, or they would find ways to make it more possible for mothers to stay at home and take care of their babies and children.
>
> The first mothers did not have babies one right after the other. This was partly because by nursing their babies in the natural way and for a long time they could not conceive right away. That was nature's way of insuring the mother-infant bond would continue for a long time after birth, long enough for a baby to fully and properly develop. But it was also because the people supported nature through their belief that all babies needed to have their mothers for themselves for a long time. And because mothers and fathers were responsible to the life they created, they did not have babies one right after the other, even if this meant the father and the mother had to alter their sexual life together.
>
> The fact that the first mothers cared for their babies in the way nature intended, and they were supported by their group to do so, permitted the development of a wonderful and beautiful creation—the human being. The first people knew a baby was not a separate person at birth. They were aware it was necessary for a mother to provide her baby with herself, or the baby could not become human. Nature, in its wisdom, had provided every baby with a mother so that, through the mother's presence, the baby could continue to grow as human. The mother, by caring for her baby for the appropriate time period and in the human way, ensured her baby would become an appropriate human being; someone who would be sociable, intelligent, caring of others, and believing every human life was special and important. You see, the difference between the people of a long, long time ago and us is that they all had real mothers, so they were all fully human.

James Kimmel's book, *Whatever Happened to Mother? A Primer for Those Who Care about Children,* can be purchased at http://www.naturalchild.org/shop/books/whm.html.

ℒ๑

The following paragraphs worthy of being read over and over again are from the e-book *Spontaneous Creation: 101 Reasons Not to Have Your Baby in a Hospital (Volume 1)* by Jock Doubleday (www.spontaneouscreation.org). This is a book about natural childbirth and the birth of wisdom and power in childbearing women:

Parental Bond

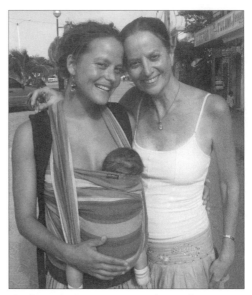

Science tells us physical contact, particularly in the first year of life, has a positive effect on children's health and wellbeing. Infant intelligence, an indicator of health, has been found to be closely correlated with a strong parental bond, specifically skin-to-skin contact in the first few hours after birth.

What exactly is it about skin-to-skin contact that can elevate an infant's intelligence in only a few hours? How can touch so profoundly affect the infant brain?

Touch is associated in an inverse way with something called "serum plasma cortisol levels." Cortisol is a steroid hormone secreted by the adrenal glands in response to stress. The more touch, the lower the levels of cortisol. The less touch, the higher the levels of cortisol. When plasma cortisol levels are imbalanced, as in the case of touch deprivation, infant brain tissue develops abnormally. Such a hormonal imbalance can even result in the destruction of previously normal brain tissue.

Czech woman Janna practicing skin-to-skin contact with her baby on the street in Tulum, Mexico, posing with the author after just having met.

If parental (especially maternal) touch affects the growth and life of infant brain cells, isn't it reasonable to conjecture that infant intelligence relies on, or is to some extent a function of touch?

This is indeed what scientific research indicates. Carefully designed studies performed over the last three decades demonstrate a clear relationship between timely, affectionate parental touch and increased infant intelligence. Researchers have found enhanced infant learning, improved language acquisition, improved reading achievement, improved memory, improved visual-spatial problem solving, and improved IQ all result from greater mother-infant skin-to-skin contact in the first hours, months, and years of life.

"You don't want your baby to be taken away from you." There are many reasons hospital staff use to justify taking your baby away from you immediately after birth—and for keeping him isolated from your loving and human touch for hours and even days at a time. The benefits of skin-to-skin contact and bonding are not recognized by today's institutional mediocrity. Separation of mothers and newborns is standard hospital practice. Touch deprivation for newborns is simply "the way things are" in medical institutions today.

The midwifery model of childbirth, on the other hand, solidly grounded in both scientific research and common sense, allows a completely different scenario to emerge. If you give birth at home with a midwife, you are able to hold your baby as long as you want to, without any "professional" interference. Parental-infant skin-to-skin contact is encouraged, especially in the precious first few hours after birth. When your newborn is allowed prolonged mother-infant contact, many advantages accrue, and elevated infant intelligence is among them.

ℰઠ

My friend, Carole Blane, is a postpartum doula and lactation consultant who practiced skin-to-skin, long-term nursing, and attachment parenting. Carole writes here about carrying your baby and skin-to-skin contact with baby, extremely important insights into the needs of the young child and mother as well.

Carrying Your Baby and Skin-to-Skin Contact
by Carole Blane

Carrying your baby skin-to-skin decreases cortisol in both baby and mother. Cortisol is a stress hormone that can damage the body. Carrying your baby increases oxytocin, the love hormone. Skin-to-skin contact provides stimulation to the skin, the largest sense organ in the body; carrying your baby skin-to-skin provides movement that is so crucial to brain development.

When you carry your baby skin-to-skin, you feel one with him/her. Babies are meant biologically and emotionally to be connected to their mothers. Until about nine months, when initial separation anxiety sets in, they believe they are still part of their mothers. It FEELS wrong to be left alone anywhere, anytime.

I carried my first daughter a lot until she was about four years old. I believe she needed to be carried that long because her need to be carried/held had not been adequately met in the early months of her life. My second daughter I carried from birth 24/7. She was "down" much sooner. I carried my third daughter skin-to-skin 24/7 for the first year of life. I did not drive. I went to the bathroom with her "in arms" and bathed with her on me. The only separation we experienced was when she initiated going to her sisters or father and I remained nearby for her to return to me at her whim.

I found it impossible to think badly about her. Thoughts like…"Please stop crying… I can't take it….why won't you sleep?" did not even cross my mind. Here was my baby still connected to me, part of me.

You can't be vain and carry your baby this way. Bodily fluids, poop, pee, and breast milk abound. There is such an intimacy and yet no embarrassment or shyness.

The practicalities of carrying your baby skin-to-skin are surmountable with some creativity. The summer was easy. I was practically naked all summer as was she. You need shirts that can accommodate two people. Most of the time, I carried her inside my shirt. She was wearing only a diaper; and then I put a sling over the two of us. No one even knew she was naked in there. I bought a "mama" coat that covered us both. We walked down the streets of Chicago in the winter with her skin-to-skin inside my coat. I wore shorts and long skirts all winter so when she wanted to be down she could still be in skin-to-skin contact with me. They were also elasticized, so as she got longer, her legs could stay against my skin inside my clothes. We kept each other very warm that winter.

Many people, my chiropractor included, were concerned. They said babies need to be down to develop strong torsos. My daughters' bodies are solid and firm. They are all athletes and have remarkable upper body strength for females. Having to hold themselves upright makes their spines supple, flexible, and very strong.

People might believe it's coercive and that you're holding your baby against his or her will, or they wonder how you know when to let go of the baby. Babies will let you know when they're ready. They slink and slither out of your arms so you must let go of them. That is what happens when the two are connected, both having instincts intact. Babies want to get down, and mothers recognize and satisfy this need.

Babies who have this connection to their mothers do not have to expend time and energy worrying about where their safety is. They can utilize all of their resources for learning about the world.

The most remarkable aspect of this closeness I found was in my third child's quiet, alert state. In most infants it is fairly short, yet it is the time for absorbing their environment. She could hold eye contact with me for such extended periods to the point that I could not bear the intimacy of looking so intently into another's eyes—even at age forty. I was totally amazed at the openness, wisdom, trust and love I saw there.

Carole Blane, cell phone: (917) 407-1166
Lactation Consultant

Sandy Rzetelny was the leader of the Attachment Parenting group that completely changed my views on the mother-child relationship. I wish so much I had met her and been part of this group before having my babies, so I could have followed my instincts better and not let others influence me in my very earliest mothering. I was lucky to have finally met Sandy while my children were still young, and I could carry my son when he was 5 without feeling it was wrong. The following is from the excellent quarterly newsletter Sandy used to write, "The Maternal Instinct":

A mothers' group to which I belong came up with the following statement of our beliefs: "We believe all babies have the expectation of continuous contact with their mother, from the moment of birth through the crawling phase. Babies need to be in arms every minute, 24 hours a day even through naps and bedtime. It is babies' need and expectation not to be put down at all. They are not to be put down for trips to the bathroom, the taking of showers, or doing chores, etc. Babies need continuous contact with their mothers for at least the first three months. Carrying can be shared with others thereafter, if the baby and mother are willing. Babies need to be in arms until they initiate separation toward mobility. Babies move from one stage to the next without our intervention. Babies need as much skin-to-skin contact as can be had in this society. Continuous contact promotes self esteem, bonding, the healthiest physiological development, and the development of the maternal instinct in the mother. A held baby feels right with its world and with itself." Most of what I write about, I've learned from listening carefully to babies and children through their words and actions, and from listening to parents as they pour their hearts out, speaking of their love for their children.

In response to the question, "What are our kids missing in our civilized society?" the "Maternal Instinct's" reply is:

> For one thing, a real community to socialize with every day from birth on, peopled by joyful children and adults of all ages, including extended family. They need an opportunity to play all day outside in lots of fresh air and sunshine. Instead our kids are the unlucky recipients of a multitude of restrictions and requirements, including numerous interventions: medical, social, legal, etc. They are faced with constant separations from important people in their lives: family, playmates, neighbors, etc. (I could go on and on with the many differences between our culture and a more natural society.) All of these and more, from having to wear clothing to premature weaning, leave our babies and children (and us) vulnerable, frustrated, and aching for a sense of rightness in our homes and communities. Our children demand from us parents that we take up the slack and make up for some of the missing elements by giving our time and energy and focused attention as a viable substitute. Our kids want and need us to be present with them in the here and now. They need us to talk, chat, play, laugh, smile, work on their projects however unrealistic or silly, and be as fully involved with them as we possibly can.

Sandy Rzetelny, psychotherapist and parent educator, can be reached at 201-410-2226. She is a parent and educator who truly understands the emotional needs of infants and children.

Please note *Hygienic Care of Children* by Dr. Herbert Shelton, albeit a resource on raising children on healthful food, is very backward in terms of how it looks at children's emotional needs. Dr. Shelton believed children should be held and touched as minimally as possible, which ignores important mental and emotional needs. When reading this book, keep in mind it was written during a period when adults wanted children to be seen but not heard.

The following article about the importance of the family bed is by author

Hygeia Halfmoon, who wrote *Primal Mothering in the Modern World*. I recommend her book as must-read material:

> The greatest discovery of any generation
> is that a living soul can alter his life
> by altering his attitude.
> WILLIAM JAMES

Americans are afraid of the family bed. Since they seem to lead the way in global thinking, more and more children are spending less and less time with their parents.

Mothers, since the advent of erroneous information, dished out mostly by the medical world, have been letting their little ones cry it out at night, actually believing the idea that a baby in bed is sure to be spoiled or suffocated.

Our attitudes are the emissions of thoughts we possess, thoughts that were trained into us with the tool of fear. If the thought is wrong, the deluded attitude carries itself like the wind and pollinates with a perverted eye. A change in attitude creates a reality that honors the needs of our children while giving us the gift of family bonding. I had a glimpse of the family bed long before becoming a mother who embraces and considers sacred every aspect of shared sleeping.

My nana's house was big, but boring. My idea of a good time was a stroll—or sleigh ride, depending on the season, to the little shack just down the road.

Rundown on the outside, the inside was as bright as the morning sun. An Eskimo family made this shack their home, and what a beautiful home it was! A doll and a big bed, those were the only things I remember seeing in that tiny room...the rest of the space was filled with love. Here is where they loved, laughed, slept, played, and lived in celebration of one another.

Each day, they greeted me with smiles and hugs and laughter. We couldn't speak each other's language, but our hearts were right in tune. It was my introduction to the feeling of aloha.

One morning, I skipped down the street, looking forward to another dose of love. But everything was gone. Somehow in the night, the little shack had burned to the ground. My "family" was dead, only the little doll remained. I picked her up and breathed in the memory of the greatest love I had ever known.

When I became a mother decades later, I knew *exactly* where my little one belonged. My fondest mothering memories are straight from the family bed. Just last week, my birthday-boy eleven-year-old son served breakfast in our family bed...apples and almond butter. Then we proceeded to finish the book *Indian in the Cupboard* and begin another book about the kitten that was rescued by two caring children.

And now, I have two grandbabies joining in on the fun of the family bed.

I give thanks to those loving folks way back when, when they showed me the most important thing in life...love expressed in every way, through the night and through the day. Yes, they practiced togetherness day and night, and so do we; falling asleep to the breathing of my loved ones, feeling their warmth throughout the night, waking to their angelic faces, and surviving the pouncing of two *huge* puppies who fly in to say, "We Love You!"

If you need me, you'll find me happily lounging in the family bed.

12

Feeding Baby Uncooked Foods

*"The fault of children's ill-health can be directly traced
to the threshold of parenthood."*

Celia Horowitz

B ecause life's healing power so easily manifests when eating raw vegan foods, I think all parents should have the right to raise their children in the most nutritionally, mentally and emotionally beneficial way. It is crucial to get this information disseminated to the public so more parents will have the knowledge to make wise decisions for the future health of their precious young. When others try to intervene and take away our true instincts as parents, it can only hurt the children. It is imperative parents understand the needs of their children, and follow the instincts true to their hearts instead of being influenced by others who have not studied the nutritional, mental and emotional needs of *your* child. An organization is needed to protect parents' rights to raise their children in the healthful lifestyle they believe will most benefit the whole family. Health Liberties Network, a new organization I formed with Rhio, author of *Hooked on Raw*, will serve to protect parents' healthful lifestyle choices. See our Vision Statement on page 284.

It is fundamental that the infant receive mainly mother's milk for most of the first year of life. The child should not be given solid food to chew until there are many teeth. Another likely sign of readiness for solids is if the child isn't gaining enough weight from mother's milk alone, and requires additional food. When starting solid foods, choose a tiny piece of easily digested fruit such as a ripe banana, to avoid choking, and observe any reaction. Children who begin eating before they're ready often develop allergies. Toward the end of the first year, foods high in carbohydrates can be offered only if the child truly desires them: grapes, cut in small bite-size pieces, a well-ripened banana, ripe pear, mango, peach or melon. It is best for baby to eat mono meals (one food at a meal) as this is easiest on the baby's still developing digestive system. Some babies approaching their first birthday are not yet ready to eat solid foods, while others are ready and can't wait. Many babies are curious about foods but not yet ready to eat them until well after the first year. Babies explore the world by placing objects in their mouths, but this is not necessarily a sign that baby is ready to eat solid foods. Human breast milk will provide all the necessary nutrients, fat and protein as baby grows, and mother need not worry the older baby is not getting enough nourishment. Breast milk changes to provide for baby's nutritional needs. During the first few days of lactation, colostrum, a yellowish liquid, is secreted by the mammary glands. It is higher in protein and immune factors than milk. After this initial period, the milk gradually adjusts to become lower in protein to fit baby's needs.

When the child is ready, the first solid foods should be ripe fruits. I started my own two children on bite-sized pieces of very ripe non-starchy bananas toward the end of their first year. At the time, I had not realized they may not have been ready for it. Some people feed coconut milk to their older babies, but it's important to limit the amount because of reports that conventional coconuts imported to the United States are dipped in fungicides. The fleshy part of the coconut is high in fat, and so, should not become a big part of the regular daily diet since breast milk is still providing the necessary fat and pro-tein. Coconut water, however, is much lower in fat than coconut flesh and can be easily digested. During the latter part of the first year, a very limited amount of diluted unprocessed fresh fruit juices may be given. These juices could be 50% water and 50% juice, made of oranges, apples, melons, or pears. You can use the whole fruit and make a very simple watery smoothie after 9 months of age, but only if baby is eager. However, there is no urgency to feed foods other than breast milk to baby. Some babies don't ask for or require solid foods until closer to two years of age, yet parents have been led to think their child needs them much sooner. If the parents decide to feed other foods to the young baby under one year of age while still nursing, the juice or watery smoothie intake should be limited to not more than 3 to 4 ounces of diluted juice or smoothie in a day to ensure baby is drinking enough breast milk to provide the fat, protein, and myriad other nutrients for proper development. Juices are not considered a whole food since the fiber has been removed, and accordingly should not become a large part of your baby's diet. It's not necessary to give juices and smoothies to the young baby. Some breastfeeding mothers attending my classes have mentioned, in addition to nursing, their babies did well with green juices made with leafy green vegetables and/or green smoothies toward the end of the first year. Bite-size pieces of green leaves and vegetables are harder to chew and digest, so they shouldn't be introduced until later in the second year.

At least until the end of the first year, the baby's diet should be mother's milk. Dr. Graham points out: "Mother's milk is 50% fat by calories. A one year old fully-nursing child will take in about 1000 calories from milk, 60 of which are protein, hence about 15 grams. This supplies more than enough protein for the child to demonstrate the fastest growth spurt in the complete human growth cycle. The introduction of fruits between ages one and two should total approximately 10–20% of calories, with fat intake being reduced by only a few points. As larger scale weaning occurs between ages two to three, fat from mother's milk will drop another 10–20% or more."

Between the ages of two to three, the child should be taking in sufficient calories from fruits, including avocados, and can eat vegetables in addition to the continuation of nutrients from mother's milk. Almond milk and avocados are high in fats that are more difficult to digest than those in breast milk. Wait before adding nut and seed milks until between ages two and three, and soaked nuts and seeds until after age three because of possible allergies to nuts and the greater digestive capacity they require. When you begin feeding nut milks to your child, the number of nuts should be strictly limited. The simplest nut milk consists of 15 almonds soaked overnight in one liter of filtered water. Blend the nuts with the soak water on the following morning, and then strain. There will be enough for the rest of the family to enjoy too. Beyond age three, the child will continue to incorporate solid raw foods, including a variety of nutrients from live fruits, leafy greens, vegetables, and ground up soaked nuts and seeds, with increases in total fat intake occurring during growth spurts and times of high physical activity.

Dr. Graham says, "Under age five, children still require plenty of fat, but more than the percentage of fat found in mother's milk would be too much fat. When children begin eating solid foods, their overall fat intake is likely to remain close to 50% for a year or two, or even longer, depending on when/if they are forced to wean. When children reach the natural weaning age, at roughly 5–6 years or so, the percentage of their fat intake should begin to drop."

Children I've known who were eating a sufficient variety and quantity of raw vegan foods have grown extremely well. Often, the child's height mirrors the height of the parents, but there are many variables. In case your child seems not to be thriving on raw vegan foods, or appears weak and lethargic and/or is consistently losing weight, then the assistance of a qualified health professional should be sought.

The first time many children are cajoled to eat cooked food, they turn away from it in disgust, and their bodies attempt to get rid of it by throwing it right out. Unfortunately, the first foods given to baby make impressions that become a permanent part of the child's memory. Even children who were transitioned to raw vegan foods at a very young age will often still recall the tastes, sensations and textures of cooked and processed foods.

Victoria Boutenko, in her article "The Imprinting of Eating Habits," writes:

> Lifelong food preferences start to develop while a baby is still in the womb. The strongest pattern for future food preferences is formed during the age of 9 to 18 months. At this time, everything connected with food intake leaves a strong imprint on the child's brain. Also, the baby is tasting everything with his mouth: toys, shoes, body parts, everything. Simultaneously, the child is memorizing the experiences of his mother and father eating, what they're eating, what they're feeding the baby, and their emotional reaction to the baby's consumption of these foods. While the unsuspecting parents believe the child doesn't comprehend much that is happening, the child is forming food habits for a lifetime. Whatever his first tastes, textures, smells and sights of food are, he will crave them for the rest of his life, especially in moments of distress.

> I remember how I was feeding potato chips with cola to my older son while taking pictures of him and being amused at how cute he looked. If only I had known those "cute moments" would compromise his health, I would never have done that.

> Even worse than seeing my children suffering from sickness was feeling completely helpless several years later when they began persistently to demand unhealthful foods. By the time I realized healthful eating contributed to health, I was unable to change my children's junk food preferences. It took a long time, and several life-threatening illnesses to correct the patterns that had been instilled in them as babies.

The strongest positive impression on your child's brain will be left by him/her watching his/her parents eating fruits, vegetables and other healthful foods. Having our children crave grapes and cucumbers will surely aid them in their lives, don't you think?

The Boutenko family website is: www.rawfamily.com

According to Ruth Yaron, author of *Super Baby Food,* a 4 to 7 day waiting period is recommended after the introduction of each new food in order to enable the mother to avoid any possible reactions to a single food. Although her book is vegetarian, not vegan, it has many excellent parenting tips that can also be used with a raw vegan diet. She also advises giving baby only 2 or 3 bits of finger food at a time so he or she doesn't have an overfull mouth which can cause choking. If a young child under three years old is fed grapes, berries, or celery, these must be cut into small enough pieces so even if baby doesn't chew them at all and swallows them whole, they won't become lodged in the throat. Ruth Yaron explains you should "always watch your baby carefully while he is eating, and never turn your back or leave the room. Use his mealtimes as quality times to bond with your beautiful baby. Never let baby eat unless he is seated in an upright position. Lying on the floor, or eating while walking or running may also cause choking. Emphasize to your children to take small bites and chew carefully and thoroughly before swallowing."

I continually chewed with my babies and watched them imitate me. Frequently, I would pre-chew the food a bit before putting it before them.

If your child reacts to a solid food by developing diarrhea, constipation, a rash, fussy behavior or other reaction, then continue nursing and wait before giving more solid pieces of fruit until the child is ready.

As your children grow, you can juice green vegetables with them. The apple is a fruit that goes well in a vegetable juice and sweetens it. Beets would be harsh on the child's digestive system and should be avoided.

Many parents give nut milks to their young babies and some believe it is all right to substitute these nut milks for mother's milk. Although some children seem to do fine with the nut milks, they are more concentrated and not as easy on some babies' developing digestive systems. I recommend only mother's milk throughout most of the first year, and then the introduction of fruit toward the end of the first year of life if baby is ready. Nut milks and solid soaked nuts and seeds should not be given until later.

Mother's milk contains no starch. Mother's milk is made up of the simple carbohydrate of sugar. The baby has difficulty digesting starch prior to the age of three. Most children under age three or four do not secrete enough of the salivary enzyme ptyalin, or the pancreatic enzymes necessary to digest starch. Babies who eat cereal grains and legumes will often have indigestion, colic, constipation, colds, hives, diarrhea, problems with tonsils and adenoids, poor dental development and other even more severe problems. I recall when he was about one year old, I began to give my son some grains in addition to the bananas he was eating. He had many colds, ear infections, colic, indigestion and poor development of his primary teeth. His first teeth were not fully developed. I believe the poor dental development was a result of drugs in the IV when he was hospitalized at five weeks old as well as the later consumption of grains (prior to age three) when his body was not yet ready to process starch. His secondary teeth were big and beautiful due to the mineral-rich fresh fruits and vegetables we were eating. When he was a young infant, he was frequently ill with chronic ear infections. My diet while nursing was largely cooked and processed starches and cooked vegetables. When I would take my son to various pediatricians, they would treat the symptoms instead of figuring out the cause. Please read *The Cure is in the Cause* by Dr. Ruza Bogdanovich to understand why treatments never solve the problem and only temporarily relieve the symptoms.

Dr. Herbert Shelton wrote, "Until mothers heed the laws of nature, children will suffer countless unnecessary diseases." There are a growing number of medical doctors in the United States with a strong background in nutrition, but most doctors have little understanding of what actually constitutes health. Parents need to take their children's health and wellness into their own hands, and find educators and doctors who support a natural diet and lifestyle.

When baby is ready to start eating solid foods—no sooner than the latter part of infancy, the end of the first year—these foods should be cut up in bite-size pieces for baby to chew. If the food is mashed and pureed, the child will learn to swallow and gulp without chewing, and this may persist into the child's older years.

As attentive parents, it's important to observe any reactions the baby may have, even to healthful ripe raw vegan foods. If baby is not yet ready for a specific food, the following reactions may occur: colic, vomiting, circles under the eyes, diarrhea, constipation, gas, crying, fussy behavior, and rashes. As said previously, it is best to introduce a new food every few days, or even one in a week. That way you can more readily observe any allergic reaction.

Jarred foods for baby? All of the sealed, ready-to-eat, jarred baby foods in stores, even if organic, are heated at high temperatures. The inorganic minerals in these dead foods, devoid of vital nutrients, are poisonous to baby. Since baby can't utilize them, she/he has to find a way to detoxify these poisons. The amino acids, vitamins and enzymes are destroyed by high temperatures and oxidation. These vitamins and proteins begin to be destroyed at 115 degrees Fahrenheit. In addition to the high temperatures, most of these pureed jarred baby foods oxidize on the shelves—valueless to your child.

When the baby is well into his or her second year of life, he or she can chew on small pieces of apples, oranges, berries, squash, celery, cucumbers, carrots, avocados or sweet red peppers (green peppers are not yet ripe). Leafy greens, more abundant in minerals than fruit, are beneficial to introduce at a young age. An excellent way to include them would be in green smoothies—leafy greens blended with pieces of fruit. When fruits are served without blending, they should be cut into small bite-size pieces.

Sprouts, such as sunflower greens and clover sprouts, add protein and calcium, and can be added later in the second year, or whenever the child seems ready. Solid nuts and seeds should come later as they require thorough mastication in order to be digested. Some children naturally begin nursing less after one year of age, but others, like my children, continue to nurse as much or more for quite some time. Avocados can provide additional fat for children nursing less frequently. My own children were still avid nursers into their second and even third year, still receiving fat and nutrients from my milk. As the child grows older, raw nuts and seeds and nut and seed butters (such as almonds, sunflower seeds, flax seeds, walnuts, pecans, Brazil nuts and pine nuts) can be added for increased fat, minerals and protein. Nuts and seeds should be soaked overnight to begin germinating them, thereby inactivating enzyme inhibitors that would impair digestion. Most importantly, be sure your child is eating plenty of fruit to provide the glucose and calories for energy needs and plenty of greens in salads and green smoothies for mineral needs. Two to three ounces of nuts or seeds a day, or half an avocado or a small whole one, provides additional fat. There will be times during growth spurts when your child will want more food and more of the higher protein and fat foods, so be sensitive to those times, and let your child be the guide. Always have an abundance of fresh, ripe, organic fruits and vegetables available as well as some soaked nuts and seeds.

Hybrids are fruits or vegetables that have been cross-bred by farmers, such as seedless grapes, seedless watermelons, corn, carrots, and beets, even seedless bananas. Some people believe hybrids rob the body of minerals and cause mineral depletion. Others feel these hybrid fruits and vegetables remain loaded with valuable nutrients and should not be avoided, and every plant has become a hybrid over time. If you can find watermelons and grapes with their seeds intact, that would be the best nourishment, but don't limit your child's diet by avoiding healthful foods even if they are hybrids. Seedless grapes are certainly a healthy choice compared to packaged and processed foods. We need to have a great variety of fruits and vegetables available to our children to make the diet interesting and delicious.

If you prepare a fruit puree or pudding for the young child, blend it quickly in a blender or Vita-Mix and serve immediately to prevent loss of vitamins and minerals through oxidation.

It's best not to establish fixed mealtimes. Instead, permit your growing child to eat when hungry. A baby or child who is forced to eat when not hungry will be overfed. Overfed babies often display difficulty sleeping. All children need to attend to their own physiological balance. Their natural clocks will let them know when they're hungry. When experiencing growth spurts, they will know to eat more of the higher caloric fruits and to eat more avocados, soaked nuts and seeds. Note: when nuts and seeds are soaked overnight, they become easier to assimilate.

A child should not be fed when tired, emotional or ill. When Gabriela didn't feel well, she would drink water and go to bed, sometimes for two or three days. She would always wake up happy, refreshed and feeling wonderful. Marco would do the same, except he liked to drink diluted orange juice. Although my children have rarely been ill, they have the knowledge of how to take care of themselves if that happens. Medication has not been an option in their lives because we have always looked at symptoms as a clue to the cause of what might be afflicting the body. For any problem that may occur in the human body, there is always a cause. At the age of 18, Gabriela was in a serious car accident. She was bruised and had severe stomach pains. We went to the doctor to make sure she didn't have internal bleeding or a concussion. Following this very traumatic incident, she knew exactly what her body needed. She went to sleep and fasted on water for a few days, until she felt much better.

Children who eat predominantly raw vegan foods tend to heal more quickly than those who don't, and I have seen this in my children and other children brought up on raw foods. Sometimes my children's friends would be sick, but we didn't mind being near them at that time. I believed my children were internally clean and strong, and I felt completely comfortable having them play with children who were not well. They never got sick or "caught" anything from anyone else. I don't believe the germ theory holds for children who have attained internal cleanliness. The hot water bottle was our soothing remedy for any ache or pain, whether a headache, stomachache or foot ache. Although infrequently needed, it was nice to have the hot water bottle since medication was not an option for us.

After the child has decided to wean, there is no need for any kind of milk. When the dairy industry foists the belief that cow milk is needed, it's to increase their tremendous profits. Milk from another species is known to cause health problems, such as asthma, mucus, colds, ear and throat infections, and is linked to many diseases such as various forms of cancer and osteoporosis that abound primarily in countries that consume cow milk. Aside from breast milk, fruit is the easiest food for baby to digest during later infancy.

In his book, *Food for Life*, Neal Barnard, M.D. explains, "Aside from the colic-inducing proteins that bother many children drinking cow milk, it is a common cause of allergies." He reports, "Immune responses to milk proteins are implicated in insulin-dependent diabetes and even in sudden infant death syndrome." He also says, "Children need to grow, but they do not need high-protein foods. The 'protein deficiencies' our parents worried about in impover-ished countries were the result of starvation or diets restricted to very few food items. Protein deficiency is extremely unlikely on a diet drawn from a variety of plant foods. Excluding animal proteins will actually help the body retain calcium." Dr. Barnard points out, "Childhood is a time when dietary habits are established—habits which exert a lifelong effect. Children who acquire a taste for chicken nuggets, roast beef, and French fries today are the cancer patients, heart patients and weight-loss clinic patients of tomorrow." He also talks about the more gradual growth of vegetarian children, which concurs with my ob-servations of my own and vegan children in general. Many vegan children will initially grow more slowly but will catch up later on. Interestingly, breastfed babies grow more slowly than bottle-fed babies. Dr. Barnard concludes, "It may well be that nature designed the human body to grow up more gradually, to reach puberty later, and to last longer than happens for most of us raised on omnivorous diets."

I once heard a speaker talk about "gigantism" in our population. He was referring to the children, teens and adults who grew abnormally large on a diet high in animal protein. I was aware many large children of our times were born of small parents, and I wondered frequently if this was related to diet. My son grew more slowly than other players on his athletic teams, but according to both our pediatrician and our family physician, Dr. Joel Fuhrman, he was growing appropriately according to his growth chart. My son began to catch up with many of his friends after he had reached fourteen.

Although both of my children did grow at a slower rate than their peers who were eating animal food, the pediatrician assured us they were following a normal growth pattern. He also supported our nutritional and home-schooling choices. It was helpful to take my children for a wellness checkup to doctors who supported a healthful vegan diet. Our pediatrician told me the parents' physical stature is the greater determining factor for the child's eventual height.

Dr. Joel Fuhrman, author of *Eat to Live*, says, "Most Americans are not aware that the diet they feed their children guarantees a high cancer probability down the road, and that eating fast-food meals may be as risky as smoking cigarettes. It is difficult for parents to understand the insidious, slow destruction of their child's genetic potential and the foundation for serious illness that is being built by the consumption of fast-foods." He adds, "Twenty-five percent of children are obese today, setting the stage for obesity as an adult and early heart disease. Cancer is a fruit-and-vegetable-deficiency disease. Vegetables and fruits protect against all types of cancers if consumed in large enough quantities, and the most prevalent cancers in our country are mostly plant-food deficiency diseases. Studies on the cancer-reducing effects of vitamin pills containing various nutrients (such as folate, vitamin C and E) show only a slight benefit, most showing no benefit, and occasionally studies show taking isolated nutrients is harmful." He also points out vegans have such low cholesterol levels that they almost never get heart attacks. He includes much research showing those who avoid meat and dairy have lower rates of heart disease, cancer, high blood pressure, diabetes and obesity.

During the first year of life, baby has big growth spurts which will be signaled by increased nursing. Although these growth spurts can vary according to the individual child, author Ruth Yaron presents a schedule many babies seem to follow: "The first growth spurt occurs about a week after birth, the next at 3 weeks, then 6 weeks, and then at about 3 months. After about 5 or 6 months, you may notice your baby is eating less, which may be because he is growing at a slower rate at this time or because of teething pain. Another growth spurt begins between 8-10 months of age. You may notice an increase in baby's appetite when he begins crawling and walking, an effect of his using more energy. When he begins his second year of life, his growth rate again decreases and he will consequently eat less."

My two children nursed more during teething, not less, but this may have been because of the increased need for bonding and emotional support during this time.

A healthy baby should not be regulated on how much to eat. Baby will automatically stop eating when full as long as he or she is eating natural, whole raw vegan foods. When the child is allowed to eat refined and processed foods, overeating most often results. The child will become malnourished, and because of cravings and lack of nutrients in the food will not be able to listen to the body's special way of signaling it has had enough to eat.

Some mothers feeding their children healthful raw vegan foods were concerned their babies were not gaining weight. Nursing set on a strict schedule rather than according to baby's demands, limiting the quantity of baby's food, or his emotional needs not being met in some other way could all be reasons for inadequate weight gain.

The quantity of food my children ate would vary daily. The amount of breast milk they asked for would also vary when they were still in the nursing years. Normally, when they were toddlers and began showing interest in certain activities, nursing would decrease on some days. There were other times when nursing was sought frequently throughout the day. My children, with outstretched arms, would say, "Come mommy," which was very easy when we were out in public. People may have thought they just wanted to be picked up, but I knew it was nursing time.

During their first two years, my children would often nurse frequently throughout the night. This is much easier when mother shares sleep with her young nursing child. If a mother chooses to discontinue nursing during baby's first year, giving raw foods, nut milks, and juices as a replacement, problems may arise. As I have emphasized, this can prove inadequate for young babies. Mother's milk supplies all the protein, fat, vitamins and minerals the baby requires, and it's an absolute necessity for as long as the child desires, and essential during the first year of life. Many infants may not be able to digest the fats and proteins in the replacing almond or sesame milk. Any child weaned too early from mother's milk may develop problems with digestion and lack of growth. It is imperative that the introduction of solid foods not decrease baby's nursing during at least the first eight months. In the latter part of infancy, solid foods should supplement mother's milk rather than replace it.

It's important to let your older baby or child eat when he or she wishes and not to react if he/she chooses not to eat. Never force baby to eat. It would throw off baby's self-regulatory mechanism. Forcing causes great harm to the child. If you have a variety of healthful foods in your home, then the healthy baby or child will not starve, so there is no need to worry. Your child will have certain food preferences, and that is all right. Over a month's time, there will be an accumulation of all the necessary nutrients on deposit. My son went through a phase when he only wanted bananas. I remember panicking quite a bit, only later to learn this was very normal. Fruits are similar to mother's milk in a number of ways. The child should be presented with a variety of foods, including leafy greens, but his/her choices should be respected. A child also may eat more at one meal and less at another, but this will balance out.

Raw vegan foods are rich in water. Watermelon is 90% water. All fruits, even the heavier more filling varieties such as avocados have a high water content. All vegetables contain high water content. A child eating this way will most likely require less drinking water, but purified water should always be made available. According to Ruth Yaron, "Getting enough liquid is as important for a baby as for an adult, maybe even more so because a baby's body is made up of a higher proportion of water than an adult's. You must make sure your baby gets enough liquids from water or food to prevent dehydration, especially on hot days. Besides helping the kidneys, water is needed by baby's body to replace that which is lost through the urine, feces, sweating, evaporation, and breathing (as seen in cold weather)."

Many people who decide to go 100% raw may have some symptoms of detoxification for a short period. Permitting these symptoms to occur without using medicine to treat them will result in improved health. As their digestion has not been aggravated for so many years, babies and young children will have fewer or no detoxification symptoms when transitioning to raw foods.

13

Teaching Your Child How to Eat

"Nature will castigate those who don't masticate."
HORACE FLETCHER (1849–1919)

There was earlier discussion on the importance of chewing for improved digestion. From his book, *The Power Eating Program: You Are How You Eat*, by Lino Stanchich: "Creating quiet, relaxing mealtimes is an integral part of healthy eating. This peaceful mealtime atmosphere, along with proper chewing of food, is as important for health as what we eat." Lino Stanchich elaborates: "Talking while eating tends to send the energy from the mouth to your throat or brain, creating a separation of energy in the body and disrupting the digestion process. We receive much less energy from the food when we expend the energy by talking." He has observed: "People who talk while eating often need larger quantities of food and experience more frequent indigestion. It is best to practice silence while eating or to speak as seldom as possible between bites. Turn off your television and telephone as you eat. Many people find soft music very relaxing at mealtimes." He feels if you must talk during meals, discuss topics that are positive and pleasant as negative topics will charge the food with negative energy as it gets digested, and this negative energy will go inside you: "If you charge the food with thoughts of strength, joy and appreciation, then the same will become you."

In *Quantum Eating*, Tonya Zavasta explains: "Concentrate only on eating whenever you are eating. Let this principle become your mantra. The organ involved in eating is the same organ used for talking. Don't use your mouth for both at the same time. Social eating leads to overeating and impaired digestion.

Being psychologically present when you eat is the key to liberating yourself from hunger. When you eat and socialize at the same time, your awareness of eating diminishes. You'll quickly feel hungry again. Eating is personal. You can allocate other times for family gatherings. Teach children to eat in silence and gratitude, concentrating on the moment. Use books - not spoons - to bring your family together."

Let's be grateful for our food, for today's endless bounty of Nature, to the Creator, the Cosmos, to the food itself, and to those who plant, harvest, and deliver it. We should eat only after expressing our thanks for all meals, saying grace or sitting in reverent silence to thank Nature's forces, and the hardworking farmers. These are ideas for a loving pre-meal prayer.

Prayers we have used that children will enjoy learning by heart are:

"Thank you God for the world so sweet,
Thank you for the food we eat,
Thank you for the birds that sing,
Thank you God for everything."

BY THE SCOUTS OF AMERICA

"Earth who gives to us this food,
Sun who makes it ripe and good,
Dear Earth, Dear Sun, by you we live,
Our loving thanks to you we give."

BY FRANKLIN KANE AND BETTY KANE STALEY

Chewing is an important part of the *Power Eating Program.* "Chewing strengthens our immune system and promotes rejuvenation. Chewing stimulates the release of parotin hormones which encourage the thymus to create T-cells, the protectors of our immune system. Parotin hormones are released by the parotid glands, located on each side of our jaw behind our ears. Only the chewing motion stimulates the release of the ptyalin enzyme in the saliva and the parotin hormone, both vital digestive and rejuvenating elements awaiting release into your body. The strongest animals in the world such as the ox, bull, elephant, and buffalo are plant eaters who chew their food very well. If you do not chew well you will not digest your food and will tend to overeat. The more you chew, the more powerfully you will transmit your food into energy."

Lino recommends chewing 50 times a mouthful, but if you want to produce strong energy and really activate your digestive power, then chewing at least 100 times is necessary. He says if you have any ailment or need above average energy, even more times of chewing is needed. www.macrobioticconsultation.com. Lino comes from an orientation which goes back to times when the only available food was grains and root vegetables, predominantly rice, in the mountains where Japanese monks lived. These starchy foods require longer chewing for the starch to be digested in the mouth by ptyalin, produced by the salivary glands. Since we are now living in times when we can get fresh food no matter where we live in the civilized world, we no longer need to eat only starchy grains and vegetables. We can eat non-starchy fruits and green vegetables. Lino's chewing recommendations deal primarily with starchy grains and vegetables.

Everyone's in a desperate hurry, even shoveling food down, without enjoying the glory of chewing, and the subtle flavor changes as the food is well chewed. The old adage: "Chew your liquids, and drink your foods!" commands the food be chewed until liquefied by the action of chewing and the saliva. This is especially applicable to almonds. Pecans, walnuts and seeds are softer, but even when soaked, they need to be chewed for a long time, as do salads. Obviously, when following the raw foods lifestyle, the number of chews will vary significantly when ranging from watermelon to celery to nuts. Even blended foods and juices should be well mixed with the saliva through adequate chewing.

Most of our food, and the food we provide for our children, should be served at room temperature so as not to chill the stomach and stop the gastric juices from flowing, creating indigestion. Some people put everything in the refrigerator. Have you ever tasted a refrigerated tomato? It loses its taste and is difficult to eat. It's best to eat more perishable fruits such as berries, grapes and cherries soon after they're picked or purchased. When stored for subsequent use, they need to be refrigerated. Perishable fruits such as berries should be taken out of the refrigerator at least thirty minutes prior to eating to bring to room temperature.

Overeating is harmful to the body. It creates an imbalance that takes blood away from the brain by bringing it to the lower digestive organs instead, interfering with clarity of thought. Chewing thoroughly as well as deep relaxation through meditation will help us to eat less. Eating with chopsticks can also help to slow down eating.

જી

Eating During the Day

Here is a brief list of the benefits of eating during the day while avoiding eating at night.

Whoever has practiced this powerful rejuvenation and health technique cannot stop extolling its virtues:

■ Digestion is strongest when the sun is highest;

■ Deep, sound sleep is essential to good health. When we eat at night, we force the digestion of this food to happen during sleep, thereby diminishing the sleep's focus on cleansing and healing;

■ The energy gained through eating in the morning and early afternoon can be used productively throughout the day, but when eating at night, the energy is not used for physical activity and accumulates as fat during sleep;

■ We are awake to the beautiful colors and tastes of fresh foods when we can see them in daylight. Owls and bats will feel differently.

■ We can eliminate waste more perfectly in the morning when not eating the night before;

■ The rejuvenation and healing benefits of daylight eating are amazing and must be experienced to be believed.

To learn more, please read *Quantum Eating* by Tonya Zavasta and *The Daylight Diet* by Paul Nison.

14

Personal Care Products for Children

"If you can't eat it, don't breathe it."

DR. ALFRED V. ZAMM

Powders and other personal care products are toxic to baby's skin and internal health. Sixty percent of the chemicals in the products we put on our children's skin begin circulating in their bloodstream within minutes. Babies and growing children are much more susceptible to injury and harm from these chemicals. I used to think it was safe to buy personal care products from health food stores, but upon further research, I found out many products are not safe at all. To be certified organic, foods are under strict regulations, but there are absolutely no regulations for labeling personal care products "organic." The products flaunt words such as "natural" and "organic" in big lettering on the front label, but if you scan through the tiny words listed in the ingredients section usually found on the back label, you will see many words that look like they belong in a science experiment. And that is basically what you and your child will be when using these products on your skin. Toxic ingredients in skin care products can cause tumors, reproductive complications, biological mutations and skin and eye irritations. Personal care products for babies, even those labeled "Natural" or "Organic," are often loaded with toxic chemicals. "Natural" fragrances in shampoos and lotions have been linked to cancers.

Foods with higher fat contents hold toxins. Such high fat foods are meats, dairy products and fish. As consumers, we need to carefully examine what we purchase: our food, our personal care and cleaning products as well. Many top brand toothpastes display the warning: "Do Not Swallow." We should not use any personal care product we would not be able to eat.

It is best to avoid products containing chemicals, artificial colors and fragrances. Look for products that state, "NO ANIMAL TESTING," that contain non-irritating vegetables, fruits, herbs, and natural scents. Terressentials, a company located in Middletown, Maryland, believes strongly that personal care products should be totally chemical-free, so they make their own. Their website is www.terressentials.com.

I washed my children with nothing more than warm water. We purchased shower filters from the Waterwise Company to remove harmful chemicals, and then bathed the children in the purified water, without using anything else on their skin or hair. Both children grew up having clear, silky-smooth skin. People commented about their glowing skin and clear eyes, which I attribute to the use of water significantly reduced in toxic chemicals, and a raw food lifestyle rich in high water content foods that allowed for a clean internal body. When they grew to be teenagers, it became difficult to keep them away from using some of the toxic personal care products, due to their buying into peer pressure and falling for advertisements that specifically targeted them. I was able to get them to use cruelty-free products because of their love for animals, but many products not tested on animals still contain some toxic chemicals as well, albeit usually less.

Many people are not willing or ready to use water only, and feel they need soaps, shampoos, deodorants, etc. to feel clean and smell fresh. Teenagers especially want to use these products because of extensive advertising targeting their age group.

Studies have demonstrated a relationship between the chemical parabens, used in antiperspirants and other cosmetics, and its presence in breast cancer tumors. The article "Five Types of Parabens Detected Intact in Human Breast Tumors" by Suzanne M. Snedeker, Ph.D. of Cornell University Sprecher Institute for Comparative Cancer Research was published in *The Ribbon*, Vol. 9, no. 1, Winter 2004. Betty Kamen, Ph.D. and Dr. Michael Rosenbaum also report the connection between parabens and breast cancer in "Parabens and Antiperspirants" (www.naturallyhome.com/articles/parabens.shtml).

The ingredients used by Terressentials are gentle oils such as jojoba, sunflower and coconut, as well as essential oils and herbs such as calendula and chamomile. It is not necessary to wash your child's hair frequently or to bathe them every day. Taking a bath every other day and washing the hair no more than once a week is sufficient. My son didn't want to bathe every day as a young child and we didn't force him. When he was eating totally raw vegan foods, his body always smelled delicious. Terressentials reports the following information in their brochure "Protect Your Little Angels":

Why do you need to study labels on body care products? The 1993 National Academy of Sciences (NAS) report "Pesticides in the Diets of Infants and Children" included recommendations that : all sources of pesticide exposure be considered when attempting to reduce your child's pesticide exposure. The NAS report concluded that in the absence of other factors, direct carcinogens are more potent in rapidly growing animals and that infants and children are subject to rapid tissue growth and development, which will have an impact on cancer risk. Children's bodies are small and because they do not have an adult's ability to detoxify and excrete toxins, they absorb proportionally higher doses of toxins per unit of body weight, which means their organs may suffer permanent and irreversible damage more quickly because they are not fully developed. Chemicals in body care products have been linked to reproductive problems in both women (e.g. endometriosis and the increasingly early onset of puberty in young girls) and men (e.g. falling sperm counts and congenital birth defects of the reproductive organs) and to some cancers. Many synthetic chemicals have also been linked to developmental deficiencies and learning disabilities in children. The National Toxicology Program (NTP) recently found repeated application to skin of some of the chemicals listed by the FDA- diethanolamine (DEA), or its fatty acid derivative cocamide DEA- induced liver and kidney cancer. NTP also emphasized DEA is readily absorbed through the skin and accumulates in organs, such as the brain, where it induces chronic toxic effects.

Companies have sprouted up producing nontoxic personal and home care products. The Environmental Working Group reports the European Union is focusing on creating safer cosmetic and personal care products for its people, and as a result, major companies are reformulating their products to be safer for European standards. However, these same companies are not yet planning to sell these safer products to consumers in the United States. Therefore, it's always necessary to study the ingredients listed on every package. Although the consumer may choose not to buy the product after finding one or more toxic ingredients listed on the label, not all the ingredients are required to be listed. Purchase products that list only plant-based ingredients, not petrochemicallybased. For example, mineral oil is a petrochemical, but olive oil, coconut oil, jojoba oil, aloe, etc. are plant-based. Nontoxic personal care products can be purchased at Paul Nison's website at www.rawlife.com, David Wolfe's website at www.sunfood.com, Rhio's website at www.rawfoodinfo.com, Tonya Zavasta's website at www.beautifulonraw.com, Hippocrates Health Institute's website at www.hippocratesinst.org, Live Live and Organic at www.live-live.com, and High Vibe Health and Healing at www.highvibe.com.

Because children are more susceptible to toxins than adults, we need to be especially careful about what they inhale and what we rub onto their skin. Problems from synthetic "fragrance" reported to the FDA have included headaches, dizziness, rashes, skin discoloration, violent coughing and vomiting, and allergic skin irritation. Exposure to fragrances can affect the central nervous system, causing depression, hyperactivity, irritability, inability to cope, and other behavioral changes. Are you aware manufacturers are not required to include the ingredients for fragrance chemicals on product labels? Babies can't tell you they're experiencing a headache or lung tightness when you use powder with synthetic fragrance. Synthetic chemicals pollute the earth in their manufacture, and they pollute your body and your home. If they don't benefit you and cause harm to your children, why use them?

Make sure to study the ingredients of any personal care product you purchase. Here is a list of only some of the very toxic chemicals found in personal care products: fluoride, ammonium laureth sulfate, decyl polyglucose, cyclopolymethicone, cocamide DEA, lauramide DEA, sodium lauryl, laureth sulfate, cocoamidopropyl betaine, olefin sulfonate, disodium cocoamphodiacetate, PVP copolymer, polyvinylpyrrolidone (causes kidney damage and thesaurosis of the lungs), EDTA, soy, wheat or oat (hydrolyzed) proteins, MSG, methylparaben, propylparaben, butyl parabens, diazolidinyl urea, tricolasan, quaternarium 15, sodium benzoate, FD and C color and synthetic fragrance.

Many women, even raw foodists, continue to color their hair with toxic products. Many products sold in health food stores appear to be natural, but contain toxic chemicals. The labels will emphasize herbs or organic ingredients, but there are still toxic ingredients in these hair coloring products. After 11 years of eating exclusively raw vegan foods, and after a two-week water fast, I decided to stop using poisons to color my hair. I felt the water fast was beneficial to help me expel old medications I had taken years earlier. Why would I want to continue taking in poisonous products when it's something over which I have control? Even though my intentions are always to avoid toxic materials, I don't always have control of them in the air I breathe. I certainly do have control of the food I eat, and the products I use on my skin and hair. I now use natural, organic henna for hair coloring. My hair has filled in where it was starting to thin from the chemical dyes. There are organic henna products. A good quality organic henna product I've used is the Anthony Morrocco Method (www.morroccomethod.com). It takes a long time to rinse off the earthy henna, but it's definitely worth it to have a natural, non-toxic result. The advantage of not coloring the hair at all is being able to experience the likely return of its natural color after a period of enjoying the raw food lifestyle. The chemicals in skin and hair products enter our bloodstream within minutes. Pregnant and lactating women need to be especially aware of this danger.

In addition to protecting ourselves, it's also important to check labels of all products to make sure they are not tested on animals. Many personal care products mean torture and even death for unfortunate laboratory animals.

As we are growing with our families, we're confronted frequently with many personal choices for our children, our home and our lawn care. It has been reported that many cancers in humans are a direct result of exposure to carcinogens in the environment. The brains and nervous systems of children are much more susceptible to nerve poisons as their bodies are not yet completely developed. Their livers and kidneys are not able to detoxify and eliminate specific chemicals as rapidly as adults. Children breathe in a larger volume of air and have a larger skin surface area in relation to their lighter body weights and therefore they take in proportionately greater amounts of pesticides than adults. Household cleaners, personal care products, paints, plastics, and oven and carpet cleaners are some of the most poisonous products used inside the home. Today there are many alternative nontoxic products that can be used. The organic lawn care industry is growing, and there is no need to use dangerous lawn and garden pesticides. Children are playing outside and breathing in these toxic products. For years, my husband has used only organic methods to take care of our lawn, and we have noticed our lawn looks as good as and sometimes better than other lawns on which pesticides and harmful fertilizers are used.

Plastics present another danger. Plasticizers are chemically known as phthalates. They have been known to cause breast cancer and are major endocrine disruptors in the body. Plastics that are frozen or heated are extremely poisonous, as dioxins from the plastic will then more readily leach into the liquid or food and can be lethal. Be careful of plastic toys and teething devices. Many children will mouth their toys. Plastic toys should not be purchased because young children will put them in their mouths. They can contain phthalates and Bisphenol A, that are in many plastic materials. The leaching of BPA bisphenol, the chemical used to harden the plastic used in manufacturing baby bottles, becomes even more dangerous when the bottles are heated. The toxicity of these materials can cause abnormal development.

There are many good alternatives to plastic toys that are not hazardous to your child's health. These items may be purchased at stores selling solid wood toys and items with non-toxic finishes. Solid wood toys are a good choice. A couple of mail order companies offering non-toxic items for children are: Nova at www.novanatural.com; 877-668-2111 and Babyworks at www.babyworks.com; 800-422-2910.

Most canned goods have a lacquer lining containing plastic. Cans contain BPA-containing plastic, and canned food is sterilized at 250 degrees, leaching plastic into the food or beverage inside. This is a considerable exposure for those who eat canned foods. It's advisable to use glass, wood, or ceramics for food storage. The use of glass jars and bowls for storage is best.

For cleaning the house, I use vinegar, baking soda and water. Baking soda and water work well for cleaning floors, toilet bowls, and as a drain cleaner, performing as an excellent replacement for ammonia based cleaners. Vinegar and water make an excellent cleaner for bathrooms, glass surfaces, linoleum floors and drains. Borax works well as a bleach to brighten, whiten and add a clean scent to clothing. Bon Ami is a nontoxic product that can be used to clean the bathroom and kitchen. Today, thanks to increased consumer awareness, there are also many nontoxic, biodegradable, non-animal tested cleaners from companies such as Seventh Generation, Gaiam Harmony, and Ecover. There is no need to use poisonous chemicals inside or outside of your house. Exposure to lawn and garden pesticides can increase the risk of leukemia, cancer, non-Hodgkins lymphoma, soft tissue sarcoma (lung cancer), kidney damage, genetic defects, asthma and respiratory disorders, learning, developmental and behavioral disorders. Organic lawn care is highly recommended. Three important websites by environmentalists Patti and Doug Wood: www.ghlp.org (The Grassroots Healthy Lawn Program); www.grassrootsinfo.org (Grassroots Environmental Education); and www. howgreenismytown.org Other useful websites: www.envirolink.org; www. rachel.org; www.checnet.org; www.igc.org/panna/resources/advisor; www. foodnews.org; and www.pesticidefreezone.org. Books I recommend are: *Prescriptions for a Healthy Home* by Paula Baker-Laporte, Erica Elliott, John

Banta and Lisa Flynn, *Homes that Heal and Those that Don't,* by Athena Thompson, and *The Nontoxic Home* and *Home Safe Home: Protecting Yourself and Your Family from Everyday Toxins and Harmful Household Products,* both by Debra Lynn Dadd, who also lists details of finding nontoxic hotel rooms: www.debraslist.com/athome/athome.php?id=26. Other recommended reading: *The Household Detective Primer: Protecting Your Children from Toxins in the Home,* and *CHEC's Guide to Environmental Childproofing.*

Children spend most of their time indoors. Indoor toxicity is vast, at a far greater level than toxicity outdoors. Commercial cleaning products containing such lethal ingredients as ammonia, benzene, dioxins and chlorine need to be avoided at all costs. Phosphates are hormone disruptors and also need to be avoided. Studies have shown pesticide residue in mothers' blood. Brain cancer has often been associated with pesticide exposure. As Dr. Alfred V. Zamm says in his book, *Why Your House May Endanger Your Health,* "If you can't eat it, don't breathe it."

Chemicals, such as chlorine, can be inhaled as well as absorbed into the skin while taking a shower. It's very important to use shower filters. Children love to go swimming, but most pools are highly chlorinated, and your child will absorb this poison. If you start when they are young, by getting your children excited about going to the beach and freshwater lakes, maybe the toxic swimming pools can be avoided as much as possible. Some pool owners successfully dechlorinate and remove other toxic chemicals from the water in their pools by using special systems. Our friends in Costa Rica enjoy swimming only in fresh water holes, by waterfalls, rivers and in the ocean.

It is also important to dress our children in nontoxic clothing such as organic cotton and hemp. Synthetic materials don't allow the skin to breathe. See more information about beautiful natural clothing at: www.gonaturalbaby.com.

A useful practice to begin as a family is dry brushing for adults, children and babies. I never realized its importance until I stayed at American Yogini with my daughter for five days, where we experienced a dry brushing workshop with Mary McGuire-Wien. Mary says that for pregnancy, dry brushing can help to remove stretch marks. In addition to diet, this can also significantly help children with immune problems. It helps to activate the lymphatic system and increase circulation. She recommends making dry brushing a healthy daily habit, just like brushing or flossing one's teeth. There are special super-soft brushes for the most sensitive skin, and very little pressure is needed. Babies love it. Remember to brush toward the heart. Followed by a massage with some sesame oil, this can be soothing and cleansing to both adult and child. See www.americanyogini.com for different sizes and textures of Merbin brushes.

Crucial information on the hazards of cell phone usage is presented by Dr. Joseph Mercola (www.mercola.com). In the following article, "Are Cell Phones More Dangerous than Smoking?" Dr. Mercola presents the results of new studies that need to be acted on immediately to prevent serious health problems, especially for growing children:

> Award-winning cancer expert Dr. Vini Khurana has concluded that mobile phones may kill far more people than smoking or asbestos. The latest study, which is being called the "most devastating indictment yet" for the safety of mobile phones, draws on growing evidence that using handsets for 10 years or more can double your risk of brain cancer. Professor Khurana reviewed more than 100 studies on the effects of mobile phones, and concluded that "there is a significant and increasing body of evidence for a link between mobile phone usage and certain brain tumors." "We are currently experiencing a reactively unchecked and dangerous situation," he added. Earlier this year, the French government warned against the use of mobile phones, particularly for children. Germany also advises people to minimize handset use. Khurana urges people to avoid using mobile phones whenever possible, and believes that governments and the mobile phone industry must take immediate steps to reduce exposure to this radiation. If nothing is done, Khurana believes the rate of malignant brain tumors and the associated death rate will rise around the world within a decade, and by then it may be too late to intervene medically.

Dr. Mercola adds: "Professor Khurana based the notion that cell phones are more dangerous than smoking on the following logic: 3 billion people use cell phones worldwide, which is three times more than the number of people who smoke. Of course, smoking doesn't immediately show any deadly signs either. But wait a decade or so, and the evidence is there right before your eyes. According to Khurana, the 'incubation time' or 'latency' (the time from the start of regular mobile phone usage to the diagnosis of a malignant solid brain tumor is around 10-20 years. In the years 2008-2012, he says, 'we will have reached the appropriate length of follow-up time to begin to definitively observe the impact of this global technology on brain tumor incidence rates.'

There is VERY solid evidence that the number of brain tumors will increase to 500,000 per YEAR in 2010—and this will double to 1 million every year by 2015 if the causes are not addressed. Folks, this is the real deal and represents an impending health care crisis."

Dr. Mercola goes on to say: "I am absolutely convinced that the explosion of cell phone usage around the world is a major contributor to a host of diseases ranging from autism to cancer to insomnia. You are fortunate, though, as you are receiving this information today, while there is still time to circumvent some of the damage. Please do not wait another 10 years for the 'definitive' link to be found and publicized in the mainstream circles before you take action to protect yourself, and your children, from the electromagnetic radiation and information-carrying radio waves emitted by cell phones and many other wireless devices. If you're looking for some type of indication that cell phones are causing you harm, consider that all of the following ailments have been scientifically linked to information-carrying radio waves: fatigue, headaches, sleep disruptions, altered memory function, poor concentration and spatial awareness, Alzheimer's, senility and dementia, Parkinson's, autism, and cancer. These modulated information-carrying radio waves resonate (vibrate) in the same frequencies as many of your cellular receptors; frequencies of a few to a few hundred cycles per second. These are biological frequencies and, unlike ionizing radiation (X-rays), which you can tolerate in small doses, there is NO dose of these radio waves that are safe. They cause damage at ANY dose, no matter how low. This concept is called zero threshold, and that is precisely what you have with cell phones, most portable phones, and WiFi routers. These information-carrying radio waves can stimulate or confuse your cellular receptors, causing a whole cascade of pathological consequences that can culminate in fatigue, sleeplessness, anxiety, neurological decline, and ultimately cancers. The reason why children should NOT use cell phones is because they have developing nervous systems and thinner skulls than adults, making them especially vulnerable to this type of damage."

"Information-carrying radio waves are all around us — especially from cell phones, but also from WiFi, WiMax, BlueTooth, and other wireless devices. And you are likely receiving exposure to them 24/7. Remember, kids should NOT be using cell phones. As a parent, it's up to you to protect them from this avoidable risk. Assuming you do choose to use a cell phone for more than just emergencies, here are the tips to increase your safety level (for cell phones and other radio-wave exposures):

1. Limit the amount of time you spend on a cell phone or cordless phone.

2. Use a wired headset to limit your exposure to the cell phone — ideally, an air tube headset that conducts sound but prevents any radiation from traveling up the wire to your brain. Also, make sure the wire is SHIELDED, which prevents it from acting as an antenna that could attract more information-carrying radio waves directly to your brain. Wireless BlueTooth headsets should be avoided.

3. Limit your exposure to WiFi routers. Find out where they are located in your work environment and stay away from them.

4. If you have any land-based (non-cellular) portable phones, do NOT use anything other than the 900 MHz phones, as the Gigahertz phones stay on continuously, blasting you with information-carrying radio waves 24/7.

5. Use the speakerphone instead of putting the phone to your ear; this is probably one of the single most important steps you can take other than not using your cell phone.

6. Limit calls inside buildings.

7. Use your cell phone only where the reception is good. When the reception is poor, your phone has to work harder, and therefore emits a much stronger radiation signal."

Dr. Mercola points out that cell phones, which work due to electromagnetic waves, are just one way cancer can be caused through impairing and weakening the immune system. Children also get cancer from numerous other sources: heavy pollution, bad food, hereditary factors, vaccines, from the fact that the parents didn't take the care to protect them from toxins during and before pregnancy, and many other contributing factors.

15

Children's Exercises and Ventilation

"Nature is the original church. Worship there daily."
ALAN COHEN

Carrying the infant benefits him/her in several ways:

- His/her head, neck, and shoulder muscles steady the body, creating stronger torso mobility.
- The torso and core muscles become stronger.
- Physical responses are regulated.
- The vestibular system, controlling balance, is toned.

The two-week old infant can make attempts to copy your funny facial expressions. Infant massage can be beneficial for baby. Adoptive parents, unable to nurse their baby, can use infant massage as a way to bond with their child. The book I recommend is: *Infant Massage: A Handbook for Loving Parents*, 3rd edition, by Vimala Schneider McClure, Bantam Books.

It can be challenging for new mothers to find time to exercise, but if you carry your baby all day and go for brisk walks while carrying him/her, you will enjoy the dual benefits of walking and weightbearing exercise. Walking while carrying baby also offers her/him an excellent opportunity to fall asleep.

Because Gabriela and Marco grew up on raw vegan foods with an abundance of energy, it would have been difficult for them to sit in school all day. As homeschoolers, we were able to be outside a lot, getting exercise and doing

145

fun activities while camping, exploring nature, hiking, and participating in outdoor sports. After eating raw foods for months or years, parents, and especially their children, become aware of how much lighter and more energetic they feel due to ease of digestion. Once, I watched Marco playing basketball with his friend, a good athlete. Although the friend played basketball quite well, he tired easily and needed to take frequent breaks, whereas Marco would go on endlessly. Marco participated in many of our town's team sports. Many observers, including coaches, remarked on his stamina and endurance. Both Gabriela and Marco developed muscle easily. Even when they were young and smaller than other children their age, they were extremely agile and strong, eating fruits, vegetables, nuts and seeds.

Children love to be active but today's epidemic increase in obesity has resulted in children living a sedentary lifestyle. From the time their children are very young, parents need to be excellent physical role models by getting their children involved in activities which provide exercise and enjoyment. Hiking, bicycle riding, running, climbing, skating, swimming, skiing, tennis, team sports, dancing, martial arts and boating are only some of the physical activities which keep us in good shape.

Yoga is also extremely beneficial for children. Many yoga studios now include classes specifically for children. Parents can take certain yoga moves from yoga videos, and practice them at home with the whole family.

Jingee and Storm Talifero describe some wonderful exercises for growing children in their e-books that I highly recommend (available at www.thegardendiet.com).

It is important that baby, child and adult have a well-ventilated room all year round. In the winter, if the room gets chilly, use heavier blankets. The growing child needs fresh air day and night. It is also important to be outdoors in summer, fall, winter and spring for fresh air, sunshine, and exercise.

I once had an experience that amazed me insofar as how healthful and healing the ocean air can be. I went to the beach with some friends. Several days prior to the beach trip, I had incurred a serious cut to my left eye from a contact lens. I had rested and kept my eyes closed for a good part of a few days, but my eye continued to be very red, swollen and painful. At the end of the day at the beach, my eye was almost completely healed. According to Dr. Timothy Trader, plankton is the number one oxygen-giver on this planet, and therefore the freshest air is at the beach.

Mountain and forest air is also very health-giving. According to Dr. Alfred V. Zamm in his book *Why Your House May Endanger Your Health*, "The best place is either to the oceanside, in an area where sea breezes blow inland constantly, or high in the mountains. The mountains, in fact, with their heavier concentration of negative ions and relatively pollution-free atmosphere, make the best all-around choice for a homesite."

We need to get our families outdoors hiking, camping and playing together, skating outdoors in winter, and swimming at the beach in summer. As they grew older, I focused on getting my children involved in wilderness-survival programs. Through working with wilderness and natural history instructors in programs such as The Primitive Kids Club, Common Heritage Skills, and The Children of the Earth Foundation, we found people passionate about the outdoors, further instilling our children with understanding, appreciation and love of Nature and animals. We spent much time outdoors with friends, camping in mountainous areas and learning about Nature and Native American ways from the wilderness instructors with whom we worked. The children spent years building debris huts and other primitive shelters in the woods, making mats out of cattail weeds, playing nature awareness games, making nature observations, carving spoons and bowls out of fallen pieces of bark and wood, gathering tinder and making their own fires using native bowdrills, and using all of their senses to perceive the world around them as they roamed the woods and forests.

We took Permaculture Gardening classes from a young woman who had studied permaculture on farms around the world. Gabriela, Marco and I were filmed for a show called "Teen Kids News," since we had been invited to do a special segment on homeschooling. They were interviewed about their daily lives, and then the camera crew followed us and other homeschooled children to a big garden where the children worked with Heather Stewart, who enthusiastically involved them in permaculture gardening while she explained what they were doing. The show aired nationally on CBS and Cable Television.

A wonderful family camp I recommend is called "Camp Common Ground," located in the beautiful surroundings of Starksboro, Vermont. Common Ground Center is a family friendly, attachment parenting, vegetarian retreat center offering rentals and family camping programs. Family friendly beds for co-sleeping are available. From our personal experience at Camp Common Ground, a raw vegan diet is easily accommodated (Common Ground Center,

473 Tatro Road, Starksboro, VT 05487, Phone: 800-430-2667; info@cgcvt. org; www.cgcvt.org).

It has always been my goal to have my children involved outdoors, with family and friends. My husband also loves the outdoors, participating in team sports, and has played many of them outdoors with the children. We have chosen to take our family vacations each year in the middle of winter, so that we could go to a beautiful sunny spot where we could be outdoors. One of our favorite trips was hiking in the rainforests of Costa Rica where we spent most of our time outdoors.

16

Caring about the Creatures
Who Share Our Planet

"From an early age, I have abjured the use of meat, and the time will come when men will look upon the murder of animals as they look upon the murder of men."

LEONARDO DA VINCI

*"People get offended by animal rights campaigns. It's ludicrous.
It's not as bad as mass animal death in a factory."*

RICHARD GERE

Dr. Gabriel Cousens reminds us, "Pythagoras once said, 'as long as we're eating meat, we'll never have peace.' When you eat meat, you take on that violence and fear. The blood contains the soul of that being. Many great rabbis, including Jesus, were vegetarian."

As your child grows, make outdoor activities in nature a priority, and your child will have a strong connection to animals, and the plants and trees around him or her. I believe when we choose to be vegan and not harm animals, we gain a closer connection with them. I remember as a young child watching my father Sol sit for hours in the backyard with squirrels approaching him, and eating nuts out of his hand. I always felt they clearly understood his connectedness to animals.

When my daughter Gabriela was eight, she went to a nature and hiking oriented day camp for two weeks. The camp questionnaire inquired if she had any pets. She wrote, "Oh yes, I have chipmunks, squirrels, groundhogs, skunks and all sorts of other animals." She considered the beautiful free wild animals that live their lives the way they were meant to be lived, to be her pets. For many years, our pets were all the wild animals we enjoyed observing

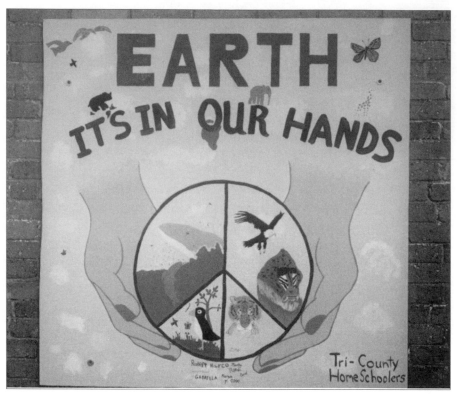

A mural dedicated to improving the environment for all creatures, "Earth: It's In Our Hands," painted by Marco, Gabriela and Karen Ranzi along with other homeschool families of Tri-County Homeschoolers - The mural was given as a community service project to The No Harm Store of Nyack, New York in 2000.

outdoors. At one point, Gabriela cried desperately that she wanted a dog, and we did get her a dog. If you do have an animal as a house pet, it's necessary for the animal not to be alone, or at least to be with another animal. Because we were homeschoolers, our dog had us at home a good part of the time, especially when the children were younger. There was also a big yard to roam freely, and organic raw foods were prepared.

It is important for children to visit some of the people and organizations active in helping animals. We volunteered for a wildlife rehabilitator for many years, a compassionate woman who rescued, rehabilitated and hoped to re-lease most of the animals back into the wild. We went on rescue missions with her, and helped her to rehabilitate many hurt and suffering animals. I still recall the memorial service she had for one of her beloved rescued creatures, a deer she rescued after an auto accident. Her love and care for all creatures had a great impact on us.

Our friends Linda and Scott Murray of New Mexico joined me in becoming avid animal rights activists. In 2000, we accompanied them on a trip to film an interview with the president of United Poultry Concerns, Karen Davis, Ph.D., at her fowl sanctuary in Virginia. We were deeply touched to see Karen's dedication and passion for promoting respectful treatment toward chickens and turkeys. Her publication, "Poultry Press," is available at www.upc-online.org. If you can't go for a visit, United Poultry Concerns sells many books and videos, some that are very valuable for children. Some of these are listed in the Appendix. Following our visit to the sanctuary, we went to PETA (People for the Ethical Treatment of Animals), an organization that works endlessly to eliminate animal abuse. These experiences help children to build a strong conscience and understanding of veganism. This one spiritual act, veganism, would end torture and pain for other souls who share the planet with us.

The Farm Sanctuary, an organization that rescues farm animals and provides a safe haven for them to live out their lives, has sites in California and New York. We went to visit and volunteer for the Farm Sanctuary in Watkins Glen, New York. Holding chickens and cleaning the chicken house, placing hay in the sheep barn, petting pigs and feeding turkeys were some of the chores that gave us a closer connection to the animals. The Farm Sanctuary also has internship programs for teenagers.

I was never able to comprehend how a baby chick project could be used to demonstrate the chicks' growth and development to children. They are taken from their mother, and an unnatural environment of lights is used to warm them. People may think it's fascinating for children to watch the baby chicks, but it is not natural for the chicks to wake up not being protected by their mother's feathers and warm body.

By not eating animals and products made from them, nor abusing animals in any way, we open ourselves to beautiful relationships with the creatures of the world. How wonderful to share this with our children! Why should we relate to dogs and cats but not care about cows, pigs, turkeys, ducks and chickens? A neighbor who loved her dog and cat once told me she felt guilty about eating farm animals and products made from them, but she just didn't have the discipline to give up eating meat and animal products. "Each year approximately 26 billion cows, pigs, chickens, turkeys and fish, each a unique individual capable of experiencing happiness, joy, loneliness, and frustration, are killed to satisfy America's appetite for animal flesh, milk, and eggs" (www. chooseveg.com). Every day, more than ten million animals are killed in the United States for food. I have heard author and lecturer Matthew Grace emphatically express: "What if 'filet mignon' were called 'Dead Cow?' Maybe then people would listen. Methane gas is given off by livestock and is destroying the ozone in the atmosphere. Pesticides and drugs are in the meat. And we are the only species on our planet who drink the milk of another species."

Every year on the weekend following Thanksgiving, we have a big Thanksgiving Celebration at our home to cherish the life of the beautiful turkey at a horrific time when millions of turkeys have been slaughtered. We adopt one or two turkeys from the Farm Sanctuary of Watkins Glen, New York, encouraging others to do the same. We pay for the turkey's care and food for the year at the shelter. We call our gathering the "Thanks Living" celebration.

I've shown documentary videos about the cruelties humans inflict on animals: *Eating*, produced by www.RaveDiet.com is a powerful movie about nutrition and animal cruelty. It's important to expose others to the realities and devastations of the slaughterhouse, factory farming, the fur trade and other animal abuses. *The Witness* and *Peaceable Kingdom* were produced by Tribe of Heart: www.tribeofheart.com; *Awakening of Wyndell Stames* by Scott Murray is a film exposing animal industry torturing (email: tbamerica@taosnet.com or call 505-741-0180). The world will continue to have wars and violence as long as we continue this holocaust on the animal world.

Many years ago, a boyfriend of mine told me my animal rights activities were a waste of time. My participation in demonstrating against fast food chains, the fur industry and many other animal cruelties were seen by him as useless because, as he put it, "How many animals could I realistically help?" Years later, when I read the following anecdote, I knew why I was so determined to fight for animal rights, even if it were only to save one animal at a time:

Starfish

As the old man walked down a Spanish beach at dawn, he saw ahead of him what he thought to be a dancer. The young man was running across the sand, rhythmically bending down to pick up a stranded starfish to throw it far into the sea.

The old man gazed in wonder as the young soul again and again threw the small starfish from the sand into the water. The old man approached him and asked why he spent so much energy doing what seemed a waste of time. The young man explained the stranded starfish would die if left until the morning sun.

"But there are thousands of miles of beach, and miles and miles of starfish. How can your effort make any difference?"

The young man looked down at the small starfish in his hand, and as he threw it to safety in the sea, said, "It makes a difference to this one!"

— ANONYMOUS

Inside my favorite metal frame, engraved with animals, the saying is: "The Goal of Life is Living in Harmony with Nature." I believe by eating the raw vegan food given to us by the Creator and spending time in Nature, we can live a more spiritual and divine existence. A treasured plaque contains a quote by Albert Schweitzer: "By respect for life, we become religious in a way that is elementary, profound and alive." Belief in the connectedness of all creatures and love for Nature is very deep and spiritual, deeply religious. I thank my grandmother and my father for passing this down to me. Although it is obvious, many people are blinded to this truth.

Gabriela was eight when she wrote "Why I'm a Vegetarian" for a second grade school paper:

Why I'm a Vegetarian

It's not healthy for us to eat animals. Because they are given drugs and shots. And by being vegetarian you can live a longer life. And our bodies are not meant to eat meat and dairy. Our intestines are different from the carnivores. And meat and dairy can cause heart disease and cancer. It also is important to the animals. Baby calves are taken away from their mothers. Dairy cows are overworked all day for their milk that's supposed to be given to their babies. They are put in narrow stalls where they are separated from their loved ones. The chickens' beeks are cut off and they are squished in little cages. After that, they cut open their throats and hang them up alive on conveyor belts. Slaughterhouses are terrible places where animals are very scared. Some places like the Farm Sanctuary help animals. They take in animals that have been injured or left alone. On Thanksgiving my family adopted a turkey from the Farm Sanctuary. His name is Tolstoy. We are very happy he was not a Thanksgiving dinner. Instead he had his own Dinner.

AND BY BEING VEGETARIAN YOU CAN MAKE A WORLD OF DIFFERENCE!!!

At age 12, Gabriela wrote:

MY LIFE AS A VEGAN by Gabriela Ranzi

It all really started with my great grandmother, who was sick in 1921 and given six months to live. She was advised by her brother to read books about becoming a vegetarian, and later a vegan. I am a proud descendant of my great grandmother, and my grandfather who has lived his life as a vegetarian as well, and my mother, who became a vegetarian at age seventeen. I am vegan for three reasons:

1. I love animals and I don't want to eat them. I also want to be healthy.

2. The animals that are eaten in the United States of America are shot up with hormones. And we are just not meant to eat animals. The human intestine is about 25 feet long and very twisted. The lion's intestine is very straight and very short, which means that when the lion eats meat it goes directly through its body and out in a short time. But if a human eats meat, it takes days and even weeks to digest.

3. I also want to save the environment. All over the world the rainforests are being cut down to put cattle there for meat. All of the trees that are being cut down are causing global warming on our planet. Soon we won't be able to breathe because we need to breathe the air that the trees produce. I recently went to Switzerland and I saw miles and miles of corn, and it's all for the cows!!! With all that corn, we could feed all of the hungry people on this planet and still have some leftover. I love being a vegetarian and a vegan. Because I help the animals and I have spoken for them, I also feel I have helped the world.

In 2009, Gabriela continues to write on her beliefs about "Veganism." As a college student majoring in Global Environmental Studies, she completed a paper titled "Environmental Vegetarianism," discussing all aspects of dietary and environmental abuses and how they directly affect the future of the planet.

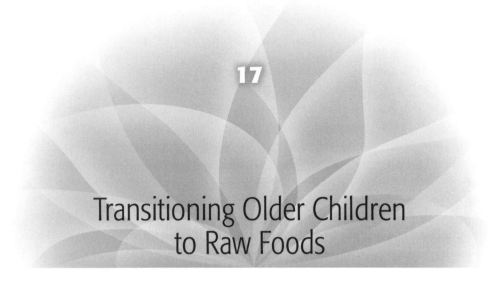

Transitioning Older Children to Raw Foods

"Let food be your medicine, and medicine be your food"

HIPPOCRATES

"A good basic rule is—Everything you eat and drink should come from
a garden, tree, bush or the grocery produce section. Make sure it's organic.
If you sprayed a can of Raid on an apple, would you eat it?"

JINGEE TALIFERO, THE DAILY RAW INSPIRATION FROM JINGEE AT WWW.THEGARDENDIET.COM

Transitioning older children to the raw food lifestyle can be daunting. I only learned over time with the unfortunate mistakes I made with my own children that this transition must be done gently and with love. You as the parent need to start off as the example. If you set a good example yourself, your actions will speak louder than words. You will be teaching your children it is all right to be different and to live what you believe to be the truth. Only through educating yourself will you become confident raw plant foods are scientifically and nutritionally optimal. You are then a very powerful example. If one of the parents is still eating unnatural and unhealthy foods, the children will be influenced by that parent. It would be most beneficial for both parents to read and understand the importance of healthful raw vegan foods and to support each other toward a healthy lifestyle, as the nutrition given to developing children's bodies will either enhance or have a negative effect on their health and future wellbeing.

You might begin by talking to your child about young people who have triumphed over illness and disease. For example, both children of the Boutenko family (see their books referenced in the bibliography) overcame illnesses after switching to raw vegan foods. My son Marco overcame asthmatic symptoms, ear infections and chronic allergic rhinitis after changing to raw vegan foods. Prior to making this dietary change, pediatric allergists' tests revealed he was allergic to many foods, pollens and animal hair. His wheezing and gasping during the day became even worse at night. Some improvement was noted after giving up processed foods. But following the change to live foods, the allergies and asthmatic symptoms were relieved within a year, and he no longer had allergies to any healthful foods, or pollens or animal fur. It was so obvious that ease of digestion had a lot to do with healing. A number of children eating mainly raw foods have made remarkable improvement in their abilities to focus and learn. Fresh fruits and vegetables with their high water content exit the body quickly. Live foods are easily digested, taking from 20 minutes to 5 or 6 hours to digest, whereas cooked foods can take several days to digest. These cooked, denatured, slow transiting foods with their low water content cause constipation. The body wants chlorophyll, glucose and enzymes, found in fruits and vegetables, and when those needs are met, the system operates the way it was intended. Dr. Douglas Graham states: "Health is the natural state of everything on this planet, and your body, if given the proper chance, will always go toward health. When the kidneys and liver are overloaded, toxemia levels rise. At a certain point, the toxemia level reaches toleration, and then you get symptoms." We need to nurture and care for ourselves and our children to avoid this toxemia toleration level and to have the health we desire for our families.

In the book *Disease-Proof Your Child—Feeding Kids Right*, Dr. Joel Fuhrman writes about healing children from A.D.H.D. (Attention Deficit Hyperactivity Disorder) through high nutrient plant foods.

A.D.H.D. may also disappear or diminish when a child is removed from a pressurized, competitive institutional environment and has the chance to learn through following his or her interests. See the Homeschooling chapter. A.D.D. (Attention Deficit Disorder) and A.D.H.D. are often unrealistic labels, which can be unfair interpretations of different ways of behaving. Each child might be taken care of in a way that makes that particular child shine. The established method of trying to make all children fit through a certain production system and drugging all of those who don't will have future consequences for us all.

As a certified speech pathologist working with learning disabled and autistic children for over 30 years, and as a teacher of "Creating Healthy Children" classes, I've observed children suffering from A.D.D., learning disability or autism spectrum disorder improve their overall health and ability to focus and learn.

Improvements can be expected when animal foods including dairy, processed foods, and gluten are excluded, and when fresh fruits and vegetables predominate. Additionally, permanently stopping the administration of all vaccines containing many dangerous chemicals that affect the nervous system is strongly recommended. Parents attending my classes have been able to witness their children heal from A.D.D., learning disability and autism by adopting these measures. Some parents have also had success with detoxifying their children from heavy metals through use of the hyperbaric chamber. Dr. Tim O'Shea, author of *The Sanctity of Human Blood*, observes successful results with his autism detoxification protocol.

Animal-based foods are loaded with growth hormones, often leading to abnormal growth and obesity. Many North Americans are wary of raising children on raw plant foods because, upon examination, some vegan children may weigh less or be smaller than those raised on the standard American diet. However, it's really the overweight and obese children who need to be scrutinized more carefully. It's not the parents who are taking care to feed their children Nature's food who are risking their children's health but those who unwittingly feed their children fast foods. The latter are victimized by ignorant peer pressure and advertising. Studies show the high sugar content in processed foods contributes to the elongation of the bones—children become taller but their bones are weaker. From the article, "Secular Changes in Size and Maturity: Causes and Effects" by Robert M. Malina in the Monograph of the Society for Research in Child Development: "Overweight and/or obese children are generally taller than their age and sex due to the addition of refined sugar from processed foods and beverages." Additionally, a Harvard University researcher found girls who drink soda more than triple their chances of breaking a bone, especially among more active girls. High amounts of phosphorous in soda are also linked to bone loss.

Jingee Talifero emailed this letter to the editor of the *New York Times* in May 2007:

> "You cannot create and nourish a robust baby merely on foods from plants" writes Nina Planck in "Death by Veganism," an article in Monday's paper. That is not a fact. I have four robust children who have eaten only foods from plants since conception. See photos at www.TheGardenDiet.com where I sell my eBooks "The Garden Diet," "Raising Raw Vegan Children," and "Raw Pregnancy, Ecstatic Birth."

Science says humans do better without animal products. Why are children different? Because we like fat babies! Not long ago if babies didn't have extra fat they would be less likely to survive famine or hard winters. These problems don't exist in our overfed society, yet the aesthetic endures. A more relevant question is why did these parents receive such strong punishment when obese children die daily and their parents go free?

JINJEE TALIFERO

Even increasing the diet to 60 to 70% raw plant foods can make an amazing improvement when processed and refined foods are eliminated.

Rick Philip, who writes for www.vegetarianteen.com, became a self-taught raw foodist as a teen in Florida. While living in a family who formerly followed the standard American diet, he got interested in animal rights through Internet sites, and quickly became vegan, bypassing ovo-lacto vegetarianism. He soon embraced raw vegan foods and explains how they changed his life, helping him to conquer food addictions and depression (see his articles later in the book). His motivation and passion for learning health, nutrition and animal rights eventually influenced his family as well.

My son Marco noticed over the years that he could eat a lot more food than some of his friends, but they often gained excess weight while he didn't. He remarked to me that he realized this was related to the difference between what he regularly ate and what they ate.

When eating largely cooked and processed foods, the taste buds become altered and unable to appreciate the taste of natural fruits and vegetables. The altered taste sensations of cooked foods, and the sauces needed to disguise them, cause us to ignore the true reason for eating—to provide nourishment to the body. A short time after I had begun eating exclusively raw foods, my sense of taste became heightened. For many years, I've been reveling in the glorious choices I have of delicious fruits and vegetables with some nuts and seeds. When children begin to eat increased amounts of fruits and vegetables, they too will begin to desire these natural foods.

In transitioning children to raw vegan foods, you will encounter a number of issues that may cause some difficulty in the process. Some of these issues involve dealing with relatives, social pressures, school lunches, holidays, and your own insecurities if you are not completely confident in the raw foods lifestyle. In order to deal with these issues, you need first to be knowledgeable in the science of raw vegan foods. When you feel confident in your choice, then you will be able to deal with any difficult situation that should arise.

Obtaining support from others who are following a healthful raw foods life-style will provide additional security.

Most processed and packaged foods contain highly toxic, and consequently addictive, substances which may be initially difficult to remove from your child's diet. Many processed foods contain Monosodium Glutamate (MSG), which gives extra flavor to the food but will inevitably cause health problems. MSG is often hidden in the ingredients in items which can sound healthful such as *natural flavoring, hydrolyzed vegetable protein (hvp)*, or *natural spices*. The manufacturers of MSG are aware of the addictive nature of this substance. Food from restaurants, fast-food chains, and store-bought packaged and pro-cessed foods usually contain enormous amounts of MSG, negatively affecting the developing brain and nervous system, killing off brain cells that will not regenerate. Artifical flavorings, designed to stimulate the salivary glands in such a way that healthful foods would no longer have taste in comparison, of-ten create brain fog and numbing. MSG, which has been called an excitotoxin, is contained in some baby foods. It causes an addictive reaction, so the baby will want more. Recommended reading includes the books *Excitotoxins* by Dr. Russell Blaylock (a neurosurgeon who researched the detrimental effects of toxins such as MSG and aspartame on brain cells), *Chemical-Free Kids* by Allan Magaziner, D.O., Linda Bonvie, and Anthony Zolezzi, and *The Slow Poisoning of America* by John Erb. Upon giving up foods containing the extremely toxic MSG or aspartame, improvements have repeatedly been noted in the ability to concentrate and learn. Positive emotional and behavioral changes have also been observed. When children give up foods containing potentially harmful chemicals and excitotoxins, they will experience more poise and ability to concentrate. Drugs often administered to A.D.D. and A.D.H.D. victims will become unnecessary when children eat unadulterated natural foods.

If your child is receptive, examining and discussing ingredients are impor-tant. Pointing out that sodium is salt content, and explaining the chemicals, colorings and fat sources will educate your child. One day some years ago, I took my children into the supermarket and we played a game, calling our-selves "Supermarket Sleuths." We examined packaged foods that had hidden dairy products as well as MSG. The children were surprised to find so many of the processed, packaged foods had all sorts of hidden labeling.

Life in all species is universally intelligent and programmed for survival. Many parents have asked me why their children develop acne, severe rashes, constipation, diarrhea, or vomiting. All these health problems are almost al-ways related to ingesting low quality foods. After eating harmful substances, the body seems to adjust while working very hard to eliminate the toxic ingredients. But Nature never really adjusts to harmful substances. It only learns how to store them in order to preserve life for as long as it can.

The best way to transition toward eating healthful raw vegan foods is by replacing snack foods with fruits and vegetables. Some parents are successful with introducing delicious fruit smoothies. Children will eat if they are hungry, so there is no need to worry about them not getting enough to eat. Remember a 100% raw vegan diet is excellent, but any steps toward that objective will be beneficial. Make special treats such as delicious raw ice cream, cakes, cookies and pies to bring and share at birthday parties and other celebrations. While others used to think our children should share in the sugary cakes and treats offered at parties, I continued to make them my own special treats, explaining once they begin eating refined sugar and flour at so many gatherings, they will inevitably crave it all the time. Now 21, my daughter expresses gratitude that I didn't give her the junk food offered at so many parties in her childhood. After the switch from snack foods to fruits and vegetables, begin transitioning your children to the least harmful of the cooked foods while at the same time adding more fruits and vegetables. The introduction of more fruits and vegetables while eliminating animal products and processed foods will create a vast improvement over the standard diet of most children.

Don't badger children to follow food combining principles unless they are interested. At first, I tried to teach my children to properly combine their foods when at home, but they showed no interest in it, and it wasn't fair for me to impose food combining principles. However, by setting a positive example by the food you serve, they will learn the idea that a harder-to-digest nut paté will not be followed by fruit. If your children show interest in eating all or mostly raw foods, they will be so far ahead in the future. They may food combine naturally after a time of listening to their own bodies while eating foods adapted to our physiology, but if they choose not to, just be thrilled they are eating more healthfully. Their younger, hopefully less damaged digestive systems work better than ours. At some future date, they may grow more interested in proper food combining.

Hygeia Halfmoon, author of *Primal Mothering in a Modern World*, wrote: "Like a house built with a substandard foundation, a child who grows his body without the optimal foundation will find his house weak and unable to serve him for a lifetime as intended."

As children become teenagers, some may perceive pressures to conform, especially from peers. If you, as parents, continue to show a firm conviction that this way of life is the most natural and healthiest, your children may very well embrace it. In the families I've observed in which both parents had incorporated raw vegan foods and lived a healthful lifestyle, the children were more likely to stay on the same path. When it is made into fun, and the family creates delicious food together, the children will enjoy it. Perhaps your spouse may be interested if you ask him or her to eat raw foods for just two weeks, or even to start with just one day. It's important to help your child understand which foods are health-giving and not to be afraid of the diseases publicized in the media. By setting an example, your child can help teach others to optimally nourish their bodies.

Your child may suffer consequences after eating candy, cookies, other re-fined and processed foods, hotdogs, etc. These foods cause unnatural cravings which throw the body off balance. If the child has eaten any unhealthful foods, these will be circulating in the bloodstream, and the body will encounter dif-ficulty in cleansing properly.

Even more alarming is the Swedish nutritional study, completed at the University of Stockholm, revealing when starches form a golden-brown crust, after being heated at high temperatures, they undergo a chemical reaction forming a carcinogenic plastic known as acrylamide. Foods in this group in-clude French fries, chips, breads, biscuits, cereals, crackers, pizza, and pasta dishes baked at temperatures over 256° Fahrenheit. Many articles regarding acrylamide have been published by the World Health Organization, the U.S. Food and Drug Administration, and other agencies concerned with health and may be found on the Internet.

Fresh vegetables most children on the standard diet shun will eventually be loved by children who are eating them, and they will crave salads. The clean taste buds prefer the tastes of natural foods as they were meant to be eaten—unadulterated, unprocessed and unheated.

Some suggestions for the less harmful cooked foods would be steamed sweet potatoes, steamed vegetables, whole grains such as millet and quinoa, steamed squash, vegetable soup, and split pea or lentil soup. If the child is not willing to give up bread and pasta, then the switch from white flour products to whole grain breads and pastas would be an improvement. One example of an upgrade over the allergen "wheat" is the whole grain gluten-free brown rice pasta, Tinkyada. Orgran organic rice and corn pasta is another wheat and gluten-free food and would also be a good choice during transition. Wheat-free sandwiches and wraps filled with salad are good transition foods—stuff bread or wraps with tomatoes, lettuce, cucumbers, sprouts, shredded carrots, and homemade dressings or spreads. Although cooked foods are acid-forming, if your child eats at least 70% to 80% alkaline-forming green vegetables and fresh ripe fruits and 20% to 30% acid-forming foods (the less harmful cooked foods), this will insure a healthful blood pH, moving toward greater alkalinity. Although raw foods are optimal, all steps in that direction will be extremely beneficial. When eating predominantly cooked foods, the body becomes malnourished because it is deprived of nutrients. When changing to predominantly raw foods, there may be an initial healing crisis if the person is healthy. Mouth sores, rashes, diarrhea, headaches, bad breath, body odor and bladder infections are some ways through which the body detoxifies. Diarrhea also acts to dispel toxic debris. The longer cooked and processed foods have been eaten, the greater the percentage of body fat, and the more that drugs were taken over the years, the more prolonged the transition period will be.

Because many children habitually eat white flour and white rice products, other more healthful and nutritious foods are diminished or completely eliminated. Studies report these white foods cause significant damage to the body and may be the cause of type 2 diabetes and cardiovascular disease.

The most difficult addictions to give up are to bread and pasta. The chemical reaction to cooked starch in the body acts similarly to a drug and causes a sedating effect. Eating a lot of cooked starches during the holidays used to make me feel weak and lethargic afterward, even to the point of experiencing difficulty getting up off the chair. As a long-time raw foodist, I now have energy following my meals, even on holidays! Cooked foods wear out the adrenal glands. The adrenals will get a good rest on raw food. When eating simple raw foods, emphasizing fruits, leafy greens and vegetables, you will notice many health benefits including improved digestion, increased energy, decreased heart rate, reduced body odor, less thirst, increased mental clarity, reduced or no mucus in the throat or head, ideal weight, and the best quality nourishment.

Dr. Douglas Graham explains in *Grain Damage*:

> Every indicator points to grain consumption as a major health threat. In spite of advertising's insinuations to the contrary, the popular trend of eating whole foods cannot apply to...breads..., as grains require a great deal of processing just to become edible. Bread simply does not exist in nature.

There are, however, small grains that become more alkaline-forming and digestible when soaked and sprouted—quinoa, amaranth, and millet to name a few, but some have found preparations using these grains hard to digest.

The processed and cooked starches in pastas and breads can only provide empty calories since their enzymes and vitamins have been destroyed by heat, and their minerals have been removed in the refining process. Pastas and breads are acid-forming, devoid of electrical charge or life force and require cooking and processing in order to be eaten. A diet consisting for the most part of cooked starches can cause Candida, chronic fatigue, diabetes and an array of other physical problems. Many Candida sufferers have been advised they must give up all fresh fruits in the effort to alleviate Candida. Often, it's not the fresh fruits by themselves that cause this problem, but combining them with refined sugars and starches at the same meals—eating fruits with grains (such as fruits and cereals, fruits and pancakes, fruits and bread, even fruits with whole grains). Once the refined and processed sugars and starches are eliminated and fruits are eaten on an empty stomach and alone, rather than combined with grains, the fruits can easily be digested and their healthful nutrients can be assimilated. Pastas, breads and chips are so de-mineralized, regular consumption of these processed foods does not permit enough minerals such as calcium to be absorbed.

Temporarily giving up fruits and gradually adding them back has been offered as a solution for Candida problems. Not combining fruits with nuts or grains has also brought good results.

Many people, including children, get tired and stressed in the winter from cooked food. When I first started eating 100% raw foods in 1995, I did feel very cold for the first two winters, but afterwards I had no problems with the cold. Moreover, I felt I could tolerate the cold better than when I was eating cooked food. Although my body temperature is normally lower than that of people who eat primarily cooked food, I've been able to get through the winters easily for many years while enjoying the simple raw foods lifestyle. I also notice the intense heat and cold don't bother me the way they did years ago, although I do prefer hot summer days when I can dress very lightly. Once, my family went far below ground to visit a crystal cave, but we hadn't brought along enough warm sweatshirts. I gave mine up and was the only one with a sleeveless shirt in this icy environment. I noticed it getting colder and colder as we walked deeper into the cave, but it didn't affect me as much as I thought it would. My tolerance for cold had significantly improved. I also notice a huge difference as far as being comfortable in cold weather when I exercise adequately throughout the winter. Years ago, I would clam up and stay inside all winter, feeling chilled, having no desire to get outside to exercise until it got warmer. Now, I go hiking whenever I can throughout the winter. Exercising in combination with raw vegan foods have made the winter months much easier for me. For many years, I used to suffer from cracks or sores on the corners of my mouth during winter, but once I began to eat significant amounts of leafy greens along with other raw foods, it never happened again.

The following article on the effects of cooked food on the body is titled "Can We Eat Raw Food in the Cold Climate?" by Victoria Boutenko from the December 2004 Raw Family Newsletter:

Many ask about being able to stay raw in a cold winter climate. When any impure substances get into our blood through the walls of the intestines, they irritate our adrenals, the endocrine glands located above the kidneys. The adrenals immediately begin to produce epinephrine, norepinephrine and a variety of steroid hormones. These hormones stimulate our sympathetic nervous system, which is why we feel awake at first. They also force the heart to beat faster and to pump greater amounts of blood through the body, which makes us feel warm. This feeling doesn't last long and we pay a high price for it. After 10 to 15 minutes our body gets exhausted from performing extra work, the heart requires rest, the nervous system becomes inhibited, and we feel tired, sleepy and even colder than before.

However, we remember only the feeling of getting warmer after eating cooked food and repeat such stimulation again and again. This harmful practice wears the body out, and by the end of the winter many people feel exhausted and depleted.

Winter after winter of eating quantities of cooked food doesn't help the human body to withstand cold weather better. On the contrary, weakened adrenals eventually won't be able to work properly even at warm temperatures. If you truly want to feel warm during the cold season, a raw food lifestyle is an inevitable choice for you. During your first "raw" winter, you may experience some cold due to the weakened adrenals, so put on an extra sweater, take a hot bath, or do some pushups. If you will continue staying raw, your adrenals will rest and recover, your capillary circulation will improve, and your nervous system and your heart will naturally strengthen without any artificial stimulation.

In a year, you will tolerate cold better than ever before. My family is now enjoying our eleventh "raw" winter without feeling any discomfort from the cold. We jump into icy-cold mountain rivers year round for enjoyment. In fact, that is how we celebrate Christmas and New Year's Eve. We always sleep outside under the rain or snow. Sergei, my son, goes snowboarding sometimes wearing only shorts. My daughter Valya rarely wears socks. Igor, my husband, loves to take snow baths. We strongly believe staying on a raw food diet has helped us to feel comfortable in any weather and not to feel the cold.

ॐ

Even though winters become easier to bear when eating raw foods for a few years, I still feel human beings are meant to live in a tropical climate, especially in winter. Our family has traveled to a warm climate for a few weeks every winter—to a place where we can get good sunshine and be out in the fresh air for many hours of the day, and we're hoping to buy land there to eventually spend the entire winter. We could live all year round in the tropics without heating or air conditioning, while also having fertile land for gardens and fruit trees. This would be our best chance to become self-sustainable. Many say they love the cold weather, but if they're spending their time indoors with the heat set high, in reality, they're trying to recreate a place of warmth. By spending the majority of our time indoors, we're depriving ourselves of oxygen. Spending time outdoors for just a few months of the year is not nearly enough.

In his book, *Raw Foods Bible,* Dr. Craig B. Sommers has a chart titled "Thermal Properties of Foods." This chart includes warming, neutral and cooling foods. Some of the warming foods listed include: basil, burdock root, cabbage, collard greens, cauliflower, coconut meat, dill, fennel, papaya with seeds, nuts (pine nuts, walnuts, pecans), parsley, sprouted quinoa, rosemary, rutabaga, and seeds (pumpkin, sunflower, sesame). He mentions pecans are "very warming."

During the initial switch to raw vegan foods, your child may always be hungry. It will take some time to get used to feeling lighter. Animal products and cooked starches provide a full feeling. After they're eliminated, there may be a period when your child wants to eat constantly. In a few months, this will change. During growth spurts, your child will naturally desire to eat more. During the transitional phase, there are many raw food recipe books that can recreate the feeling of the more filling cooked foods. However, these recipes are not meant to be daily fare, as reliance on them will not maintain optimal health.

It would be better not to name our meals "breakfast, lunch, dinner" as this will make the child feel it's necessary to eat even when not hungry. The body will derive the most benefit from natural whole foods only when truly hungry. Most people think true hunger is felt in the stomach, but, essentially, it is felt in the throat. Were we to eat only when truly hungry, our digestion would work better, and we'd be healthier. We would also learn to trust our own bodily intuitions. Natural whole food would taste superbly delicious if eaten when truly hungry. Many eat for other reasons, including fatigue, emotions, and adaptation to overeating. Because sitting down to dinner is important to my husband as a means of bonding, I've explained to our children, "You're invited to sit with us, but you don't have to eat if you're not hungry."

Not every meal needs to contain different foods. Salads can be eaten as a meal or for two meals every day. Salads can be made with different ingredients each day, and dressings can be varied or not used at all. Creating new salad recipes is so much fun!

Adding vinegar to salads can be problematic. The consumption of vinegar (acetic acid) can cause thyroid problems. Vinegar is extremely acidic. The adrenals depend on phosphorous which is depleted by vinegar, and this will affect every gland in the body. Additionally, vinegar stops digestion.

The more we got used to eating raw foods, the simpler were our meals. As you can see from the recipes we liked, they were not very complicated. Marco, as an older teenager, still loves banana splits as a special treat (simply bananas sliced lengthwise topped with pureed strawberries).

For transitioning children, vegetables can be made more appealing when accompanied by a delicious dip. My kids liked a tahini dip. Made from ground sesame seeds, tahini is rich in protein and calcium. I would also add water, lemon juice, chopped tomatoes and fresh herbs (dill is my favorite). They also liked to dip veggies into a homemade guacamole or freshly made salsa. We made up some of our own simple recipes and searched for other simple recipes from books such as *The High Energy Diet Recipe Guide* by Dr. Douglas Graham, *Hooked on Raw* by Rhio, *The Raw Gourmet* by Nomi Shannon, *Eating without Heating* by Sergei and Valya Boutenko and others.

Some of the many advantages your children will experience after three months of living on predominantly or exclusively raw foods: absence of eye, ear, nose, throat or sinus infections, increased energy and attention spans, enhanced ability to process information, a heightened sense of ease, comfort, harmony, and perception, no hyperactivity, strenghtened immune systems—fewer colds and no diseases, enhanced athletic capability, increased brainpower and intellectual curiosity, emotional poise and a greater range of expressivity.

General Tips to Remember

1. Try different textures. For example, a child may not like green leafy vegetables but may enjoy them in smoothies, soups or dips.

2. Keep fruits and vegetables around the kitchen in pretty baskets and brightly colored bowls. Children will find the varied colors of the foods in their everyday environment attractive.

3. Name the foods you make with lively or catchy titles! My kids created their own recipes, even from the time they were very little, and then gave names to the recipes:

   BAT (Banana, Apple and Tahini)—by Gabriela and Marco Ranzi

4. Kids love using equipment—A saladacco for making veggie pasta; a snow cone maker by the Pampered Chef for making ices from fresh fruit juice; a small juicer (such as Krups or The Healthy Juicer); a mini food processor; the Champion Juicer for making all sorts of recipes (especially banana ice cream); a dehydrator (not for everyday use, but nice to have for making transitional food—I recommend the Excalibur 12-tray dehydrator). The fresh orange, strawberry or watermelon ices made with the snow cone maker made for great birthday breakfasts for years when lots of kids slept over at our house. They looked forward to cranking out their own fresh fruit juice ices. The cold fruit ice is not the best for the stomach, but for the birthday parties, it sure beat bagels.

5. Play restaurant—Let your kids be the Raw Food Chefs!—Our children loved setting up counters, and preparing smoothies, veggie pasta, fruit and veggie platters, and beautiful salads. They often used a doorway as their ideal place to set up their restaurant. The ironing board or a small table was the counter. Even when we traveled, we bought food for them to prepare meals for us in our hotel room, and my husband and I would be the customers, paying them for our meals.

6. The raw foods movement is growing. Inspire your children by bringing them to raw food potlucks organized in many cities, or to other raw foods events growing all across North America and in other areas around the world. Or start a raw foods support group or potluck in your own vicinity.

   There are wonderful festivals such as The Raw Spirit Festival (www. rawspiritfest.com) organized by Happy Oasis, and The Vibrant Living Expo in Fort Bragg, California, organized by Cherie Soria, or raw food retreats, some listed on page 430. I am willing to travel to present my classes titled "Raw Food Fun for Kids," and "Creating Healthy Children."—Contact me at www.SuperHealthyChildren.com. Sonja Watt offers a raw food family camp in Germany, and can be reached at www.rawfunfamily.com.

7. Make sure your child eats whenever he or she desires during the day. Some fat is an important ingredient for a growing child, particularly during growth spurts. Nuts and seeds and fatty fruits such as avocados can be mixed in with other foods such as green leafy vegetables. Children should have easy access to fruits and veggies during the day.

8. Move your child gradually toward raw foods. Each week add more fruits and vegetables. Learn some recipes your child will love!

9. Don't be surprised if your child wants to eat the same food for periods of time. Marco ate bananas for periods of time from ages 3 to 4, and called himself "Monkey." However, it could easily be observed: the longer he ate the natural diet, the more he moved toward eating a variety of different food, including lots of green leafy vegetables.

10. Be extremely cautious of dried fruit. It can wreak havoc on the teeth. Dried fruit is less harmful on the teeth if it is mixed into a food, such as a smoothie or sauce. Teeth should be brushed immediately after eating dried fruit alone. This should be an occasional treat and not eaten frequently as part of a daily meal.

11. Organize nature trips for your children, especially if they're growing up in a fast food, materialistic suburban or urban environment. Take trips to forage for wild edible plants, to organic farms, and animal sanctuaries. Let your kids and their friends touch the animals, pick wild edibles and get their hands dirty in the Earth's sacred soil! They will feel a sense of connection to the earth and animals. Make hiking in nature a part of your daily life. Let your children see you are connected to nature and the creatures who live in the wild. Get a copy of Peter Ragnar's book *Alive and Well with Wild Foods*. The book comes with a deck of colorful photos of edible wild plants, making it accessible for children to use for collecting wild foods. Although wild foods are loaded with nutrients, we must take caution to identify them correctly before eating. Do the annual "Walk for Farm Animals" to support the Farm Sanctuary, a rescue and rehabilitation farm with sites in New York and California. There are walks for the Farm Sanctuary in many major cities across the country. My daughter Gabriela and I walked for the farm animals in New York City with about 200 people. She saw we are not alone in our concern for farm animals. We also volunteered for the Farm Sanctuary, helping with the feeding of the animals and cleaning the barns. In July 2008, Gabriela and I visited Oregon to hike

the mountain trails of the breathtaking Sky Lakes region with Sergei Boutenko (www.HarmonyHikes.com). Sergei served only delicious raw foods during the four days the thirteen hikers explored this beautiful environment. I was so thrilled my daughter and I were eating healthfully with other healthseekers while enjoying sunshine, excellent exercise, pure air and water, and scenery that relaxes and calms the mind. We swam in pristine lakes, surrounded by the comraderie of others desiring a healthy lifestyle for physical, emotional and spiritual wellbeing. I highly recommend hiking with Sergei Boutenko for families with older children, teenagers or young adults. In June–July 2009, Gabriela interned with Katrina Blair, founder of Turtle Lake Refuge, a non-profit organization in Durango, Colorado. Its mission is to celebrate the connection between personal health and wild lands. Turtle Lake Refuge offers a "Local Wild Life" lunch made with locally grown, wild harvested and living foods (www.turtlelakerefuge.org).

12. Try as often as possible to serve food in special ways. I use a heart-shaped cake pan to prepare special treats on Valentine's Day. I purchased a ridge-shaped cutter from The Pampered Chef to make decorative trims on cucumbers, peppers, cantaloupes and carrots. The attractive design makes the dish more artistic and fun. Kids like attractive and fun designs in food, so why not use these tools for making fun shapes with raw foods? I also have many different cookie cutter shapes and holiday designs for making live cookies, cakes and other treats.

13. In her book *Rawsome*, Brigitte Mars recommends taking kids to the produce section of the grocery store and each week asking them to pick out a food of each color of the rainbow that they would be willing to eat. Remind them that just because they did not like a particular food, at say, age four, as they get older, they will like more foods. They will love to tell you, "I'm bigger now. I like spinach."

14. Brigitte offers the following tips for keeping raw foods fun: "Almost all children like sweets and to deny them will only cause arguments. Be sure to provide homemade raw sweet treats. Make fresh frozen treats from blended watermelon, or the juice of oranges or apples. Freeze some carob almond milk for 'fudgeysicles.' It is fun to create theme meals: a jungle meal, for example, or a meal from a particular country. Then watch an educational video or read a story about that region."

15. Traveling with your children provides an excellent learning experience and creates family bonding time. We were always able to find fruits and vegetables during our travels to Central and South America and Europe.

In each place we visited, we encountered people who understood the benefits of eating fresh fruits and vegetables. On our visit to Colombia, South America, on a main street in Bogota, we were handed a book titled *Frutoterapia* by Albert Ronald Morales, explaining the therapeutic value of 104 fruits that give a wonderful life potential. Costa Rica is the place where many raw foodists are setting up retreats and communities. It's an ecologically progressive country and the people are very friendly. In Tulum, Mexico, my husband went to a small shop to buy freshly squeezed orange juice for us. The owner of the shop told him of an experience he had while working in the markets of Veracruz, Mexico. He had observed an old, weak horse with patches of missing hair. He noticed the horse started to eat the scraps of peels and pulp leftover from the juice stands and partially eaten green vegetables people had been throwing away at the market. He observed the patches of missing hair had filled in and the horse had grown beautiful, thick shiny hair, and developed a strong, muscular physique. The man decided to open his own fruit and vegetable store featuring fresh juices where he could explain to others the amazing benefits of fruits and vegetables.

It was easy to find non-toxic eco-hotels in Costa Rica and Mexico due to the peoples' heightened ecological awareness. In certain parts of Europe, it was sometimes easier to find salads than fruits, but it was not difficult to find raw foods. The difficulty in traveling occurs when you're presented with foods your family doesn't eat at home. Because I didn't want to isolate my children from other peoples and cultures, this was impossible to avoid. However, I know parents who have raised their families on raw foods, and are simply accustomed to these offerings but know how to respond in a way that not only doesn't insult the person making the offer but, at the same time, doesn't put children in a position to eat unnatural foods. Gabriela tells me in order to live healthfully in the future, it will be necessary to move to a more tropical place where fresh produce grows nearby, as the predicted fuel problems, distances from the source, and high cost may make it difficult to buy it in areas where it is trucked or flown in. Additional local greenhouses during winter months may help to solve these problems.

16. Make family fun with food—My kids are always laughing about my love of food, saying I usually have some sign of it left on my face, like

greens left over from my raw green soup or blended salad on my mouth or a piece of mango on my chin. One time, a prize for best costume was awarded at a raw food potluck and dressup party in Manhattan. My kids jokingly said, "I bet the prize was a durian." Funny enough, it was. Use of puppetry with young children is an excellent way to introduce them to the concepts of a raw food lifestyle and to encourage discussion of healthful living topics in a non-threatening play situation.

17. Read some excellent children's books to your kids about health, nutrition and vegetarianism (See Healthy Lifestyle and Respect for Animals—Books for Children on page 421).

18. I feel the most important thing we as parents can do is to talk about Nature and how animals live in the wild. They don't own stoves to cook with, they don't drink the milk of other species, and they don't get the diseases domesticated pets can get. When your child eats something unnatural and doesn't feel well afterwards, this is your opportunity to ask if the food came from Nature or if it was made in a factory. If the child is open to discussing this, you can further elaborate on the resulting digestive problems from the unnatural food and how it caused the ill feeling.

19. Hanging beautiful fruit and vegetable pictures, especially in the kitchen, will show your children the food you cherish. Bowls of glass or ceramic fruits and vegetables also create a colorful display in any room. I have a lovely memory of visiting the Corning Glass Museum in Corning, New York with my children many years ago. It was just before Mother's Day, and Gabriela and Marco very sweetly purchased a whole bowl of glass vegetables to give me as a gift.

20. It may help to feed your children a meal just before attending a birthday party. If they have eaten enough, they may not be as tempted to eat the party food. Make sure to bring plenty of delicious raw food treats to share.

21. Gabriela, Marco, and their friends loved the treasure hunts I created for them with written messages that sent them all over the house and yard. For example, I would start them on the hunt with a note that read: "Go to the place where plants are grown." They would go to the garden to find another note sending them to the next location. After the tenth message, they would find their treasure, usually a favorite fruit or something usable for a special project, such as colored pencils.

When an infant is born, it has no food addictions. Nursing, and later raw vegan foods, support the baby in living a natural, free life in which the child will develop appropriately in each stage—able to listen attentively to his or her body, knowing what to eat, when, and just how much. If a child is raised on processed and refined foods, these bodily intuitions often vanish and are suppressed by food addictions.

Several years ago, when I spoke on raising healthy children at "The Living Now Festival" near Buffalo, New York, I met a very intuitive family. The father described how his child led him to some empowering life changes: first to homeschooling, then to vegetarianism, veganism and finally to raw foods. This teenaged son, initially raised on conventional processed foods, now brings a bag of raw foods with him wherever he goes. He set the example for his family, and they soon followed him. It was amazing to me that this boy had such a strong intuition about which paths to follow in order to lead a life of truth for himself, and then for his family. (Read about Sean Kimmel and the Kimmel family on page 260 in the raw family section).

Obesity has developed into an overwhelming epidemic in the United States. Children are overweight, or even obese, following in their parents' footsteps. "Worldwide, over one billion adults are overweight," according to the World Health Organization (WHO): "An estimated 66 percent of U.S. adults are either overweight or obese," according to the Centers for Disease Control and Prevention. "In addition, about 17 percent of children and teens are overweight. Overweight children and teenagers are more likely to become overweight or obese adults compared to their normal weight counterparts. Obesity is a major risk factor for heart disease, type 2 diabetes and some types of cancer." The CDC reports the following results on their website:

> Results from the 2003–2004 National Health and Nutrition Examination Survey (NHANES), using measured heights and weights, indicate an estimated 17 percent of children and adolescents ages 2–19 years are overweight. Overweight increased from 11 to 19% among 6–11 year olds between 1988–94 and 2003–2004. Among adolescents aged 12–19, overweight increased from 11 to 17% during the same period.
> http://www.cdc.gov/nchs/products/pubs/pubd/hestats/obese03_04/overwght_child_03.htm

The CDC website presents "The Healthy Aging Project" that includes recommendations involving key measures: regular physical exercise, healthy eating, and discontinuing tobacco use.

In a study conducted by Dr. Gabriel Cousens of The Tree of Life Foundation, a non-profit religious organization, a research survey focused on babies and children raised on vegan diets of 75–100% raw food, with a research database encompassing birth to age eighteen:

> Preliminary findings are clear that a live-food diet is completely safe. Live food kids are average or above in height and weight as compared to the "normal" standards.

> The preliminary summary of this study shows about two thirds of the children on a live food diet are average to above average, and all children are above the lowest 10th percentile in height and weight as measured by The National Center for Chronic Disease Prevention and Health Promotion.

> It's important to note the height and weight of these children are in these ranges without being influenced by the stimulating effects of growth hormones to which the majority of non-vegan children are exposed. It is interesting to observe that the National Center for Health and Statistics 2001 shows the average weight for children "has doubled" while heights have remained the same. This suggests we have a serious obesity problem in U.S. children.

> The preliminary conclusion of our data is a live food diet has no major positive or negative effect on height and weight. None of the children in the study have a score above the top 90th percentile or below the lowest 10th percentile. Therefore, the children fall into the middle 80% of normal height and weight.

> These findings are documented on www.treeoflife.nu.

Our meals were quite simple as Marco and Gabriela were growing up, although we did create special new recipes a few times a week. In our first two years on raw foods, I found many recipes for dehydrated raw dishes that deliberately mimicked cooked foods in that much of the water content was removed. Although I spent hours preparing these recipes, Gabriela and Marco didn't like most of them. Perhaps they intuitively knew raw foods should be allowed to keep their water content, varying in whole raw foods from 70% for avocados to 96% for watermelons. Eventually, raw dehydrated dishes became a far less frequent event, limited to parties and special holiday occasions. Although enzymatic activity that would have been destroyed by heat is preserved in dehydrated dishes, they are largely a complex effort to satisfy emotional attachment to the cooked foods of the past rather than a move toward more healthful eating. With their dense textures and "filling" feeling reminiscent of the heavier cooked foods, dehydrated dishes provide a transition for those new to raw foods, but, in my experience, raw foods enthusiasts eventually will prefer fruits and vegetables with their water content intact.

Most days, we ate fruits high in water content in the morning. Marco enjoyed melon smoothies, especially blended Galia melon juice, which was very cleansing for him when he was recovering from chronic allergies, mucus and wheezing. Gabriela especially loved mango mush in the morning (2 apples blended with 1 mango) or honeydew melon cubed. Sometimes they would both want only freshly squeezed orange juice (make sure your child rinses the mouth after orange juice to avoid tooth decay and discoloration), or Marco occasionally liked fresh orange juice blended with fresh organic strawberries in season. Other times, Gabriela would ask for a sliced orange and Marco would want a bowl of pineapple, mango and blueberries. Or Marco would ask for two large pink grapefruits cut in half with the individual sections sliced so he could eat them with a spoon. Both children have always loved a good smoothie, either in the morning or later in the day. Marco loves 2 bananas, strawberries (7 to 10) and one cup freshly squeezed orange juice; or one banana, one chopped mango, strawberries or raspberries, and orange juice. Gabriela made up a smoothie of bananas (2), frozen strawberries (7 or more), a teaspoon of almond butter and water. Since 2004, leafy greens have been added to smoothies to enhance the mineral content. Sometimes a green juice would be the first nourishment of the day, usually consisting of half a cucumber, 2 to 3 stalks of celery, 3–4 leaves of kale, 3–4 leaves of Romaine lettuce and half an apple. Gabriela especially loved to use the small Krup's juicer when she was a young child. Harvey, Gabriela and I have enjoyed green smoothie recipes, especially after reading Victoria Boutenko's book, *Green for Life*. Sometimes we were able to get tasty exotic fruits. Marco has loved mameys, monstera deliciosa (a long, bizarre looking fruit that tastes like a pineapple-banana combination) and cherimoyas. Gabriela enjoyed a bowl of papaya—especially delicious when we visited Colombia and Costa Rica. In the summertime, when fruits are absolutely at their most delicious, the children loved cherries, nectarines, peaches, apricots, grapes, plums, berries, and melons. We would often bring fruit with us as a treat when visiting friends. Some children unacquainted with our food choices would ask questions about the fruit. One child in particular would eat as much of our fruit as he could because he rarely was given fruit at home. Another child did not know the difference between strawberries and cherries and had no idea about the color of the inside of a pineapple. His diet consisted entirely of processed, refined foods and animal products, but he showed interest in more healthful foods when we introduced them to him. This child told his parents he no longer desired meat but his decision was met with resistance.

Frequently Gabriela and Marco would ask for "BAT" a little later in the day (noon or early afternoon), made of two mashed bananas mixed with a scoop of tahini and topped with the bitesized chopped pieces from one whole apple (BAT = Banana, Apple and Tahini). On cold winter days, they would like

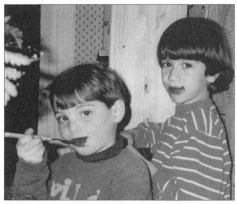

Spencer Corwin and Marco Ranzi enjoying raw berry pie and the effect it has all over their mouths at a raw family potluck at our home in 1997.

to have BAT in place of cereal in the morning. Fresh apple sauce was also enjoyed (two fresh apples blended with some soaked raisins or a few dates with a sprinkle of cinnamon). Gabriela would eat a Gala apple every day in season. We wouldn't buy cherries in winter or apples in summer because food tastes so much better in season. Dr. Douglas Graham (in his book *The 80/10/10 Diet*) and Brigitte Mars (in her book *Rawsome*) have excellent charts listing when fruits and vegetables are in season in the United States. However, if our children would ask for a certain food to bring to a party or a friend's house, I would almost always buy it for them, even if out of season, because they were already eating so differently from the other children at the party. I also knew it was better for them to eat an out-of-season live food than for them to want the toxic, junk party food. Bananas, tropical in origin, are always in season and were enjoyed by the children year-round. I'm not sure if they would have stayed with the raw food lifestyle if not for the versatile banana—great in smoothies, ice creams, banana splits, puddings, cakes and pies, eventually to be enjoyed just as is.

From my experience of having eaten sun ripened bananas directly from the plant in Costa Rica, I learned the force-ripened variety, available in the Northeastern United States where I live, bears no comparison to plant-ripened bananas. Bananas ripened on the plant had a richer color, a smoother texture, a heavenly fragrance and a sweeter taste.

After eating raw foods for nearly a year, we all began to crave more veggies. We often had salads or veggies with dips midday, and always had big, varied salads later, incorporating different vegetables and tasty homemade dressings.

Salads can be greatly varied with changes in the vegetables that are added to the green lettuces. We made salads of Romaine, green leaf, red leaf, Boston or butter lettuces, sometimes shredded kale, adding 3 to 4 toppings that changed daily—cucumbers, tomatoes, cherry tomatoes, celery, red, orange or yellow peppers, various kinds of sprouts, shredded carrots, string beans, snow peas, sugar snap peas, shredded cabbage, zucchini, yellow squash, jicama, etc. There are so many excellent varieties of fresh fruits and vegetables that salads can be completely different every day. After going on wild weed walks with "Wildman" Steve Brill and Closter Nature Center director Mark Gussen, wild edibles became part of the numerous salads we prepared. Purslane, lambsquarter, plantain, wild dandelion, stinging nettles or miner's lettuce make for tasty, vitamin and mineral packed wild green additions to any salad or smoothie. We have also enjoyed sunflower greens, broccoli sprouts, microgreens, pea shoots, and clover sprouts in our salads.

Salads are rendered unhealthful when doused with processed, bottled dressings containing vinegar and other chemicals. We sometimes used fruit dressings, such as orange and raspberries or a tomato sauce of tomatoes, sun-dried tomatoes, two dates, fresh oregano and/or basil. A good dressing could be made of acid fruits such as tomatoes, oranges, tangerines, kiwis, lemons or strawberries combined with a small amount of blended nuts or seeds, or one small avocado (e.g. one acid fruit and one type of nut, such as tomatoes with pine nuts, pecans with tomatoes). We would occasionally enjoy a tahini dressing made with raw tahini, lemon, water and ginger. On my own salads, I often sprinkle a few tablespoons of hempseeds with the juice of half a lemon. Later in the day, we almost always prepared creative salads together. As described in the general tips, Gabriela and Marco also prepared and sold many salads to us as part of their "Raw Food Restaurant." They enjoyed making stuffed avocados or stuffed tomatoes by simply scooping them out and mixing them with each other and then placing them back in the avocado or tomato shell, and serving them over a bed of greens. They loved a variety of fresh fruits and vegetables prepared very simply. Chopped fruits (cucumbers, zucchini and red peppers are considered fruits because they have seeds) and veggies such as string beans and carrots would often be enjoyed with a simple homemade nut butter (we used many from the raw food recipe books listed) or just plain. The children also loved to hang out in the kitchen with me, noshing on fresh green English peas from the pod. We made green juices sweetened with an apple or carrot for the children. I love mine just made with the greens without adding anything sweet. I make the juices in the Champion juicer or the small Krups juicer. When the children prepared their own juice, it was fun and simple for them to use the Krups juicer, a small juice machine very suited to children. This juicer may no longer be available, but The Healthy Juicer is another lightweight, easy-to-use juicer young children will enjoy using (www.healthyjuicer.com).

When the children needed a lunch to bring to outside activities, I would pack some of the following: whole fruits, fruit salads, nori rolls, dehydrated nut and seed crackers or cookies, raw dips with chopped veggies (carrots, string beans, red peppers, celery, etc), blended tomato-basil soup (from *The Raw Gourmet* by Nomi Shannon), gazpacho (from *12 Steps to Raw Food* by Victoria Boutenko or *The High Energy Diet Recipe Guide* by Dr. Douglas Graham or *Rawsome* by Brigitte Mars), salads with homemade dressings on the side, live ice cream (made with frozen bananas, mangos, carob powder and some dates processed in the food processor with the "S" blade and then placed into an ice cream container to bring to a party—needs to be kept in the freezer), dehydrated veggie chips (from thinly sliced zucchini and sweet potatoes), dehydrated at 95° in the Excaliber dehydrator until slightly crunchy, coleslaw (made from shredded green and red cabbage, shredded carrots, finely chopped red peppers and one or two tomatoes with a dressing consisting of a mashed avocado and a lemon), Ants-on-a-Log (celery stalks filled with almond butter, and raisins dotted on the top), guacamole and chopped veggies, and occasionally, homemade trail mix.

In summer, the children enjoyed preparing banana ice cream from frozen bananas (kept in glass dishes in the freezer). We also sometimes added frozen strawberries or frozen mango chunks, all put through the blank plate of the Champion Juicer. I often poured any leftover smoothie into popsicle molds which were also welcomed by my children and their friends on hot days. I always felt content knowing their snacks were made of fresh fruits or vegetables.

As you can see, this lifestyle is never boring. Limitless varieties of fruits, vegetables, nuts and seeds can be eaten in different combinations every day, if you so choose.

When she was ten, Gabriela expressed happily, "I love to eat apples, bananas, tomatoes, red peppers and all types of vegetables. I also love mangos, oranges, pineapples, dates, raisins, strawberries, honeydews, almonds, sunflower seeds, and many other fruits. I do face challenges though. One day, when we went to the bank, the lady there asked us if we wanted a lollipop. My brother and I said 'No, thank you.' It's hard for me to understand why people are always offering candy and junk food to us kids wherever we go."

For birthday parties, the children would help me make raw cakes and candies. I would use recipe books to create raw cakes and pies. These were acceptable for special occasions, but not as a daily food because they were usually filled with excessive amounts of nuts, seeds and dried fruits. We also had a great time with lots of fun party activities. Marco and Gabriela had lively birthday parties for fifteen years. Each year at Marco's parties, all his friends delighted in and still remember the indoor piñata-banging competition and the outdoor sports. The piñata didn't contain candy but was filled with toys and coins. Even at Marco's eighteenth birthday party, the piñata was filled with masks and miniature basketballs. I would also squeeze fresh oranges or blend a small watermelon the night before the party and freeze the juice in round containers. The next morning the children who had slept over would love to crank snow cones from a little machine I bought from *The Pampered Chef*, and watch the colored ice fall onto their plates. At most of their friends' parties, bagels were served for breakfast. Although frozen fruit is not ideal for digestion, it's definitely a winner when compared to the processed starches and animal fats usually served for birthday breakfasts.

In addition to eliminating health and overweight problems, the joy of the live food lifestyle is that it frees you to do things that interest you. Many mothers I know spend hours in the kitchen chopping and cooking. Eliminating the cooking process and simplifying food preparation frees moms to spend more time with their families. During my first few years on raw foods, I thought I had to make a big complicated raw food meal for dinner each evening in order to get the needed variety of nutrients, but later, I came to understand eating simply and varying the food over the days and weeks is the best way to feed a family. Healthful raw foodism is not about recipes. If anything, the ideal would be to get away from complicated recipes. Perhaps they're wonderful for the first few weeks or months after switching to raw, but if the passion for recipes continues, the simplicity of the lifestyle becomes labor intensive—enslaving rather than liberating. Is the dehydrator going to replace slaving over a hot stove? The enzymes might still be intact, but the digestion will never be simple, and our ability to heal will be continually compromised by complicated, time consuming digestion. Let's get used to the deliciousness of the foods by themselves or in simply combined recipes. It reduces so much stress involved with the time and effort it takes to prepare a big meal. Instead, parents and children can plan and prepare lovely, simple raw food meals together.

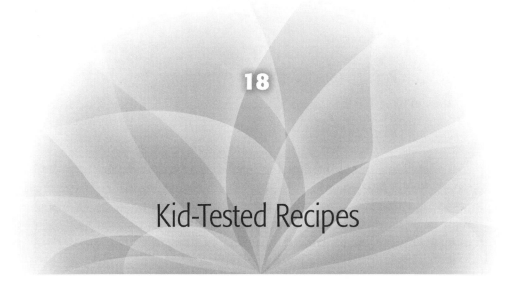

Kid-Tested Recipes

"If we could live on uncooked food alone, we should be saving so much time and energy, as well as money, all of which may be utilized for more useful purposes."

MOHANDAS K. GANDHI

Some of the following are recipes Gabriela and Marco liked, some simple and others slightly more time consuming, but many within the children's abilities to participate. Other recipes here were lovingly provided by friends and top raw food chefs for you to enjoy with your family. Recipes requiring dehydration and made with large amounts of nuts, seeds, and oils, and the more complicated recipes are best eaten in small portions and are excellent for sharing at special celebrations and holidays. Daily living should be kept simple, focused on fruits, leafy greens, and vegetables—the easiest foods to digest.

Raw honey, listed as an ingredient in three shared recipes, is not a vegan product. All of these recipes taste delicious without adding sweeteners.

Enjoy the following recipes in your everyday lifestyle or for use on special occasions. Raw food recipes are to be adjusted to individual taste. It's not as if the soufflé will fall or not rise if the ingredients aren't in exact proportions.

Banana Fun Pops *by Karen Ranzi*

1/4 cup pine nuts
5 bananas
water to process

Process 1/4 cup of pine nuts in the food processor, add 5 bananas until smooth. Add a little water if needed to process. Pour into paper Dixie cups and freeze. After an hour, place a wooden craft stick in the middle of each pop. Freeze for at least 5 hours. This is still a favorite at holiday time with my older children as well as their friends.

Orange Ice *by Karen Ranzi*

Oranges

Juice a bunch of oranges, place in round containers and freeze. The next morning place the ices in a snow cone maker like the one from The Pampered Chef, and let the kids crank out the ice. This is a big success at sleepover parties. I contacted The Pampered Chef only to find out the snow cone maker has been discontinued. It is possible to find this wonderful piece of child-friendly kitchen equipment from another company. Students in my classes have been able to find them in some large department stores. I don't recommend eating frozen foods frequently because they hamper digestion. This is a special treat for birthday parties or other special occasions. Children love it, and it is awesome compared to the typical birthday party food. Other fruits can also be juiced or blended. Try watermelon or strawberries!

Ants-on-a-Log *by Karen Ranzi*

Celery stalks
Almond butter
Raisins

Spread almond butter on celery stalks and dot with raisins. Try other nut butters as well. Marco liked pistachio butter made with raw unsalted pistachios and celery in the food processor.

[Peanuts are legumes, not nuts. Peanut butter is almost always roasted and contains aflatoxins—one of the most potent toxic molds that occurs naturally.]

Marco's Strawberry Splash *shared by Marco Ranzi*

Juice of 2 oranges   2 bananas
Flesh of one orange   10 strawberries, fresh or frozen

Juice 2 oranges, add one orange and 2 bananas and 10 strawberries (fresh or frozen), some water (depending how thick you like it) and blend in a Vita-Mix or blender. Marco ate this smoothie every morning for years. Sometimes we also added a chopped mango to it and/or a scoop of goji berries.

Emerald Smoothie *shared by Gabriela Ranzi*

1 banana
1 mango peeled, pitted and chopped
6 or more Lacinato kale leaves
2 cups of water

Chop banana and add to blender with chopped mango. Add kale leaves to blender with water. Blend until smooth.

B.A.T. (Banana, Apple and Tahini) *shared by Gabriela and Marco Ranzi, inspired by our friend, Beth Corwin*

[One serving]

2 bananas
1 apple
1 teaspoon raw tahini

Mash two bananas, mix in a scoop of raw tahini, and top with small, coarsely-chopped apple pieces. My kids ate this yummy cereal replacement for many years. In summer, we would substitute the apples with peaches or nectarines. My husband Harvey likes to add a little water to give it a looser consistency.

Toona *from "Hooked on Raw," shared by Rhio (www.rawfoodinfo.com)*

3 cups walnuts, soaked overnight (or for at least 3 hours)
3 cups carrots (chop first, then measure)
1/4–1/2 medium onion
1 cup chopped celery
1/2 cup parsley or cilantro

1/2 cup fresh basil (other fresh herbs, such as dill, can be used in place of
   basil for a slightly different flavor)
2 oz. lemon juice

Drain and rinse walnuts. Cut the carrots into chunks and measure out
three cups. Process walnuts and carrots to a paté through a Champion or
Green Power juicer with the blank in place. If you don't have one of these
machines, process in a food processor until smooth. You may have to add a
few ounces of water. Set aside in a bowl.

Cut the celery into 1-inch pieces so you don't end up with long strings,
then pulse chop onion, celery, herbs and lemon in a food processor until well
chopped. Add to the carrot and walnut paté and mix well. Serves 6.

[Gabriela and I have loved eating a nice scoop of Toona with a big leafy
green salad. This colorful dish is great for potlucks.]

Stuffed Tomato *shared by Gabriela Ranzi*

1/2–1 avocado
Tomato
Juice of half a lemon or one lime

Mash one half to one avocado in a bowl. Cut along the inner edges of a
tomato and scoop out the pulp. Add the tomato pulp to the mashed avocado,
add lemon juice to taste, and fill the empty tomato with the mixture. Gabriela
grew up relishing this simple recipe.

Cashew Lasagna *The idea for this recipe was given to us by Ana Inez Matus, Natural Hygiene educator from Pennsylvania.*

1/2 cup raw cashews
2 tomatoes

I don't recommend eating cashews frequently because of the chemical
process used to remove the shell. This heat process removes a toxic liquid
between the inner and outer shells. If you do want to purchase better quality
cashews, they are available at www.sunfood.com, www.naturalzing.com and
www.livingtreecommunity.com. A further reason healthseekers often avoid
cashews is their excessive amounts of Omega 6 compared to Omega 3, but
they are tasty in this dish and can be used as a transitional food.

Using the S blade in a mini food processor, grind 1/2 cup of cashews
until it looks like parmesan cheese. Thinly slice two large beautiful tomatoes

and prepare by placing one tomato slice on the plate, then a thin layer of cashew cheese, then another tomato and then cashew cheese again. Make as many layers as you like. Gabriela and Marco were preparing this dish when they were videotaped for a show called "Highlighting Vegetarian Children" for Nickelodeon Kids News.

Macadamia Dressing *inspired by Dr. Douglas Graham, author of* The High Energy Diet Recipe Guide

> 3 ounces soaked raw macadamias
> 3–4 ounces water
> Juice of one lime

For a large leafy green salad—Make a dressing with 3 ounces of raw macadamias blended with 3 ounces of water and add the juice of one lime. This dressing comes out white and smooth and looks like sour cream.—Another one of Gabriela's favorites for many years. The dressing is simple and quick to prepare, and we would share the dressing on a beautiful, large salad.

Creamy Cucumber Dill Dressing *shared by Karen Ranzi*

> 2 Tablespoons pine nuts
> 1 1/2 cups cucumbers, peeled and chopped
> 2 stalks celery
> 2 pitted dates, soak for 1/2 hour if not soft
> Juice of 1/2 lemon
> 1/2 cup fresh dill, chopped

Blend all ingredients and pour onto leafy green salad.

Nori Rolls *by Karen Ranzi*

> Untoasted Nori sheets
> Raw nut butter, nut or seed paté or avocado
> Shredded lettuce
> Cucumber julienne
> Tomato, chopped
> Sprouts (We like clover sprouts and sunflower greens)
> Variations: shredded carrots, red pepper strips

There are numerous ways to make delicious Nori Rolls. The raw food recipe books have fantastic recipes to try. On busy days, we would just place a thin strip of raw nut butter or mashed avocado on the raw nori sheets, then lettuce, cucumber julienne, chopped tomatoes, and sprouts, and roll them up. Try different veggies such as shredded carrots and red pepper strips. Delicious nut patés or just veggies also make wonderful nori rolls.

Sometimes, we would wrap Rhio's Toona into a lettuce leaf for a great wrap. Large lettuce or cabbage leaves also make wonderful wraps filled with mashed avocados and veggies, or nut butters and veggies, or homemade dips and veggies, or raw nut or seed paté and veggies.

Ice Cream *by Karen Ranzi*

Bananas, frozen
Variations: frozen mango, peaches, strawberries, pineapple,
    raw organic carob powder*

Banana ice cream is made with frozen bananas placed through the champion juicer with the blank plate in. Other frozen fruits such as mangos, peaches and strawberries can be added for a special treat. We sometimes add frozen pineapple chunks. Occasionally we will add raw organic carob powder, especially for parties. Yummy! I keep frozen fruits in covered glass dishes in the freezer. I used to freeze the fruits in plastic bags, but research has shown dioxins from the plastic can be released into the food, especially during freezing or heating.

*Carob is a delicious fruit with a similar taste and color to chocolate but it doesn't contain any caffeine or theobromine. According to Wikipedia, "The carob tree, Ceratonia siliqua, is a leguminous evergreen shrub or tree of the family Leguminosae (pulse family) native to the Mediterranean region. It is cultivated for its edible seed pods. Carobs are also known as St. John's bread. According to tradition of some Christians, St. John the Baptist subsisted on them in the wilderness. A similar legend exists of Rabbi Shimon bar Yochai and his son."

Apple Sauce *by Karen Ranzi*

2 apples	Dash of cinnamon
3 dates	Water to blend

Young children especially love this. Chop two apples with three dates and add a dash of cinnamon, add enough water to blend until smooth. Serve immediately!

Fruit Puree—Mango Mush *created by Jean Oswald*

1 mango
2 apples

In a blender, puree any combination of fresh ripe organic fruits and create delicious puddings. Marco and Gabriela have always loved Mango Mush, a simple combination from Victoria Bidwell's *The Health Seeker's Yearbook*. It is a combination of 1 mango blended with 2 apples. Be sure to serve immediately as nutrients are lost quickly after pureeing.

Rise and Sun Shine *created by Jean Oswald*

1/2 inch thick pineapple circle and chopped pineapple
Orange sections

A wonderful display that children love, this recipe was donated by *The Health Seeker's Yearbook*: Slice off a perfect half inch thick pineapple circle—to be used as a "sunburst." Then place orange sections around the sun to make the sun's rays. Set a small bowl of pineapple chunks and orange sections nearby to eat after the sunburst is gone.

Mexican Salsa *shared by Victoria Bidwell, author of* The Healthseeker's Yearbook

4 cups pureed tomatoes
Juice of 2 lemons
Juice of 2 limes
2 red bell peppers, chopped
4 celery stalks, diced
4 tomatillos, minced
Salad Mix:
1/2 cup each, shredded red and green cabbage
10 cherry tomatoes
1 cucumber, sliced
1 kohlrabi, diced

Mix pureed tomatoes with the following: the juice of 2 lemons, the juice of 2 limes, chopped red bell peppers, diced celery stalks, and minced tomatillos. Add this to the salad mix.
The Healthseeker's Yearbook. www.getwellstaywellamerica.com

Blueberry Pie *by Karen Ranzi*

Banana slices
One pint fresh blueberries
7–10 soaked dates
Dried shredded coconut

Line a 9" pie plate with banana slices. Blend blueberries with soaked dates and pour the mixture over the sliced bananas. Decorate the top with sprinkles of dried shredded coconut. Chill for two hours in the refrigerator until it jells from the natural pectin in the blueberries—another big success at get-togethers and parties.

Cucumber Dogs *by Karen Ranzi*

One cucumber
One mango, diced
One tomato, diced

Slice cucumber in half lengthwise, scoop out seeds, and make an indentation in each half of the cucumber. Fill the indentation with the mango and tomato mixture.

Banana Splits with Strawberry Sauce *shared by Marco Ranzi*

Two bananas, sliced lengthwise   One cup fresh strawberries

Slice bananas lengthwise and place them on a plate facing up. Blend one cup of fresh strawberries to the consistency of a syrup, and pour over the open-face bananas. Marco likes it in this simple way, but other treats may be added such as shredded coconut.

Brazil Nut Wafers or Pancakes *from "Hooked on Raw," shared by Rhio*

2 cups Brazil nuts, soaked overnight   Cinnamon
3 bananas (or 2 ripe plantains)   Filtered water

Rinse and drain Brazil nuts. Put Brazil nuts in the blender with just enough water to cover. Blend, adding more liquid if necessary, until you have a smooth batter. Don't make it too thin. Then blend in bananas, adding cinnamon to taste. Pour the batter in the shape of round cookies, or larger for pancakes, onto dehydrator trays lined with Teflex sheets. Dehydrate at 95 degrees Fahrenheit.

[When we made these pancakes, we dehydrated them overnight to be ready in the morning. Rhio also makes them as a cookie recipe and recommends dehydrating them for one or two days. She tops the pancakes with blueberry jam]:

Blueberry Jam *shared by Rhio*

One pint fresh or frozen blueberries
1/4 cup soaked dates

Blend the blueberries and dates until smooth. It can be used as a pancake or cookie topping and covered with delicious diced mango.

Little Macs *shared by Living Nutrition Magazine*

Handful macadamia nuts or raw macadamia butter
One cucumber, sliced into thin discs
Small tomatoes, sliced into thin discs

Grind up a handful of macadamia nuts in a coffee grinder until the consistency is fine and doughy (or use raw macadamia butter). Scoop the mac "dough" onto a slice of cucumber, top with a tomato slice and another cucumber slice.

Super Salad *by Karen Ranzi*

Large bowl of chopped dark green lettuces such as Romaine,
    Boston, or Red Leaf
Big handful of a variety of sprouts (sunflower greens,
    broccoli sprouts, clover sprouts, pea shoots)
3–4 Roma tomatoes or chopped cherry tomatoes (or heirloom
    tomatoes when in season)
1–2 stalks of celery chopped and/or 1 cucumber sliced
Juice of half a lemon
1/2 an avocado or a small whole avocado, peeled, pitted
    and avocado flesh cubed
Handful of whole dulse, soaked for 15 minutes and then chopped

Mix all solid ingredients in a large colorful salad bowl, then add the lemon juice. This is one of my very favorite meals.

Joel's Blended Salad *shared by Joel Brody*

1/2 ripe avocado
6 leaves of Romaine lettuce
Handful of baby spinach leaves
1 large cucumber, sliced
3 celery stalks

Blend the cucumber briefly, and gradually add baby spinach leaves and Romaine lettuce leaves. Use the long celery stalks to push the leaves toward the blades. After the mixture begins to turn over in the blender, add 1 inch long pieces of the celery to the blended mixture, and blend briefly. Add 1/2 avocado for a creamier mixture, or use the sliced avocado as a garnish. Vary the proportions of ingredients according to taste and availability. Raw recipes are more interesting when they turn out differently each time.

Guacamole Wraps *by Karen Ranzi*

2 ripe avocados
2 Tablespoons chopped fresh cilantro
1/2 tsp. cumin
2 Tablespoons fresh lime or lemon juice
Romaine lettuce leaves

Mash the avocados. Add cilantro, cumin and lime or lemon juice. Top with homemade raw salsa or tomatoes, soaked sundried tomatoes and/or sprouts. Fill each leaf with the guacamole mixture, roll it up, and place a toothpick through it to keep it closed until ready to eat.

Zucchini Linguini with Tomato Sauce *by Karen Ranzi*

Use a saladacco to create the linguini from the zucchini or yellow squash, and then add this simple sauce:

4 medium zucchini sliced into linguini-like pasta

Sauce:
2 large or 3 medium ripe tomatoes (vine ripened if you can get them)
6 sun-dried tomatoes (without sulfur dioxide)
2 dates
7 fresh basil leaves

Blend the sauce and stir into the zucchini linguini.

Summer Tomato-Basil Soup *shared by Nomi Shannon, author of* The Raw Gourmet

This has been another favorite of my daughter Gabriela for years. She especially loved it when I made it from big, ripe, juicy, local organic heirloom tomatoes in the summertime.

3 cups tomato puree
(6–8 medium tomatoes)
(see note)
1/4 lemon, peeled and seeded
1 avocado
Large handful of sunflower or buckwheat sprouts
2 Tablespoons chopped fresh basil
1 Tablespoon chopped onion (optional)
Additional sprouts
Basil flowers

In a blender, combine the tomato puree, lemon, avocado, sprouts, basil, and onion. Blend and pour into serving bowls. Top the soup with sprouts and basil flowers. Serves 2.

Note: To make the tomato puree: In a blender, break up the chopped tomatoes until you have a 3-cup yield. The tomato puree should be chunky, not silky smooth.

[We have made it without the optional onion, and it was excellent.]

Family Green Smoothie

shared by the Evans-Mear Family (Laurie and Jeff, Stephanie and Julian)

2 cups water
1 ripe banana
4 celery ribs without the leaves
4 parsley sprigs
4 dandelion leaves
6 lettuce leaves
One heaping Tablespoon golden flax seeds
(We grind them at home for freshness and lower expense)

Blend all ingredients and enjoy!

In 2006, Laurie Evans wrote:

Laurie consumes this amount by herself, at least five times a week for breakfast. Stephanie, age 20, and Julian, age 16, often drink a glassful in the morning.

If the banana is ripe, it's delicious. If it's not ripe, it doesn't taste good. The above recipe is the standard as the ingredients are available in winter. The parsley and dandelion vary depending on the season and availability.

When berries or mangos are ripe, they may be added to the smoothie. We add only enough greens, or as many as possible, so that the smoothie is still sweet enough to enjoy. When we buy the greens at the farmer's market, they have a very different taste from the greens we get in winter that are shipped from great distances.

We got the original recipe from Dr. Douglas Graham—water, banana and celery. Jeff is a tri-athlete and avid biker. Julian is also an avid athlete and biker. Dr. Graham suggested the banana and celery instead of Gatorade (which we wouldn't use anyway).

Jeff has this green smoothie every morning for breakfast. He makes 60 ounces, has half for breakfast and the rest for lunch. He also adds Nutiva raw hemp powder. As an athlete, he felt he wanted more protein.

When we travel, we usually have access to a kitchen. We take the ingredients with us, and make the smoothie even when away from home.

We make the smoothie in a Vita-Mix because it's fast, easy, and the vegetables can be put in without being cut into small pieces. If we make this when traveling and use someone else's blender, we cut the celery into very small pieces not to overheat the motor. We are planning to buy a good small blender with which we can travel.

The following four delicious recipes are shared by raw food chef, Chrissy Gala:

Super Smoothie *shared by Chrissy Gala*

1 1/2 cups water
Handful of greens (kale, spinach, Swiss chard)
1/2 apple, peeled and cored

1/2 small orange, peeled
4 Medjool dates or other dates (optional)
2 Tablespoons chia seeds

Combine all ingredients in a blender and blend until smooth. Serve in a glass or drink straight from the pitcher.

Magic Wands *shared by Chrissy Gala*

4-6 celery stalks
Filling:
2 carrots
2 apples
2 tsp cinnamon
Topping: handful of raisins (optional)

Combine filling ingredients in a food processor and blend until smooth. Stuff celery sticks with filling and top with raisins. Enjoy!

Zucchini Roll-ups *shared by Chrissy Gala*

2 zucchini, peeled with a wide peeler
2 carrots
1 daikon radish

1/2 red bell pepper
1 celery stalk
1 avocado, sliced thick

Slice or julienne carrots, radish, pepper and celery. Place a few pieces of each on zucchini slices with 1 piece of avocado. Allow some veggies to stick out of the sides of zucchini. Roll zucchini tightly over sliced veggies and secure with a toothpick. Serve with your favorite dressing or dip.

*Note: Vary ingredients to make your own roll-ups by adding sliced fruit or your favorite sliced vegetables.

Cheesy Kale Chips *from my original "Goddess Chips," shared by Chrissy Gala*

2 bunches kale, de-stemmed and torn up

Cheesy Sauce:
1 cup red bell pepper
3 Tablespoons lemon or lime juice
1 cup macadamia nuts
2 Tablespoons water or more to turn mixture over

Place kale in a large mixing bowl. Combine red bell pepper, lemon or lime juice in a high-speed blender or food processor, and blend until smooth. Add macadamia nuts and a little water, 2 Tablespoons at a time to turn mixture over. Blend until smooth, but still very thick. Pour over 2 bunches of torn kale and coat well. You want this mixture really to adhere to the kale. Eat as a salad, or place kale onto a paraflex sheet, on top of a mesh dehydrator screen, and dehydrate for 2 hours at 115 degrees and then 3 hours at 110 degrees. You'll need to use two trays. Rotate kale occasionally to dry uniformly.

Chrissy Gala is a Regenerative Foods Chef and resides in Sedona, AZ. She teaches live food certification courses, regeneration lectures and workshops, and hosts healing retreats and monthly potlucks. www.LiveFoodEnergy.com

My friend Nancy (who writes for the Raw Family chapter) prepares recipes her three girls love. The following two are among her kid-tested recipes:

Blueberry or Mango Cream *shared by Nancy Durand-Lanson*

   1 cup blueberries (frozen makes ice cream) or fresh mango
   1 Tablespoon raw almond butter
   1 Tablespoon raw honey
   1 Tablespoon lemon juice or a whole lemon peel or lemon flavor (if using lemon peel, slice off only the outer part of the peel as the inner part can be very sour)
   1 teaspoon vanilla (optional)

Blend all ingredients. We have eaten these two creams like crazy, just as is or on top of fruits, or as a frozen pie (I add 1/2 cup of coconut butter in the preparation of the pie to make it creamy). The above recipe also works well with pears and as a fruit dip.

Squash Soup *shared by Nancy Durand-Lanson*

"I usually get buttercup or butternut squashes, but it's good with all the squashes."
   1 1/2 cups of squash,
   1 1/2 cup of celery root
   1–2 tablespoons of almond butter
   Water to cover (warm or cold)

Put the squash and celery root in a blender with almond butter and warm water. The water should just reach the top of the vegetables. Blend until it is very smooth and eat just like that.

Energy Soup *shared by Lillian Butler and Eddie Robinson*

(2 *cups*)

2 leaves Romaine lettuce
4 leaves dark green kale
1 zucchini squash
1/2 avocado
1 cucumber
1 cup sprouts of choice
1 Tablespoon dulse flakes
3/4 cup water

Cut up vegetables. Place ingredients in blender. Blend until smooth and creamy. Taste! Add additional seasonings to suit your taste. Serve immediately. Try different variations using different vegetables and leafy greens.

Lillian Butler and Eddie Robinson are health educators and owners of Raw Soul Restaurant in Manhattan where they prepare tasty, healthful, reasonably priced and environmentally conscious meals. www.rawsoul.com

Raw food chef, Eric Rivkin, talks to kids about healthy foods. He asks, "What is healthier, an apple or an apple pie?" He says that kids always know the answer. He shares the following recipes that kids in his classes love:

Yummy Roll *shared by Eric Rivkin (www.VivaLaRaw.org.)*

A filling, satisfying, healthy substitute for candy with lots of calcium and other minerals—and with a crunch!

Collard green leaf, cut into 1" strips, 6" long
Raw tahini
1 date, pitted
1 raw almond or other raw nut

Spread thin layer of tahini on a strip of collard leaf, stuff the almond into the date, and place on top of the spread tahini. Then roll up so it all sticks together. Chew thoroughly until liquid for complete enjoyment.

Fresh Fruit Kebobs or Fondue *shared by Eric Rivkin*

Pineapple chunks
Whole strawberries
Blueberries
Mango chunks
Papaya chunks
1" thick banana slices

Arrange creatively on wooden skewers for kebobs, or arrange cut fruit decoratively on a plate, and serve immediately with a fruit glaze, crème or dipping sauce.

Fruit Glaze *shared by Eric Rivkin*

Blend until creamy:
1 pint strawberries
2 pitted dates
Orange zest

Pour over fruit salad or use for kebobs.

Goji Coconut Cream Sauce *shared by Eric Rivkin*

Super yummy and super high in vitamins, minerals, and antioxidants. Use by itself, or as a dressing or dip for fruits, veggies or salads. If you can't get the kids to eat their greens, just try this as a dressing.

1/2 cup Tibetan Goji berries, soaked (include soak water)
1/2 cup raspberries or blackberries
1 cup young coconut meat
2 pitted dates
1/2 teaspoon orange zest (optional)
Enough coconut water to turn over in blender

Blend in a high speed blender until creamy. Keeps up to 3 days in refrigerator. For an incredibly exotic dessert variation, substitute mango for the raspberries, and add 1 banana, 1/4 teaspoon cinnamon, 1/2 teaspoon vanilla, 1 Tablespoon grated ginger, and blend without added water.

The following two fun recipes are by Jackie Graff, a raw food chef based in Atlanta, Georgia (www.rawfoodrevival.com)

Freaky Fruity Rollups *shared by Jackie Graff*

4 cups strawberries or any fruit of choice

Place strawberries in blender and blend until smooth. Pour onto teflex sheet and spread evenly. Dehydrate for 8 hours or until completely dry. Peel off the teflex and cut into pieces and rollup.

Hint: To avoid wasting fruit, especially when too ripe, make rollups.

[Whenever eating sweet dehydrated fruit or other dehydrated snacks, brush teeth immediately afterwards.]

Nana's Power Packed Green Pudding *shared by Jackie Graff*

2 collard leaves with stems
3 kale leaves, stems removed (kale stems tend to be bitter)
2 bananas
2 mangos

Blend ingredients well with a Vitamix to make the texture very smooth like pudding. Taste it to make sure it tastes sweet, and if needed add more fruit. Some toddlers may not be used to the taste of greens without the sweetness of some fruit.

Jackie and Gideon Graff are widely known for making some of the best tasting raw food recipes. Well-known pioneers in the Live Foods Movement, they are dedicated to teaching and promoting the living foods lifestyle for mind, body and spiritual awareness.

The following recipes were shared by Cherie Soria, founder and director of Living Light Culinary Arts Institute and author of *The Raw Food Revolution Diet*. She has been teaching vegetarian culinary arts for national and international organizations for more than 30 years and gourmet raw vegan cuisine since 1992. Cherie has personally trained many of the world's top raw food chefs and instructors and is often referred to as the mother of gourmet raw vegan cuisine.

Almond Milk *shared by Cherie Soria*

Yield: 1 1/2 cups (2 servings)

If you like the flavor and creaminess of milk, you will love this slightly sweet, pure white beverage that mimics the look and taste of its dairy counterpart. Once people taste fresh nut milks, they usually never go back to dairy milk. Sweeten it as much or as little as you like, and make it thick or thin—you will be pleasantly surprised at the possibilities.

1/2 cup whole raw almonds, soaked overnight, rinsed, and drained
1 1/2 cups purified water
2 to 3 dates, pitted (see note)
1/4 teaspoon alcohol-free vanilla extract

1. Put all of the ingredients into a high-powered blender, and blend until smooth.
2. To separate the "milk" from the almond skins and pulp, squeeze through a cloth mesh bag or a double layer of cheesecloth. Set the pulp aside.
3. Serve at room temperature or chilled.
4. The milk may be stored in a sealed glass jar in the refrigerator for up to four days.

Note: Dates vary in their size and degree of sweetness. If using larger, sweeter dates, such as medjools, you may wish to use 2 dates rather than 3.

Banana Boats on Fire *shared by Cherie Soria*

Bananas
Almond butter (see recipe, below)
Paprika

To make a banana boat, slice off 1/4 inch lengthwise straight along the middle section of the outer curved side of the banana. This will provide stability so it can stay upright as a boat on the plate. Use a spoon or apple corer to scoop out a little of the banana lengthwise on the opposite side of the sliced side to form the hollow space of the boat, leaving an inch of uncut banana at each end. Be careful not to break it.

Fill the cavity with nut butter using a spoon, plastic bag, or piping bag. Sprinkle paprika on top, to make it appear the boat is "on fire."

Almond Butter *shared by Cherie Soria*

Yield: 2 cups (12 servings)
3 cups raw almonds, soaked and dehydrated

Making your own nut butter is quick, money-saving and more health-promoting and easier to digest than the kind you can buy. If you soak and dehydrate the nuts first, as recommended in this delicious almond butter recipe, the butter will not separate and cause the oils to float to the top; plus the soaking increases mineral availability. Use it as a spread on bananas or celery.

To make Almond Butter in a food processor:
Put the almonds into a food processor outfitted with the "S" blade. Process for 5 minutes, or until the almonds have turned to butter.

To make Almond Butter in a homogenizing juicer:
Run the almonds through a Champion or Green Star juicer outfitted with the homogenizing plate.

Zucchini Hummus *shared by Cherie Soria*

3/4 cup sprouted chickpeas
3/4 cup peeled and coarsely chopped zucchini
2 1/2 Tablespoons freshly squeezed lemon juice
2 cloves garlic crushed (optional)
1 teaspoon ground coriander
1/2 teaspoon ground cumin
1/4 teaspoon cayenne (optional)
6 Tablespoons raw tahini

Zucchini Hummus
1. Combine the zucchini, lemon juice, optional garlic, paprika, cumin, and optional cayenne in a blender and process until smooth.
2. Add the tahini and process until completely smooth and creamy.
3. Stored in a sealed glass jar in the refrigerator, Zucchini Hummus will keep up to 3 days.

Enjoy served with crudités, or in Romaine lettuce boats with tomatoes and sprouts.

"Living Light Culinary Arts Institute is located on the picturesque Mendocino coast of northern California. The Living Light Center is designed to provide the latest advances in raw culinary education. The take-out deli, Living Light Cuisine to Go, offers organic raw vegan cuisine, juices, and smoothies, and our retail store, Living Light Marketplace, features healthy products for vibrant living."

For more information about Cherie Soria and Living Light Culinary Arts Institute, e-mail info@rawfoodchef.com or visit www.rawfoodchef.com.

Apple Mixture *shared by Ellen Forman*

Here's a quick and delicious recipe that our kids Dylan and Naomi love. It works as breakfast, lunch, snack or even dessert! We call it Apple-Mixture. We like to use a few red apples and a few green. Our favorites are Fuji and Granny Smith. Sometimes we like to peel the Grannys if the skin is tough. The nuts can be whichever you prefer. Our favorite mix: almonds, walnuts and pecans. It is good to soak the nuts, but if you're in a pinch use them dry.

4 apples cut up into small cubes
1/2 cup nuts chopped or pulsed in a food processor
1 Tablespoon almond butter
1/2–1 Tablespoon raw honey (can be replaced by 2 dates)
Small splash of warm water
1 teaspoon lemon juice (optional)

Put the almond butter and honey into a small bowl and add the splash of warm water. Mix well until you have a sauce. Don't add too much water, just enough to soften the honey and almond butter. The lemon juice can be added either over the apples or into the sauce.

Pour the sauce over the apples and stir in the nuts!

My friend April Schoenherr made the following three delicious dishes for a family potluck we had. Even those who were not raw foodists loved them.

Tabouli *shared by April Schoenherr*

1 head cauliflower
1 clove garlic, minced

1 bunch parsley
1 bunch mint
1/2 cup currants
1/4 cup olive oil
1 lemon, juiced
1 cucumber

Combine all but the cucumber in a food processor until almost smooth (1–2 minutes). Spoon into a bowl, chop up the cucumber and mix it in.

Cole Slaw *shared by April Schoenherr*

1 small white cabbage, chopped
1/2 red cabbage, chopped
3 carrots, shredded
1/3 onion, grated (optional)
1 apple, chopped
3 Tablespoons lemon juice
3 soaked and blended dates

Mix all ingredients together and let marinate for 2 1/2 hours. Meanwhile, make dressing:

Dressing:

1/2 cup tahini
2 dates
2 teaspoons mustard seed
1 teaspoon lemon juice
1/4–1/2 cup water

Blend all dressing ingredients together. Add to marinated veggies after 2 1/2 hours and enjoy.

Pineapple Cake *shared by April Schoenherr*

1 cup almonds
8 dates
1 teaspoon cinnamon
1 teaspoon coconut butter

Process ingredients in a food processor with the S blade and set aside in a bowl.

1 cup pecans
8 dates
1 teaspoon cinnamon
1 teaspoon coconut butter

Process ingredients in a food processor with the S blade and set aside in a second bowl.

1 pineapple—diced
8 dates
1 teaspoon vanilla
1 Tablespoon ground flaxseeds

Process ingredients in a food processor with the S blade and set aside in a third bowl.

To assemble pineapple cake: Spread the almond mix on a cake plate, then add the pecan mix on top, and then spread the pineapple mix on top of the pecan mix.

Dr. Douglas Graham and Professor Rozalind Graham share the simple daily recipes that their daughter Faychesca loves to eat. www.foodnsport.com

The following are Faychesca's Favorites:

Banana Fig Pudding *shared by Dr. Douglas Graham and Professor Rosalind Graham*

Bananas
Figs, fresh or rehydrated

Faychesca is particularly fond of a banana and figs blended together. During the season, she eats fresh figs, but when they are not available, she will eat rehydrated figs. Bananas and figs make a great pudding that she loves to have for breakfast.

Mango and Raspberries *shared by Dr. Douglas Graham and Professor Rosalind Graham*

> 1 mango, diced
> Raspberries

One of Faychesca's favorite fruit combos is a diced mango mixed with raspberries.

Salad with Tomato/Mango Dressing *shared by Dr. Douglas Graham and Professor Rosalind Graham*

> 1 head of lettuce, finely chopped   1 tomato
> 1 cucumber, finely chopped   1 mango

A salad favorite of Faychesca's contains finely chopped lettuce and cucumbers with a simple dressing of a tomato and a mango blended together.

The following raw food recipes were shared by Brigitte Mars, author of *Rawsome*.

Winter Waldorf Salad *shared by Brigitte Mars*

> 1 apple, finely chopped
> 2 stalks celery, finely chopped
> 2 cups grated carrots
> 1/2 cup raisins
> 1/2 cup walnuts, soaked overnight, then dehydrated until crunchy, about 12 hours

Toss all ingredients together and serve. Makes 2–4 servings

Raw Carob Almond Milk *shared by Brigitte Mars*

> 1 cup raw almonds, soaked overnight, then rinsed
> 1 quart water
> 3 Tablespoons raw carob powder
> 4 dates, soaked for 20 minutes

Combine the soaked almonds and water in a blender and puree. Strain the liquid through a nut milk or sprout bag into another container, squeezing the bag well. Rinse the blender and pour the strained milk back into it along with the carob powder and dates. Blend until thoroughly mixed. Store unused milk in the refrigerator, where it will keep for four to five days. This recipe can also be used to make tasty "fudgey-cicles" by freezing it.

Salsa *shared by Brigitte Mars*

Yield: about 2 cups
5 tomatoes, chopped
1 clove garlic
1/2 cup chopped fresh cilantro
Juice of 1 lemon
2 scallions, chopped
1 teaspoon chili powder

Combine all ingredients in a bowl and mix well; or, if you prefer, combine all ingredients in a food processor, but pulse instead of pureeing to make sure the salsa's consistency stays chunky.

Gazpacho *shared by Brigitte Mars*

Yield: 2 servings

5 medium tomatoes, finely chopped
1 red pepper, finely chopped
1 cucumber, finely chopped
1/4 onion, finely chopped
1 avocado, pitted, peeled, and chopped
1 cup water
1/2 cup chopped fresh cilantro
1/2 cup chopped fresh basil
1/2 cup lemon juice or lime juice

Combine all ingredients in a large bowl and toss. Pour half of the mixture into a food processor and pulse. Return the mixture to the bowl with the rest of the soup and mix well.

Karen: "My family loves Brigitte's Gazpacho recipe. I prepare it at least once a week throughout the Spring and Summer and into October. It's so delicious, refreshing, and loaded with antioxidants."

Brigitte Mars is the author of *Rawsome!* and *Sex, Love and Health.* She teaches raw food workshops with her husband of twenty-five years. She is the mother of raw actress/model/yogini, Rainbeau Mars (who is on the cover of

David Wolfe's *Eating for Beauty*). Brigitte, with her daughter, Sunflower Mars, also runs Herb Camp for Kids, teaching them about raw and wild foods and herbal crafts.

www.BRIGITTEMARS.com

Bonobo's Restaurant was founded by David Norman in 2002 to give raw foodists a well-designed centrally located oasis in Manhattan. The key to its success is simplicity and the delicious, easily recognizable aspect of the dishes. The diner can see, taste and choose the colorful food in this organic and raw cafeteria. This restaurant doesn't raise the blood pressure by using salt. I've always felt strong and energetic for the rest of the day whenever eating there. Even better, there's no danger of eating late at night since Bonobo's closes every evening at 8 p.m., but it does remain open later on some evenings to host raw food speakers and events.

The name is taken from the charming Bonobo, the brightest of apes, and the one closest to man. Bonobos are raw vegans too, and they're the only apes never to get jealous and scream at each other—they are peace-loving and never fight with each other in any way. They are always sweet and loving and show it to each other all day long with abundant physicality. They, too, don't eat after dark.

Asian Slaw *by David Norman, founder of Bonobo's Restaurant, 18 East 23rd Street, New York, NY 10010 (www.bonobosrestaurant.com)*

The proportions in these and all our raw food recipes are flexible according to taste. We make Asian Slaw in large quantities at a time. I estimated the relative measures, but this is not carved in stone. Feel free to modify to what makes sense to you. Of course, use organic, if you can:

4 full cups Napa cabbage, julienned (We use the small inside leaves as the large outer ones are used for the Napa cabbage sandwiches.) Napa cabbage is also known as Chinese cabbage.

1 1/2 cups shredded carrots

Sauce:
3/4 teaspoon each of finely minced peeled garlic and ginger
1/2 cup extra virgin olive oil or cold pressed sesame oil (we use the Flora brand)
1/3 cup freshly squeezed lemon and/or lime juice

Variation: about 2 tablespoons finely sliced green onion (white and green parts)

Wisk sauce well. Then stir in 3 tablespoons of white and/or brown sesame seeds and 2 tablespoons of black sesame seeds.

Let sit for about one hour.

Stir sauce into cabbage and carrots.

Keep cold, will last about 3 days. Serves 10

Sesame Bok Choy *by David Norman*

Baby or regular bok choy or a mixture of both. Pick a white and green bunch with firm stalks and crisp leaves, without brown streaks or broken stalks:

Slice across end, wash and pat or spin leaves and stalks until dry.

Julienne crosswise to make about one quart.

Use both the green and white parts.

3 Tablespoons black sesame seeds

one cup medium diced red, orange or yellow (or mixed) bell peppers

(We don't use green peppers because they are not ripe and are consequently less nutritious.)

Sauce:

one cup hulled (creamier) or unhulled (more nutritious), sesame seeds, or mix them

1/3 cup fresh lemon and/or lime juice

one cup pure water

one clove garlic (more to taste)

Blend sauce ingredients until very smooth in a high power blender. In the absence of a high power blender, grind the sesame seeds in a coffee grinder first. For a thinner sauce add a little more juice or water; depending on your blender—for a thicker sauce add more sesame seeds.

Stir or toss together the sauce, bok choy, bell pepper, then sprinkle in the black sesame seeds. Serve as soon as possible since the bok choy liquid will come out. Better to make a thicker sauce, if your blender can do it.

Will keep about 3 days if kept cold.

Use organic ingredients whenever possible. Serves 8

The following easy and tasty durian recipes for kids and adults were created by Cheryll Lynn and Scott McNabb from *The WELL to Excel*. Durians are native to Asia, containing delicious custard-like "pillows" which are fun to eat as a yummy treat.

Vanilla Durian Pudding *shared by Cheryll Lynn and Scott McNabb*

Makes approximately 4 servings
Equipment: food processor and knife

1 durian, pits removed
1 Tablespoon alcohol-free vanilla extract, or more to taste
1 vanilla bean (optional)

Fill food processor with thawed durian flesh that has the pits removed. Blend to an even consistency. Add 1 Tablespoon Frontier brand alcohol-free vanilla extract and blend until smooth. Taste, and add more vanilla if desired.

Optional addition: Slice a fresh vanilla bean lengthwise. Using the dull edge of a knife, scrape the seeds out of the vanilla bean and add to the mix to give it the speckled look and fresh vanilla taste.

Strawberry-Durian Pudding *shared by Cheryll Lynn and Scott McNabb*

Makes approximately 4 generous servings (depending on size of durian)
Equipment: food processor and knife
Durian – 1 whole fruit, pits removed
Strawberries – 1 to 2 cups

Fill food processor about 1/2 to 2/3 full of thawed, pitted durian. Blend until even consistency. Then, add in washed and stemmed strawberries and blend until smooth. Add more durian and/or strawberries to taste.

How to Choose a Durian:

Durians are large and spiky and need to be handled with care, but, with practice, or a pair of gloves, you can thoroughly examine the fruit to choose the best one possible. They're kept in the frozen foods section of the supermarket. If purchasing from a Chinatown street vendor, go first thing in the morning to find them still frozen.

Look for the following:

- Stem is still attached.
- Overall color is brown, or mostly brown. A little green down at the base of the spikes can be okay, but that means it's not as ripe as one with no green at all.
- *No splits!* From my personal experience, a split meant a critter got in. Although splits at the opposite end of the stem may mean that it's ripe, the fruit travels very far, and chances for critters to crawl into openings increase. I've always been able to find one I like without any open splits.
- Select a medium size durian with a balanced look. Larger durians don't always have more pillows inside. When I bought two durians, one weighing about 7 lbs. and the other about 5 1/2 lbs., after shelling and pitting, they both had nearly the same amount of fruit.

How to Open a Durian

Be careful while handling and opening a durian. Place the durian on a stable surface, and though it's not necessary, you may want to wear a pair of garden gloves. A knife with a 5 to 8 inch blade is sufficient to open a durian.

The best way to open a durian is along the fracture lines that run lengthwise from stem to base. The lengthwise fracture lines are found along the sections of the outer shell that appear to "bulge" out a bit more than other areas of the shell. Beginners may want to wear gloves and use a knife as follows: starting in the middle of the fracture line, halfway between the stem and the base, pierce the fracture line with a knife and cut lengthwise, but through no further than the shell (which is only about 1/4 inch thick, not counting the spikes) along the fracture line, toward the stem and toward the base. Spread the shell open with both hands for better access to the interior chambers. Scoop out the fleshy "pillows" with a spoon, or take off your gloves and extract them by hand. Cut through the flesh to reveal and remove the large brown pits/seeds. Place the pitted/seeded durian fruit in a food processor or blender. Add your choice of berries or vanilla and blend well, adding some water if necessary.

Alternately, a durian that is already out of the shell and pitted, can be bought in many Asian markets in the refrigerated or frozen sections. It will usually come in a clear plastic box so you can see the typical pale yellow flesh.

When ideally ripe, a whole durian can be opened by hand by simply applying pressure to the midway point of the fracture line, and the shell will easily split open along this line. Once you get the hang of choosing ripe durians, identifying the fracture lines, and working around the spikes, it will be quite easy to do this with your bare hands.

The WELL to Excell
www.thewelltoexcell.com
Copyright 2007

The Problem with Dried Fruit

Be extremely careful not to eat much dried fruit. Much of what you find packaged in health food stores is not sun-dried but cooked. As a result, it becomes acid forming and will wreak havoc on your teeth. "The Date People" in California, Tel. (760) 359-3211, have truly fresh and alkaline-forming dates for times when you do eat dates or need them for recipes.

Dried fruit is very sticky, requiring prompt brushing and flossing. We developed dental problems because we were unaware of this initially, after having switched to what we thought were more health promoting treats. Some raw foodists believe fresh organic fruit cleans your teeth and you don't need to brush. Not true for most of us. Don't take the chance of causing damage to your teeth.

Many raw food recipe books include numerous desserts containing large amounts of dried fruit which is often mixed with similarly large amounts of nuts or seeds, creating a combination difficult to digest. Had this problem been explained in these books, we would have limited our eating of these preparations to special occasions, and we would have been far more careful to brush and floss immediately after eating them. Preferably, to continue to enjoy the crunchy, nutty textures and intensely sweet/tart dried fruit flavors, this combination can appear in smaller, sporadic amounts as I've presented in some of the preceding recipes.

The Trouble with Salt

Shipwrecked sailors of yore often died of thirst: "Water, water everywhere, but not a drop to drink" goes the classic Coleridge poem, "The Ancient Mariner." Indeed, seawater is poisonous, but, even today, it is still dehydrated to get sea salt, and the water wasn't the poisonous part. Ancient Roman soldiers were paid in salt, and we still have the word "salary" to remind us, and salami—meat preserved with salt and garlic. The bacteria had to be killed or the meat would totally rot. But to use salt in the twenty-first century on raw plant foods is a step looking backwards.

When, not so many years ago, raw crops were largely unavailable in cold seasons, salt was used to kill harmful bacteria in rotting meat and cheeses and even to preserve vegetables. With today's refrigeration and rapid shipments of fresh produce, we no longer need the aging, drying, vaso-constricting, burning and blood pressure-raising effects of salt.

Raw leafy green vegetables contain adequate amounts of organic mineral salts, supplying our ideal mineral source with excellent flavor. If old-fashioned cooking compromises the minerals, salt is added to compensate for the loss of taste. Both cooking and the use of salt are part of an older, now surpassed technology since today's advancements permit us to have fresh plant foods in every season.

Salt eventually makes one look old and ugly. Because of its toxicity, it must be diluted in water in the cells, resulting in water retention. With time, the waterlogged cells begin to droop due to years of salt consumption, its consequent water retention, and gravity.

Although it's easier to give up salt at home, restaurants may be the last to abandon it because it does extend the shelf life of foods while retaining the familiar tastes of cooked fare. Once the patron is liberated from those salty tastes, he will move forward with great freedom, energy, and flexibility. He'll lament all the wasted time in his life when he was knocked out by salt. Hopefully, he'll learn from experience and never want it again. Optimistically, restaurants will respond by creating many salt-free dishes as found in this chapter. Rather than the near comatose effects salt has on dinner parties, let them be occasions for singing and dancing!

19

Can Our Families Get Enough Essential Fatty Acids from Raw Vegan Foods?

"Nothing will benefit human health and increase the chances for survival of life on Earth as much as the evolution to a vegetarian diet."

ALBERT EINSTEIN

Vegans are able to meet their needs for essential fatty acids through plant sources. For raw vegans, this includes dark leafy greens, avocados, soaked nuts and seeds, and nut and seed butters (raw sesame tahini, raw almond butter, and other nut butters). For those raw vegans who feel the need for additional fatty acids, they are also available in olive, hemp and flaxseed oils. Be sure to use responsibly produced oils which are first cold pressed and chemical-free such as those produced by Bariani or Flora. It's advisable to limit the amounts of oils as explained in the following paragraph.

A growing number of raw vegans don't consider bottled oils as viable food because they are fragmented and refined—removed from their whole food source. Dr. Joel Fuhrman writes in his book *Eat to Live*: "Our modern diet, full of vegetable oils and animal products, is very high in omega-6 fat and very low in omega-3 fat; the higher the omega-6 to omega-3 ratio, the higher the risk of heart disease, diabetes and inflammatory illnesses."

For the raw vegan, sufficient amounts of green leafy vegetables (especially spinach), which are quite high in omega 3 fatty acids, and some nuts and seeds such as walnuts, flaxseeds and hemp seeds will provide these beneficial fats. Dr. Fuhrman explains a diet high in omega-6 fat intake contributes to a DHA (docosahexaenoic acid) fat deficiency, a fat necessary to ensure optimum health. He suggests adding a few grams of omega-3 fat to your diet, such as

1 Tablespoon of flaxseeds, 1 teaspoon of flax oil, 4 Tablespoons of English walnuts (12 walnut halves) and plenty of green leafy vegetables. The darker leafy green vegetables such as Romaine lettuce, leaf lettuces, kale and spinach have an abundance of nutrients.

In the section on breastfeeding and "mother's milk being best for baby," I also spoke about formula-fed children lacking this very important nutrient, DHA. Please also refer to the section on essential fatty acids in Olin Idol's book, *Pregnancy, Children & the Hallelujah Diet*. He recommends freshly ground organic flaxseeds to pregnant and nursing mothers for adequate intake of essential fatty acids. There are also EFAs in hempseeds, pumpkin seeds, purslane, sesame seeds, pine nuts, cabbages, squash, chia seeds and all sprouts. Purslane, a wild green plant, is particularly high in EFAs and natural vegetable DHAs.

Herbalist Brigitte Mars explains in *Rawsome*: "All cells, including those involved in the production of hormones, need essential fatty acids (EFAs). These nutrients improve skin and hair, lower blood pressure and cholesterol levels, and reduce the risk of blood clots. EFAs are found in particularly high concentrations in the brain."

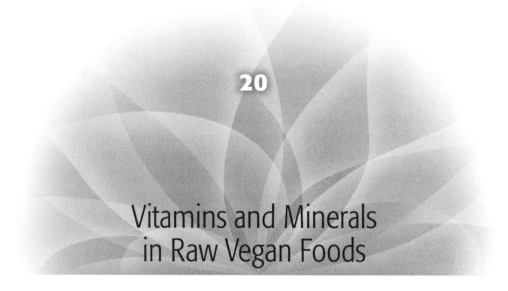

Vitamins and Minerals in Raw Vegan Foods

"There are no 'incurable' diseases. If you are willing to take responsiblity for yourself and your life, you can heal yourself of anything."

DR. RICHARD SCHULZE

I always felt secure my children and I were getting more than sufficient amounts of vitamins and minerals from eating a variety of raw plant foods.

Every plant food has calcium, and over time, this calcium adds up, especially on a diet that doesn't contain excessive protein. Animals in the wild don't go to each plant and figure out the total vitamin, mineral and protein content. An elephant and a giraffe grow into huge animals by eating instinctively, so why shouldn't the human being eat the food provided by Nature without worrying constantly about nutritional deficiencies? The animals do not own stoves, which destroy 80 to 90% of these vitamins, minerals and amino acids. They simply and instinctively know which food sources are appropriate to consume for their digestive systems. The carnivores, herbivores, omnivores and fruitarians all eat differently based on their individual digestive systems, but all know which foods will benefit them. When following the natural diet, completely eliminating processed and refined foods, the human body will be able to assimilate nutrients from the food it was meant to eat.

Most pregnant women think they need to drink milk and eat dairy products to get adequate calcium during pregnancy. However, there are far more healthful alternatives that produce vital and strong children. Green leafy vegetables, sea vegetables, oranges, sunflower seeds, sesame seeds, almonds, and figs are all known as good calcium sources, but any fruit or vegetable will provide some calcium benefits. As long as these sources are not cooked, maximum benefit will be gained. Once food is cooked, much of the minerals are lost or become more difficult to assimilate.

A diet high in protein (especially protein from animal products) leaches calcium from the bones and teeth. Countries with a high rate of consumption of dairy products have a correspondingly higher rate of osteoporosis due to calcium loss from the bones. In the United States and Scandinavia, where the percentage of dairy consumption in proportion to other foods is higher than in other countries, the osteoporosis rates are also higher than in other countries.

A well-rounded, varied raw vegan regimen, including plenty of dark leafy greens, will provide calcium in adequate amounts. Calcium cannot be utilized without vitamins D and C, pointing to the sunshine requirement for vitamin D, and fruits and vegetables for the necessary vitamin C. Iron is also plentiful in leafy greens, nuts and seeds. Greens contain iron as well as vitamin C, making them excellent foods that should play an important role in the diet. Other vitamin C containing foods, such as broccoli sprouts and tomatoes, are good to combine with the iron-rich leafy greens. Stone fruits such as peaches, nectarines and apricots contain iron as well as vitamin C. Meat contains high levels of iron, but no vitamin C to help absorb it. All dairy products inhibit the absorption of iron. Dr. McDougall explains, "Because iron is so important to pregnant women, many are convinced they need iron supplements, but iron pills have not been shown to offer any clinical benefit to the woman's health, or her baby's. They may even prove harmful to some women. Research has shown iron supplementation can inhibit the absorption of zinc from the intestines. Iron supplements can also irritate the gastrointestinal tract, causing nausea, vomiting, or constipation, and may overstimulate the production of blood. Children who have ingested their mother's iron supplements have died as a result of overdosing on iron. I doubt nature intended women or children to take pills in order to remain healthy during pregnancy."

Zinc is essential for the health of the pregnant woman and is abundant in green leafy vegetables (such as spinach), nuts and seeds (especially sunflower and pumpkin seeds). Brigitte Mars explains in *Rawsome*, ground sunflower and pumpkin seeds are rich in the mineral zinc and are excellent for kids who are slow to grow.

If you want to be sure to obtain adequate vitamins and minerals for your children and yourself, eat plenty of fresh garden salads and fresh fruits. The B complex vitamins, choline, biotin, folic acid and vitamin C are found in a variety of green vegetables, and fruits such as melons and citrus. Any plant containing seeds or a pit is considered a fruit. This would include tomatoes, cucumbers, zucchini, peppers and avocados. Vitamin A is found in yellow vegetables and fruits. Apricots, peaches and tomatoes contain generous amounts of vitamin A. Green leafy vegetables, such as bok choy, cabbage, kale, leaf lettuce, parsley, Romaine lettuce, spinach and sprouts are also some of the richest sources of vitamin A. Beware of taking vitamin A supplements. In *The McDougall Program for Women*, Dr. McDougall reports that pregnant women who take vitamin A supplements have a one-in-57 chance of having a child who suffers from a deformity of the head and face, nervous system, thymus, and/or heart.

Vitamin D is a hormone made in our bodies. A pregnant woman should take a walk daily or at least (even on cold winter days) sit near an open window for 15 to 20 minutes daily to obtain vitamin D. Those who are afraid of the sun, believing it to be the cause of skin cancer, are depriving themselves of extremely important and vital nutrients. For many years, I desired a dark tan and spent many hours under the intense sun at the beach. These excesses are damaging, but taking sun in the morning and later afternoon, even on hot sunny days, is necessary for the intake and balance of vitamin D and calcium. There are some plants also said to have some vitamin D. In her book *Hooked on Raw*, Rhio lists plants from which some vitamin D can be obtained:

Fenugreek	Red raspberry	Papaya
Chickweed	Rose hips	Agar-Agar
Basil	Sarsaparilla	Sprouted seeds
Alfalfa	Thyme	Mushrooms
Bee pollen	Watercress	Queen of the Meadow
Eyebright	Irish Moss or Carrageen	Sunflower greens
Mullein	Nettles	Wheatgrass juice

However, Rhio says, "The primary way to get vitamin D is to expose your skin to some sun everyday, whenever possible."

Folic acid is extremely important during pregnancy. Dr. McDougall discusses, "Conclusive evidence has shown folic acid deficiency in the developing fetus causes incomplete development of the spine, skull, spinal cord, and brain. Such deformities, known as neural tube defects, are the second most common major birth defect in children in the U.S. The severity of deformity caused by folic acid deficiency can be as minor as a missing patch of open skin at the base of the spine or scalp, or the complete opening of the backbone (referred to as spina bifida occulta). The absence of adequate folate in the typical American diet is particularly threatening because most pregnancies are unplanned, and because neural tube deformities tend to occur in the first two weeks of pregnancy. Thus, the quantity of vitamins you have in your blood and tissues at the time of conception is very often what determines a child's neurological health."

Symptoms of folic acid deficiency are anemia, lack of energy and lowered resistance to disease. This important nutrient is 50 to 90% destroyed by cooking.

In her book, *Rawsome! Maximizing Health, Energy, and Culinary Delight with the Raw Foods Diet*, Brigitte Mars points out folic acid helps in RNA and DNA production, and is necessary for the development of the nervous system in embryos. Some of the valuable raw foods that contain this important nutrient are almonds, walnuts, sunflower seeds, pecans, papayas, oranges, fresh leafy green vegetables (especially spinach), grapes, blackberries, cabbages, cantaloupe, avocados, and plums. All known nutrients and their raw plant sources are charted in the appendix of her book. This excellent resource clearly displays raw plant foods meet one's needs for vibrant health.

Nuts and seeds (almonds, sunflower seeds, sesame seeds, flaxseeds, etc.), green leafy vegetables, sprouts and some fruits such as cherries, blackberries and apples provide vitamin E as well as essential fatty acids. Brigitte Mars points out vitamin E is an antioxidant that improves circulation, aids tissue repair, promotes normal blood clotting, minimizes scarring, promotes fertility, and helps maintain healthy muscles, nerves, skin, and hair. Vitamin K is obtained through eating green leafy vegetables.

Because of the need for fat reduction and healing of every kind, in recent years, more and more books have been published celebrating the benefits of raw fruits, vegetables, nuts and seeds.

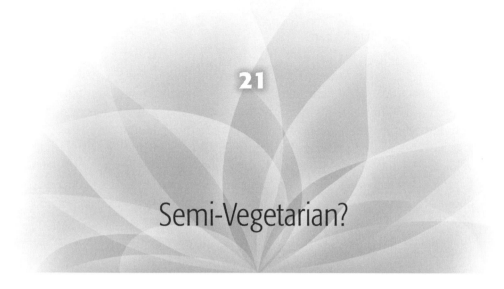

Semi-Vegetarian?

"I will not kill or hurt any living creature needlessly, nor destroy any beautiful thing, but will strive to save and comfort all gentle life, and guard and protect all natural beauty upon the earth."

JOHN RUSKIN

I've always found it interesting that some people call themselves vegetarian while still eating fish, and even chicken. In the *Random House Webster's College Dictionary*, the definition of vegetarian is: "a person who does not eat or does not believe in eating meat, fish, fowl, or in some cases, any food derived from animals." Those who say they're vegetarian while still eating animals want to feel they're helping animals, but in actuality they experience difficulty with the thought of giving up their cravings for the stimulation of meat and other animal products. They also fear the possibility of protein deprivation due to all the advertising of the meat and dairy councils.

Dr. Gabriel Cousens, in his book *Conscious Eating*, cites a study reported in *Child Development* that found a definite correlation between the amount of fish the mother ate during pregnancy and the child's brain development. The more fish the pregnant mother ate, the lower was the children's verbal IQ. Children are more sensitive to poisons than adults because their younger, more resilient bodies eliminate toxins more quickly. Adults are affected by toxins but in a less obvious way. It was also found that fatty fish can have higher levels of PCBs and pesticides than meat.

Caring parents told me they believed their autistic child was affected by the mercury in the fish the mother ate during her pregnancy.

In his book *Eat to Live*, Dr. Joel Fuhrman quotes the Seychelles Child Development Study on neurodevelopmental outcomes in children following in utero exposure to methylmercury from a maternal fish diet—background and demographics: "Higher levels of mercury found in mothers who eat more fish have been associated with birth defects, seizures, mental retardation, developmental disabilities, and cerebral palsy. This is mostly the result of women having eaten fish when they were pregnant. Researchers are also concerned about other toxins concentrated in fish that can cause brain damage way before the cancers caused by chemical-carrying fish appear."

Eliminating the Cause of Illness Can Keep Our Families Disease-Free

"In my opinion there are definite drawbacks in taking milk or meat. In order to get meat we have to kill. And we are certainly not entitled to any other milk except the mother's milk. Over and above the moral drawback, there are others, purely from the point of view of health. Both milk and meat bring with them the defects of the animal from which they are derived. Domesticated cattle are hardly ever perfectly healthy. Just like man, cattle suffer from innumerable diseases. Several of these are overlooked even when the cattle are subjected to periodical medical examinations."

MAHATMA GANDHI

There are so many situations in which disease could be avoided if people understood the true nature of the workings of the human body. Parents who bring their children to fast food restaurants are viewed with acceptance today, whereas parents who provide healthful natural foods are often frowned upon. The following information from leading authors on health and nutrition points out the reasons for disease:

From *The Cure is in the Cause* by Dr. Ruza Bogdanovich, N.D.: "Interfering with Nature isn't good, but when we go against her, that's where our problems are difficult to turn around. The damage is done in so many ways we aren't even aware of any more. We ignore it completely." The following are some explanations of immune system problems presented in Dr. Bogdanovich's book:

Today microbes and viruses can affect us differently from the way they used to because of our general weakening. Our bodies are overloaded with debris. Tuberculosis is back and spreading because drugs, antibiotics have made us weaker. Many other "new" viruses, hepatitis A, B and C for example, are on the rise for the same reason, too. The increased amounts of free radicals (cancer-causing agents) and growth hormones in the dairy foods to which we're exposed cause uncontrolled cellular growth and suppressed immunity. We have become weaker than our ancestors.

We have to pay the price now for becoming too dependent on antibiotics to knock out drug-resistant bugs our immune systems can't handle. Antibiotics have also invaded our food supply. Animals are routinely given massive doses of drugs to get rid of infections due to poor immune systems. Antibacterial products—hand soaps, dishwashing liquids, countertop scrubs, toilet bowl cleaners, body washes, etc. have flooded the market, creating new strains of bacteria by their indiscriminate overuse. This makes us more stressed and weaker.

This is all related to a confused mind/body to the point that we do not function with chemical correctness to certain impulses that are sent from the brain into the organs and glands. This is why it is so difficult to help people with multiple illnesses without looking to the real cause—the originator of the problem. It all goes back to the root of the problems that are very much related to what we put in our bodies so we can function in harmony within.

Don't heat oils or fry your food. Ask yourself: Is it natural? Is it pure? Is it whole? If it doesn't spoil, it's not natural and not good. Look for the cause of your symptom. That's where the cure is too.

I often see young children who are depleted of enzymes and can no longer digest their food properly due to lack of raw food. The liver and pancreas are designed to store enzymes if needed in case of emergency, but today that storage is depleted and the pancreas has to work much harder. This is why so many young people have health problems and allergies so early in life. Juvenile diabetes among other degenerative diseases is becoming rampant.

The body is not just one thing; it is a combination of many things. People need to realize a whole apple has a perfect balance of all elements, vitamins and nutrients, even protein. How can that apple not do the body good? But when you eat an apple pie with ice cream on top, your body has to process all that combination of stuff and isolate the things it can't use. It then stores them, causing a burden on the whole system. So in order to keep the system alkaline, it has to pull the calcium out of the bones in order to compensate for the sugar in the pie and the ice cream.

The China Study by T. Colin Campbell, Ph.D., Cornell University scientist and researcher, and Thomas M. Campbell II, is the most comprehensive long-term nutritional study ever done. I commend Dr. Campbell on his excellent research and findings represented in this book. The following comments and information are from *The China Study*:

> You pick up an issue of National Geographic Kids, a magazine published by the National Geographic Society "for ages six and up," expecting to find wholesome reading for youngsters. The pages, however, are filled with ads for Twinkies, M&Ms, Frosted Flakes, Froot Loops, Hostess Cup Cakes and Xtreme Jell-o Pudding Sticks.
>
> This is what scientists and food activists at Yale University call a toxic food environment. It is the environment in which most of us live today.
>
> The inescapable fact is that certain people are making an awful lot of money today selling foods that are unhealthy. They want you to keep eating the foods they sell, even though doing so makes you fat, depletes your vitality and shortens and degrades your life. They want you docile, compliant and ignorant. They do not want you informed, active and passionately alive, and they are quite willing to spend billions of dollars annually to accomplish their goals.

So many people believe they have no control over their health and destiny. Some women have their breasts removed if a father or mother had breast cancer. Dr. Campbell points out the causes of breast cancer are entirely different:

> The genes you inherit from your parents are not the most important factors in determining whether you fall prey to any of the ten leading causes of death.
>
> Obsessively controlling your intake of any one nutrient, such as carbohydrates, fat, cholesterol or omega-3 fats, will not result in long-term health.
>
> Vitamins and nutrient supplements do not give you long-term protection against disease.

Your doctor probably does not know what you need to do to be the healthiest you can be.

After four decades of biomedical research, including the results of a twenty-seven year laboratory study, Dr. T. Colin Campbell believes what you eat can save your life. Some of his findings include:

Breast cancer is related to levels of female hormones in the blood, which are determined by the food we eat.

Consuming dairy foods can increase the risk of prostate cancer.

Type 1 diabetes, one of the most devastating diseases that can befall a child, is convincingly linked to infant feeding practices.

The war on cancer and heart disease, which has continued for decades, is no more advanced today than it was at the beginning.

Dr. Campbell worked for ten years in the Phillipines to improve childhood nutrition among the poor. It was felt childhood malnutrition was the result of insufficient protein, particularly animal protein. However, Dr. Campbell discovered: "Children who ate the highest protein diets were the ones most likely to get liver cancer! They were the children of the wealthiest families." Their diets contained a high percentage of meats similar to the American diet.

Dr. Campbell did many years of research in China. He observed great differences in the rates of cancer in various counties of China, although the people come from the same genetic background. So the gene theory of inherited disease did not hold. He found the cancers were related to environmental factors, particularly to food intake (especially animal protein). He reported: "The death rate from coronary heart disease was seventeen times higher among American men than rural Chinese men, and the American death rate from breast cancer was five times higher than the rural Chinese rate." People in the rural Chinese counties ate significantly fewer animal products than in other counties.

In *The McDougall Program for Women*, Dr. John McDougall explains:

Once ingested by the mother, environmental pollutants can damage the genetic material, or DNA, in the cells of the developing child, causing a wide assortment of birth defects. Scientists know such defects account for much of the disability in children throughout the world, and are the leading cause of infant mortality in developed countries.

Although there are several ways such toxic chemicals can enter a woman's body—including through the lungs, skin, and mouth—the foods we eat provide by far the greatest chemical assault on the fetus. The primary carrier of such toxic chemicals is dietary fat, especially the fat that comes in meat, dairy products, eggs and fish. Grazing animals eat plants and drink water that have been tainted by industrial poisons. Usually such toxins originate in polluted rivers, soil, rainfall, or farm runoff. Once the animals eat the grass and other plants that have been contaminated, these poisons accumulate in their fat cells— the same fat cells that are later consumed by humans either as meat or milk products. A similar series of events occurs in fish that swim in polluted lakes, rivers, and poisonous parts of the oceans. Fish that swim in poisoned waters ingest the toxins, which accumulate in their fat. Fatty fish are a major source of human exposure to PCBs. Other important sources of these highly toxic chemicals are dairy products and meats.

From the article "Diet and Violence," Edwin S. Douglas, founder of the American Living Foods Institute: "What man does to animals, he does unto himself." Douglas relates the killing and consumption of animals to human aggression and violence. He also talks about mood changes that can result from refined sugars, fast foods, processed foods, and wheat:

Significant information is already available about violence as related to vitamin and mineral deficiencies. Many violent acts are related to mood swings. Modern nutritional studies point to allergic/addictive food reactions and excessive intake of refined sugar as the two major sources of mood swings. These reactions can create a constant state of inner tension which radiate throughout the nervous system. Moderate to severe depression also result from allergic/addictive reactions to food. For example, it has been noted in numerous research papers that people who have an allergy to wheat can enter a depressed state within a few hours or even days after ingesting it. Most of us are certainly aware of the "sugar blues!" Processed sugar and sugared products artificially raise the body's blood sugar level. The high is followed by an inevitable drop. When the drop occurs, an individual may experience severe irritability, frustration, anger and depression. Another possible dietary source of violence is our increased reliance on fast foods. Fast foods are almost always cooked and processed; therefore they lack the living enzymes which the body needs in order to feel really satisfied. In other words, as the amount of fast food increases, the amount of fresh, raw food usually decreases. Fresh, raw foods are needed to supply the body with essential elements not available in cooked, processed food. This modern phenomenon produces a physical state which is described as "cellular starvation."

No matter how much cooked, processed foods we eat, we still feel severely depleted and dissatisfied. Since our emotional and physical states are closely linked, this physical dissatisfaction communicates itself emotionally through frustration, anger and irritability. A toxic person generally has an acid pH level which results from the ingestion of animal proteins, refined sugars and cooked fats. These foods are poorly digested and create toxic residues which are then absorbed into the bloodstream. Conversely, the more alkaline the body, the more serene or calm the individual. Increased intake of living foods helps to create an alkaline pH level. Recent experiments with living food dietary intervention in relation to physical and psychological illness have been conducted on a small scale and produced amazing results. When the amount of cooked, processed food is decreased and the amount of fresh, raw food is increased, many chronic or non-responsive mental and physical symptoms can often be significantly reduced or even reversed.

As one can see from this crucial information, the health and future of the child are largely dependant on the mother's eating habits prior to pregnancy, during pregnancy and lactation, as the child begins to eat solid foods, and from what the child eats as he or she grows. The refined sugars, processed foods and wheat products as well as animal flesh, dairy, and eggs over time can be the cause of numerous physical, mental, and emotional problems.

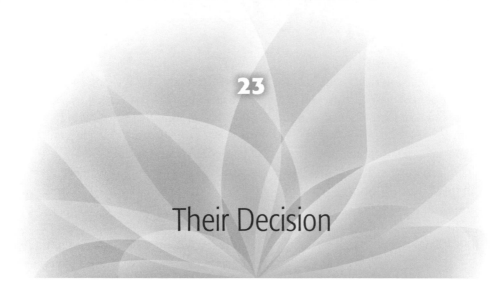

Their Decision

"The important thing is not to stop questioning."
ALBERT EINSTEIN

After eating raw foods since they were 3 and 5, my children began experimenting at 11 and 13 with eating cooked vegan foods (occasionally dairy as well). I never isolated them from activities in which they would be confronted with conventional foods, and I don't recommend isolating your family. I knew at some time the children might choose to experiment. There had been some coaxing and teasing from others about the healthful foods they ate, and then a desire on their part developed to be like their peers. What is perceived as "peer pressure" in the teen years seems intense. Marco told me of his very strong desire to "fit in" with his teenage friends. Food choices are a very important part of "fitting in," and he thought being vegetarian already "separated" him from many of his friends. Both of my children believe firmly in vegetarianism for moral reasons, but as for most teenagers, good health is just not that important an issue at this time of their lives, even though they are aware that what they put into their bodies now will determine their future state of health.

When they were young, it was easy for them because their mom was the center of their universe, and they believed the messages she gave them. Marco's ear infections, allergies, and asthmatic symptoms disappeared within a year after the switch to eating raw foods. Both children enjoyed preparing raw food dishes and loved the taste of natural foods. Over the years, they delighted in all sorts of fruit and large green salads with delicious homemade dressings, green juices, and some special raw food treats. They enjoyed preparing food and eating the results. They came along to many raw food potlucks and discussions when I led raw foods support meetings in New York City. But as the teen years approached, it became more and more difficult for them to feel comfortable with their peers. I also think they gradually grew tired of some of the raw foodists' obsessive talk exclusively about food.

One thing I have learned after living a raw food lifestyle for many years is health involves so many different aspects; raw vegan foods are definitely important, but family togetherness, a low stress environment and fun are right at the top with nutrition.

Gabriela and Marco were 5 and 3 when we switched from cooked to raw vegan foods, and they had forgotten their early childhood illnesses. However, when they do feel ill, they still know exactly how to get well... by sleeping and fasting. Gabriela has periodically returned to eating totally raw foods for several months at a time. After having visited the "Raw Family" teens for two weeks of hiking, Gabriela returned to raw foods for many months. Raw food peer support gave her the desire to stay raw. Five years later, when interning with Katrina Blair of Turtle Lake Refuge in Durango, Colorado, Gabriela was again inspired to pursue her raw vegan lifestyle through this community support. After returning home, she continued raw foods on her own incentive.

When Marco is at home, he still relishes large raw smoothies, asks for delicious fruit, and will eat celery and large salads during the week. He likes tabouli made with bulghur (boiled cracked wheat) instead of the raw cauliflower I used to use in that recipe. I include parsley, three large tomatoes and two stalks of celery in the dish to provide him with live nourishment. When he or his teenage friends want to eat sandwiches at our home, I make salad sandwiches, consisting of lettuce, tomatoes and a tablespoon of black bean spread or hummus on whole grain bread with lots of sliced carrots, celery and red pepper on the sides. Although I believe we get all our nutrients from live foods that contain all the enzymes necessary for absorption and digestion, I am willing to use whole grains and lightly cooked vegetables for them if they're not willing to eat only raw foods. I believe as long as anyone continues to eat cooked food, the addiction and craving for it will continue, but I am also no longer willing to try to coerce anyone to follow this belief if it is not his/her path. If your child chooses to remain vegan, eating fresh fruits and vegetables and some of the less harmful whole cooked foods, this is a far cleaner choice than is available to most children in the civilized world.

Throughout the years, we've had many wonderful raw food potlucks at our home, but in their teens, both Gabriela and Marco asked for cooked foods at their parties since they were friendly with many teens who weren't living the raw food lifestyle. I present a number of dishes including salads and simple live food preparations as well as some of the less harmful choices of cooked vegan foods. In saying "less harmful," I simply mean the cooking temperature does not go beyond the boiling point of 212° Fahrenheit or 100° Celsius. Although many nutrients are thus destroyed or diminished, at least acrylamide is not created as it would be with higher temperatures required for baking, frying, broiling and sautéing.

Whatever my children choose to eat away from home, I know I've provided them with the knowledge of what causes illness and what creates health to keep with them for the rest of their lives.

I think most children will eventually become influenced by the cultural values they perceive. The goal of creating raw and living foods communities around the world would be the solution to raising children healthfully and with support. I always dreamed my children could grow up in a raw vegan intentional community such as Ecoforest in Spain where they could have had adult and peer support for living a healthy lifestyle. Since most of us don't have this kind of support for a healthy live food lifestyle, we must realize at a certain age, our children may stray due to cultural pressures. As time goes on, there is a developing awareness and growth of the raw food movement within the civilized world that should positively benefit families attempting to live a natural life. By increasing public awareness that disease need not be fought with drugs but prevented through healthful eating and lifestyle, I hope eating raw foods will eventually be considered normal.

I've come to feel once we've taught our children the powerful information about raw foods, we need to let them make decisions for themselves, no matter how painful it might be for us as parents. As much as we want to lead them to do what we feel is best for them, they need to be in control, or it won't work for them in the long run. It is their path, not ours, and living in a culture in which chicken nuggets, pizza, French fries and chips are portrayed as healthful foods, teenagers will still need to find their own way without us guiding them at every step. In our society, someone eating healthful raw fruits and vegetables, nuts and seeds, was once looked at and spoken of as "weird." Today, with numerous celebrities making raw foods popular and loads of new books extolling the benefits of the raw food lifestyle, it's easier to proclaim the choice.

Letting your children make their own decisions runs into other issues—for example, do we have to cook for them daily if that is their desire? It certainly would be better for them to eat cooked, organic whole foods at home than to increase the amount of highly processed conventional foods they would eat on the outside if we should choose not to prepare cooked food for them at all. Should we then accept refined, processed foods into our homes (such as white bread, white pasta or white rice) if that is the informed decision of the older child or teenager? We must nurture their decisions while continuing to make our homes as healthful as we possibly can. It is sometimes a hard balance and frustrating to a parent who believes strongly in the raw vegan lifestyle for a healthy future. I realized over time the different issues that become involved when changing the diet. Margaret Mead's saying, "It's easier to change your religion than your diet," definitely rings true. If spouses do not support each other on eating raw foods at home, this can create significant stress in everyday family life, and there will be a much greater chance the children will want to experience the foods of the other parent's diet. It would be important to discuss these lifestyle beliefs prior to having children, as friction can arise when parents don't see eye to eye on nutrition.

When my children were still pre-adolescent and asked to eat a specific food I didn't feel was healthful, I discussed the natural consequences with them; later, I tried to coerce and even bribe them to stay with the raw vegan foods. I felt this was best for them and was worried about how much they would stray from the healthful diet that had worked so well for them for many years. I knew the more cooked food they ate, the less fresh uncooked fruits and vegetables they would eat. At a certain point, I realized they would eat unhealthful processed foods without my knowing it. I had to let go of my desire for them to maintain a healthful diet when outside the home, as worried as I was about it. I learned coercion only creates anger and defiance, and I felt this was a mistake on my part. We love our children and desire for them to be emotionally and spiritually healthy as well as physically healthy. All three aspects are connected in creating healthy children. However, in letting them make their own decision, we also have to realize the unhealthy foods they may choose to eat outside the home can create imbalances which affect mood and emotions as well as physical wellbeing. Irritability, aggression, mood swings and depression can be directly linked with cooked, and particularly with processed and refined foods, which might contain opiates, monosodium glutamate, hydrogenated oils, dangerous preservatives and colorings, aspartame and other poisonous substances, often hidden on ingredient labels.

Children who have been eating healthful vegan foods for many years will react negatively to processed and refined foods. These reactions in teenagers can be observed initially in such physiological disturbances as premenstrual syndrome (PMS), chronic acne, body odor, headaches or stomachaches, the need to sleep for additional hours, lack of energy and many other symptoms—all due to the body working hard to expel the toxic overload.

I had worked very hard to create a community of others interested in living foods among our friends so our children could share and enjoy natural foods with them, but it was mostly adults who were interested in eating this way. Food is such a social thing in all cultures, and most children eventually want to share food with their peers, especially during the adolescent years when being accepted by their peers is so important to them. One local family, longtime friends, joined us in our raw food lifestyle for a number of years. We were glad to have them living nearby to get together often to share our ideas and delicious meals. But once their children had grown up, they began to eat cooked foods as well as animal products. There were a few children in our homeschool community who were interested in raw foods, but only briefly.

We socialized with a couple of families who were vegan, living on fruits, vegetables and the least harmful of the cooked foods—steamed vegetables and grains. We felt fortunate to have these friends who shared many of our values, especially our compassion for animals. They were eating closer to nature than most people we knew.

We have many friends who've neither embraced nor even discovered a raw vegan, or even vegetarian, lifestyle. We love and cherish our relationships with them and respect their paths nonetheless; but hope springs eternal!

Both of my children have told me they believe this natural diet of raw foods is the truth about health. As a mother, I've done my best within the scope of my knowledge to give my children healthy bodies and minds. I'm at peace knowing whatever decisions they make about their lifestyles, they will remember the seeds of truth I helped plant. It can sometimes be hard for a health conscious mother to know her children may decide to eat foods which could cause problems, but if children are ever to truly understand and make a value their own, they may need to follow a different path for some time. You as the parent are the pillar—a powerful example for your children. Through you, they will always have this vital information. It's important to respect their decisions, although they may be extremely difficult to accept. At such times, it is better to focus on living for each moment, "being in the now" to avoid stress. Share other interests and have fun with your children while remaining a model for a healthy lifestyle.

On the other hand, there are some teenagers who have found the raw food lifestyle to be liberating and self-empowering, even when their parents are following the standard diet. It is normal for teens to want to try something very different from what their parents are doing.

My daughter Gabriela, now 21, is listening to her inner wisdom rather than simply following the crowd. She's comparing how she felt on raw vegan foods when growing up at home to the standard dietary indoctrination now surrounding her away at college. Questioning what she observes of everyday standard lifestyles, she came to a conscious realization—resolving to return to raw vegan foods. She has also learned the truth about the torture of animals in factory farms and profoundly understands being vegan is fundamental toward reducing global warming and healing our planet. Her return to always feeling wonderful on raw foods has given her a deep insight—fresh fruits and vegetables are the optimal "species specific" foods for humans.

We as parents need to set the raw vegan example clearly for our children. We can ask them: "Are our food and consumer choices affecting the environment and humankind in a positive way?"

Professor Rozalind Graham, who speaks so eloquently on raw vegan nutrition for health and the environment, expressed the following: "It is going to take a critical mass to bring about the shifts necessary for salvation of the human soul and true preservation of our natural world and freedom. This is through the necessity of the powerful raw vegan example. What you choose to put in your shopping cart, on your table and in your mouth is more influential to the healing of our world than any political vote you might make. If you have found the raw vegan path, then you have chosen to lead the way. Walk with strength and grace towards the creation of world peace."

24

Water, and How Much Do You Need as a Raw Vegan?

*"Water, the essential fluid on which all life depends,
has become a global garbage can."*

JACQUES COUSTEAU (1910–1997)

Humans need to eat foods with extremely high water content. Eating raw fruits and vegetables will provide this high water content. If mainly cooked or dehydrated foods or too many nuts are eaten, the water content has evaporated, and one would need to drink great quantities of water to replace it. When water is drunk along with cooked food, a pool is created in the stomach, often followed by indigestion and putrefaction. It's important not to drink with live food meals because additional water would dilute the digestive juices.

In an article titled "Distilled Water, Detoxification and Your Health," from Living Nutrition Magazine, Dr. Roe Gallo says even raw foodists need to drink water in addition to their water rich diets: "We must also drink water because most of us cannot get all the water we need from our food supply. Granted, water rich plant food is over 80% water but with exercise, heat, etc., more water is lost than can be replaced with food, unless you ate more food than needed, and then you may have the problem of excess fat. Physiology shows us that when the body absorbs excess nutrients, e.g. protein, fat or carbohydrates, they are generally stored as fat. So eating more food to try to satisfy your daily water requirement is not a good idea. You must drink water."

Eight to ten glasses of water a day are often recommended for those consuming a standard dehydrated diet, but it will vary for those on a raw food diet. Water needs, of course, will be greater for a lactating mother as she will need the extra water from raw vegan foods and drinking water to create an abundant milk supply. Availability of purified water during the day is necessary to prevent dehydration. Even mild dehydration can cause health problems, initially noted in difficulty concentrating and poor memory.

Vitamins and minerals added to sports drinks are not absorbable—the best sources for absorbable vitamins and minerals are raw fruits and vegetables, nuts and seeds.

It's a good idea to drink water or eat high water content foods just after waking up in the morning. We often become dehydrated overnight, so it would be most beneficial to drink a glass of water upon rising and then wait a half an hour before eating.

Our bodies are reported to be approximately 72% water. The average person holds about 44 quarts of water in his body, and loses about 3 quarts a day. Water is lost through the kidneys, bowels, lungs and skin, and the lost water must be continually replenished.

Dr. Graham recommends: "Drink enough water to remain well-hydrated at all times. This varies from person to person, diet to diet, based on activity levels, climate, etc. A well-hydrated person will typically urinate 9–12 times per 24 hours, on average."

This was one of the first benefits I observed on raw foods—the water and the water-rich food I was consuming would go in and come out very quickly. I've observed others not on a water rich diet don't urinate as frequently. I noticed at certain times, especially in summer, when I was getting so much water from ripe melons, fresh summer fruits, lots of delicious locally grown cucumbers and tomatoes and blended green soups and smoothies, I had absolutely no desire for extra water, and when I forced myself to drink it, I felt bloated and would be in the bathroom far more than necessary.

Tonya Zavasta, author of *Beautiful on Raw*, *Your Right to be Beautiful*, and *Quantum Eating* feels too much water in the diet can also cause harm, and might be seen in puffiness, especially around the eyes (www.beautifulonraw.com). In her book, *Your Right to Be Beautiful: How to Halt the Train of Aging and Meet the Most Beautiful You*, Tonya wrote: "A baby's perfect complexion is partly due to the fact that at birth the body is over 90 percent water. Body cells lose moisture with age. At age 75, only about a third of the body's composition is water. Raw plant foods are about 75 percent water. Fruits contain about 80% of the most biologically active water available. To continue looking youthful, eating raw food is essential. The recommendation to drink eight glasses of water a day is only valid if you consume cooked foods, which are concentrated. Simply drinking water and eating cooked food, however, does not do the trick. Drinking a lot of fluids might actually have the opposite effect on your appearance. As well as washing away waste in the blood, it washes away nutrients and is hard on the kidneys and bladder, gives a swollen look, and exhausts the glow from your face." In *Quantum Eating*, Tonya writes she does *not* get dehydrated and never drinks free water—water apart from that contained in fruits and vegetables, and she explains her position in great detail. She does drink fresh vegetable juices, green smoothies or puddings, and eats juicy fruits all of which contain more than 80% water.

The water you drink daily must be purified, or you will be causing yourself much harm by ingesting significant amounts of toxic chemicals. Most American cities and towns add at least 1ppm of sodium fluoride to the water supply. Even small amounts of fluoride are extremely toxic. Unpurified tap water should be avoided. Tap water has been referred to as a "chemical cocktail."

The EPA estimates 10% of our community drinking water contains pesticides. A 1999 Connecticut survey by The Environment and Human Health Organization found 11% of surveyed private drinking water wells were contaminated with one or more lawn and tree care pesticides regardless of whether or not the homeowner used pesticides.

In 1999, my children and I visited our town's water department to ask about the chemicals and standards, only to find out thousands of chemicals are present in our water in "regulated" amounts. I had already been using purified bottled water, but I was still alarmed because I sometimes used tap water to wash fruits and vegetables. In August 2003, I received an upsetting letter from our town's water department about a dangerous chemical in our water supply. I was shocked to learn that although this chemical, tetrachloroethylene, exceeded the standard for the level of maximum contaminant, the water department did not recommend an alternate water supply unless someone already had serious health concerns. The report said this organic chemical is a popular solvent, particularly for dry cleaning, and generally seeps into drinking water through improper waste disposal. It has been shown to cause cancer in laboratory animals such as rats and mice when animals are exposed at high levels over their lifetimes. The EPA has set the drinking water standard for tetrachloroethylene at 5.0 ppb to reduce the risk of cancer or other adverse health effects that have been observed in laboratory animals. The State standard is 1.0 ppb, which the town describes as more stringent, therefore posing little or no risk. This report was quite scary. I would not want even a drop of this noxious chemical in my drinking water, and this is only one chemical of hundreds. More recently, in 2007, we received a notice about high levels of arsenic five in the tap water. Many water filtration systems do not filter out arsenic, so an additional filter is necessary solely for filtering out this poison.

When looking for a new home, research the source of its municipal drinking water. A change in location of just a few miles might mean the difference between heavily contaminated water and nearly pollution-free water. Two adjacent towns can have completely different water sources, one loaded with chemicals and the other relatively free of pollutants.

In an article, "The Role of Skin Absorption as a Route of Exposure for Volatile Organic Compounds," from the American Journal of Public Health, 1984, the following information is provided:

> You are what you drink and bathe in! Your body is between 70% to 80% water. (Brain – 75%, Heart – 75%, Lungs – 86%, Liver – 86%, Kidneys – 83%, Muscle – 75%, Blood – 83%). Water is the key to all bodily functions (Circulatory System, Assimilation System, Digestive System, Elimination System, Temperature Control). We conclude that skin absorption of contaminants in drinking water has been underestimated and ingestion may not constitute the sole or even primary route of exposure.

> Skin absorption rates vary with the different regions of the body. Underestimated is the case of whole body immersion during swimming or bathing. The epidermis of the hand represents a relatively greater barrier to penetration than many other parts of the body, including the scalp, forehead, abdomen, area in and around the ears, underarms, and genital area. Penetration through the genital area, in fact, is estimated to be 100% as compared to 8.6% for the forearm.

> Other significant routes of absorption include oral, nasal, cheeks and mouth cavity, and eye and ear areas. These routes have been underestimated in their ability to absorb contaminants during immersion in water. Inhalation serves as yet another route. In the case of swimming or bathing, the volatized chemicals are likely to gather near the surface of the water and are readily inhaled. Absorption rates obtained from healthy adults will again tend to underestimate absorption for children or populations that are more sensitive.

Millions of Americans are made sick and thousands die each year from biological contamination of their tap water, states The Department of Environmental Protection Water Quality Inventory Reports. "In Wisconsin (in 1995), over 7.6 million people were sickened and over 12,000 killed by illnesses related to unclean water. Scientists have estimated 25 cases of waterborne illness occur for every one reported." Just because the water supply meets federal standards, it's definitely not safe from waterborne disease. Cryptosporidium (a microorganism found in cattle manure common in agricultural runoff) and giardia are not easily killed by chlorine and are often not removed by conventional water treatment.

There is much controversy about which is the highest quality water purification method, from distillation and reverse osmosis to water filtration systems to ionized water filters. I used a steam distiller for many years and then purchased bottled distilled water. Now, I have a water purification system on my sink. Questioning the safety of the tap water, even with an attached purification system, Dr. Brian Clement of the Hippocrates Health Institute recommends purifying tap water, and then further purifying it with a distillation process.

It is our natural birthright to have clean water and clean air, yet we need water filters on our showers and sinks. When I bathed in fresh water creeks, rivers, and waterholes in Costa Rica and, on another trip, in the Sky Lakes region of the mountains of Southern Oregon, my skin felt soft and refreshed. Sun, water and air bathing made me feel clean, strong, and very alive. After showering at my New Jersey home, my skin feels dry and depleted, even with the attached water filter.

We need to eat the best quality organic foods, high in water content—raw fruits and vegetables, and use only purified water for drinking, for adding to smoothies and for washing produce. Also read the chapter "Basics of Health—Water" from the book *Avoiding Degenerative Disease: The Operation and Maintenance Manual for Human Beings* by Don Bennett.

25

Genetic Engineering: How Can It Affect Our Children and Future Generations?

"Once released into the environment, unlike a BSE epidemic or chemical spill, genetic mistakes cannot be contained, recalled or cleaned up, but will be passed onto all future generations indefinitely."

DR. MICHAEL ANTONIOU

"Far from feeding the world, people are going to starve because of genetically engineered foods. More and more peasants will see their crops substituted through biotechnology."

VANDANA SHIVA, PHYSICIST AND ECOLOGIST, INDIA

Genetic engineering is a current form of biotechnology, a broad term describing processes such as cross breeding, plant hybridization and fermentation. Genetic engineering is a relatively new and rapidly developing technology that is raising much public concern. Genetic engineering focuses on the manipulation of the genetic material (the DNA) in the cells of living organisms to block undesired traits or add desired ones. The result is often called a genetically modified organism, or GMO.

It's estimated 35% of corn and 55% of soybeans grown in the United States during 1999 were genetically engineered. According to the USDA, "By 2006, 89% of the planted area of soybeans, 83% of cotton, and 61% of maize were genetically modified varieties." According to the Center for Food Safety, "It has been estimated that upwards of 60 percent of processed foods on supermarket shelves—from soda to soup, crackers to condiments—contain genetically engineered ingredients." Another common GMO Food source is dairy products from cows injected with the genetically modified hormone recombinant bovine growth hormone (rBGH). The best thing you can do for the health of your family and the planet is to stay away from dairy and processed foods, and buy only organic or biodynamic produce. This constitutes a powerful statement against GMO foods. It also supports the revitalization of the land through healthy growing practices. You can also demand the clear labeling of genetically engineered produce by contacting congressmen and senators asking for bills to support labeling of GMOs.

> *"The perception that everything is totally straightforward and safe is utterly naive. I don't think we fully understand the dimensions of what we're getting into."*
>
> PROFESSOR PHILIP JAMES

Rhio, author of *Hooked on Raw* and hostess of www.NYTalkRadio.net (providing up-to-date information on health, environmental and political concerns), is also a major spokesperson on how genetically engineered foods are produced and how they negatively impact our health and the Earth.

After learning about the threat to the integrity of Mother Nature and human and animal health posed by the genetic engineering of seeds/plants, Rhio attended numerous lectures to learn about the subject. As a layperson, she found it difficult to decipher the scientific language used by the geneticists, but she stayed the course until she had an understanding. Rhio found arrogance and greed running rampant through much of the biotechnology industry. She found what they were doing to be so shocking and abhorrent that she decided to translate the arcane scientific terminology in order to tell the story in plain English anyone could understand. Rhio reported, "Sixty-seven percent of Monsanto's sales are herbicides and pesticides."

Rhio explains, "People who eat standard American processed foods tend to be more passive, but in order to recognize the connections between food and health, one must become more conscious." She states, "Good, rich, organic soil is teaming with healthy bacteria, and when the soil is alive, the food is alive. Human interference, by artificially manipulating the very nature of Nature is altering the course of the biology of seeds and plants forever. The products of genetic manipulation, once released into the environment, cannot be retrieved because life forms (living organisms) continue on in their evolutionary path."

It is especially important for pregnant and lactating women and growing children to know the dangers of genetically engineered foods. The developing brains and nervous systems of growing fetuses and developing children are dependant on pure, fresh, wholesome foods. Chemicals and mixing genes from other animals and plants are capable of creating all sorts of problems in the evolving human body. There is no doubt we will all be adversely affected by companies altering the way Nature has provided our food.

In Rhio's article "Genetically Engineered Food Explained in Plain Language," from "Just Eat an Apple" Magazine, Spring 2004, she presents crucial information of which we all need to be aware. The following excerpt from that article shows us we need to get involved before all of our food is genetically modified:

> Out of all GE foods produced worldwide, 70% are grown right here in the USA, with Canada and Argentina making up most of the balance. Most Europeans don't want GE foods, but because of coercion from the U.S., they are accepting GE food, although they have stringent labeling and traceability requirements. Companies such as Monsanto (now Pharmacia), Dow Chemical, Du Pont, Novartis, Aventis and others have been buying up most of the seed companies worldwide. Their agenda is to CONTROL all food production by forcing the use of their patented seeds. There are counties in California that have banned the production of genetically engineered crops to protect the local economy, including its growing organic sector, and the environment.

> In contrast with normal evolution, the genetic engineering of seeds is the artificial altering, at the cellular level, of a seed's genome. When we reflect upon the way Nature has altered her seeds over billions of years, and then compare it with the modern genetic "souped up" version, it should give us all a great deal of apprehension.

> Nature, in all of her history, never crossed a fish gene with a tomato. Wouldn't you think our scientists would pause to think about what it means to alter a plant so drastically as to insert a fish gene where it has never been before? Or a pig gene into a potato? How about a rat gene into broccolini? That's not a pretty picture! And what about our right to be vegetarians if we so choose? Isn't putting a fish gene into a tomato making the tomato into an animal product? And with no labeling, how can we tell which is which?

> Why do we need plants that are altered to withstand heavy doses of herbicides? When these plants are sprayed, everything around them dies, except the target plant. What right have we to kill the diversity of Nature—all the surrounding plants, insects and animal life?

According to the Grocery Manufacturers of America, an estimated 60 to 70% of all foods in the supermarkets are contaminated with GMOs. The corn syrup in processed foods is all genetically engineered. Coca Cola is one of the biggest purchasers of genetically engineered corn syrup.

Farmers and eaters around the globe feel very strongly about this issue because for the sake of PROFIT, for the sake of milking a 20-year patent, the ecology of our planet and human and animal health are being placed at risk. And we, the people, are the guinea pigs in this giant and foolish experiment.

Rejection of GE food hit the news when starving countries in Africa refused to accept GE food for their people. They considered it too dangerous, not only to eat, but that it might also contaminate their own crops.

Rhio discusses cross pollination, a natural occurrence, but when the pollen from plants grown at farms planted with GE seeds is blown by the wind onto the plants of neighboring farms, they become contaminated and develop GE traits. If an organic farm becomes contaminated, its crops are no longer organic. She feels it should be mandated that genetically engineered foods be grown in greenhouses so non-genetically engineered crops are not contaminated by cross pollination.

Rhio discussed a study on rats that were fed GE potatoes. The rats' immune systems were damaged. Their stomach linings were affected. Some of their organs became enlarged, while other organs decreased in size.

Rhio highly recommends eating heirloom plants because their seeds will grow true to the original plant—heirloom seeds will produce plants identical to their parents.

An audio version of "Genetically Engineered Foods Explained in Plain Language" is available. For more information on GE foods, please see both the Articles and the Links sections of Rhio's Raw Energy website: http://www.rawfoodinfo.com/

For information on how to ask your representatives to co-sponsor Dennis Kucinich's GE bills, go to: http://www.house.gov/kucinich/action/summary.hm or call (202) 225-5871.

26

Modeling Emotional Poise
for Our Children

*"The grass and the trees, and the wind and the waves, and the birds and
the beasts, all sing and smile and laugh. Join in the chorus and do
what all of Nature does."*

ZOROASTER (THE GREEK NAME FOR THE PROPHET ZARATHUSHTRA)

Seeing ourselves and those around us in a spiritual light, as well as developing an evermore positive attitude toward life are fundamental to good health. Daily meditation creates a calm enabling one to better handle life's ups and downs. Even fifteen minutes of quiet time each day, closing one's eyes and focusing solely on breathing, will result in immense benefits for overall health. It is important to spend time alone every day. In a world where everyday stresses can take over to overwhelm the body, the best example we can set for our children is to find ways to show peace and calm, such as meditation, deep breathing, saying a prayer of gratitude before eating, walking in nature and adopting a tree in your yard where you sit quietly to take in your surroundings.

Modeling emotional poise for children is one of the most important things we will ever do for them. The modern-day world can be intensely stimulating. We take in a sensory overload especially through our eyes. Many people go shopping frequently to malls, big department stores and supermarkets which are extremely over-stimulating, particularly to babies and very young children. Add the stimulation from television viewing and computer use, and no wonder so many children develop ADHD (attention deficit hyperactivity disorder), and so many are suffering from severe stress.

Finding a place that provides peace for the mind and body is so essential. Most days, I go hiking in the woods at a reservation near my home in New Jersey. The trails are quiet, and I have felt most at peace there in the forest. My walks in the forest gave me the inspiration for many parts of this book. Everyone needs to find his/her own place of peace, a place to breathe clean air, think clearly and be calm. Even in the cities and suburbs, you can find a place that is your piece of peace, whether it's a hiking area, a quiet, relaxing place in a park or a beautiful tree down the street.

Starting each day with positive questions will help you to be grateful for each day:

What can you do to make this day enjoyable and fun?
What can you do today to increase your energy and mental clarity?
What can you do today to feel more connected to life and to others?
What will you learn presently that you didn't know or comprehend before?

Place affirmations and positive quotes on a frequently seen wall in your home. I've used a bathroom wall to place valuable quotes and affirmations for my children to read. I call it the "Philosophical Corner." My daughter tells me she reads everything I put up there. She is now placing some of her own positive quotes and affirmations there to be read and internalized; and my son lets me know when he really likes a particular quote. Some positive affirmations could be: I live my life in happiness and freedom, I am committed to my goals in life, I select a healthy lifestyle, etc.

The following "10 Ways We Misunderstand Children" are from *The Natural Child: Parenting from the Heart* by Jan Hunt. These 10 ways show how we hurt children emotionally by misunderstanding them; as adults, we can reverse these ten points by making them into affirmations and living by them:

1. We expect children to be able to do things before they are ready.
2. We become angry when a child fails to meet our needs.
3. We mistrust the child's motives.
4. We don't allow children to be children.
5. We get it backwards (instead of accepting our parental role to meet the child's needs, we expect the child to care for our needs.)
6. We blame and criticize when a child makes a mistake.
7. We forget how deeply blame and criticism can hurt a child.
8. We forget how healing loving actions can be.
9. We forget our behavior provides the most potent lessons to the child.

10. We see only the outward behavior, not the love and good intentions inside the child.

Reprinted with permission from the Natural Child Project. Jan Hunt is the author of *The Natural Child: Parenting from the Heart* (2001) and *A Gift for Baby* (2006); and the co-editor of the new book *The Unschooling Unmanual*. www.naturalchild.org. To purchase Jan Hunt's books: http://www.naturalchild.org/shop/books/

Author and lecturer David Wolfe once expressed: "Instead of dwelling on negative stressful thoughts, write down your goals. If you create negative thoughts about yourself, they will become real. Embrace the opposition." Another of David's phrases has helped me in stressful situations: "Turn frustration into fascination."

Many people eat for emotional reasons or when tired. Most of us eat much more than we need. Processed denatured foods often become comfort foods at times of emotional stress, and this is why so many people revert back to cooked foods during difficult times.

Mary McGuire-Wien, Director of American Yogini retreats on Long Island, New York, talks about the importance of receiving plenty of "primary food." She explains: "Children live on primary food. The fun, excitement and love of their daily life feed them, so nutrition is secondary. Primary foods feed us, but don't come on a plate. Things like love, hugs, touch, kisses, warmth, massage, meditation, fun, freedom, self-expression, tears, hot baths, nature, trees, down time, close friends, and children at play. They feed our soul, and our hunger for living. The more primary food we receive, the less will be our dependence on secondary foods. The opposite is also true. The more we fill ourselves with secondary foods, the less we are able to receive the primary foods for life."

In my observations, raw food kids seem to be calm as well as energetic in their play. Perhaps their ease of digestion due to the foods they eat is related to their low stress attitude.

In a study on "Stress and Aging," chronically stressed people were found to be biologically from 9 to 17 years older than they realized. This study, done by the University of California, San Francisco, and published in *The Proceedings of the National Academy of Sciences*, showed chronic psychological stress may lead to chromosome changes that can cause premature aging. Scientists found stressed people have much shorter chromosome-stabilizing caps than other people. These protective caps, called telomeres, shrink each time a cell divides, and when they become too short, a cell can no longer divide and it dies.

Telomere shortening is not only linked to aging, but to premature death from infections and cardiovascular disease. The study compared stressed mothers of chronically ill children and mothers of healthy children.

> "Puzzles produce a sharpening of one's ability to think."
>
> CELIA HOROWITZ

Stress makes an individual more susceptible to heart attacks, cancer and diabetes. Stress accumulates over time, causing a lack of energy, and an inability to think properly, and then the body begins to break down. Eating unfired foods high in nutrients and practicing deep breathing help to decrease stress. Just three deep breaths can reduce tension. Ten to twenty minutes of deep breathing can significantly cut stress levels, providing hormonal balance and improved sleep.

We all need to de-stress, especially for the sake of our children who take on our stressful feelings. Children enjoy happy parents who are not stressed all the time.

Jingee Talifero (www.thegardendiet.com) says: "So, how can we relieve stress? Help each other to go easy on each other, love each other. Do the same for ourselves. Take breaks, walks, breathers. Eat less. Exercise more. Steal time for our children. Nobody will ever give us that. We have to steal it in this society. This society demands every waking moment of us. But we don't have to give it up that easily. Our children are the most important part of life. And this day of their lives, this day of their growth, this fleeting moment, we will never get back once gone. There will always be money to be earned, bills to pay, and endless things to do on your list, but there will not always be young children in your life. Take time to enjoy them! You deserve it."

A number of tips will bring relaxation and calm into your life:

1. Exercise daily—moving your body burns up stress hormones, leaving you feeling relaxed and refreshed.
2. Seek support in your life by reaching out to others.
3. Eat healthful raw vegan foods.
4. Get adequate sleep to feel more relaxed.
5. Breathe deeply—inhale slowly, letting your stomach rise for five seconds. Hold, and exhale slowly for five seconds. Practice five times each day for a total of five minutes.
6. Meditate—Sitting in quiet meditation even for 15 minutes a day will create a more focused and rested mind. Silence creates an avenue for dealing with all of life's situations.

7. Develop acceptance—"Accepting whatever you cannot change" will provide a peaceful feeling in dealing with the world.
8. A loving atmosphere in your home is the foundation for your life.
9. When you and your loved ones have a disagreement, focus only on the current situation. Do not bring up the past.
10. Have family meetings to resolve conflicts. Each family member should be given time to express personal views. Do not have family meetings focusing on intense topics during mealtimes, when the focus should be on relaxation, enjoyment, and digestion.
11. Make your home a fun place to be. It's important to have a home centered on having fun times. When our children were younger, we had many game nights, drawing nights and movie nights, sometimes just with the immediate family and other times with friends. When our son was eighteen, his friends came frequently to our home for very lively, fun poker nights.
12. Pleasing melodies, especially by Mozart, have great value for children and adults alike. Music speaks in a language that children instinctively understand, and helps to mold a child's mental, emotional, social, and physical development.

It's very important to smile and laugh a lot with your children.
Regardless of the ups and downs of everyday life, there is still so much
to be grateful for, and what better contagious facial expression is there
than a smile? What sound is more cheering than laughter?
A magnet on my refrigerator maintains.
"55 Smiles per Hour."

ℰ❧

Obesity Understood – Now and Forever Impossible on Fresh Fruits and Vegetables

Whereas diets don't work in the long run, the lifestyle improvements detailed throughout *Creating Healthy Children* offer lifelong health benefits that include ideal weight. The life in our foods communicates with the life in us, but, unfortunately, this vital aspect is lost once foods are heated and processed. White, refined foods are addictive—their eaters will endlessly eat more in an effort to find that spark of life that has been removed from these foods, ironically to give them shelf life.

Children will most likely not be obese when their parents read books such as *Creating Healthy Children*. These parents will teach the health promoting aspects of fresh fruits and vegetables to their children. When foods are whole, ripe, fresh and organic, they contain vitamins, enzymes and minerals that satisfy us, as well as the essential fiber that keeps us full, but this will never be an incapacitating full feeling such as that following the standard Thanksgiving dinner. Feeling full on fresh foods is simply being free of hunger, satisfied, and energetic.

Animal foods are devoid of fiber, but the essential fiber in all fresh vegan foods has powerful cleansing benefits. When food is refined, processed, denatured in packages, its nutritive characteristics are sadly no longer intact, and the eater will not be satisfied and remains with the feeling of craving something. In an attempt to obtain essential nutrients, the craving for more will persist, but refined foods will always lack what the body needs—overeating of nutritionally empty foods ensues and becomes habitual.

The results of such "empty" eating habits are vitamin and mineral deficiencies, and obesity. In addition to being unaesthetic, obesity lays the groundwork for myriad diseases.

Whenever there is excess body fat, there is an accumulation of toxins in the fat cells that must be diluted in water. The fat cells thus become bloated, heavy, and all bodily functions become more difficult, resulting in diseases based solely on eating disorders; in reality, the disorder is nothing more than the empty food that has been destroyed by heat, chemicals, and many processing techniques before arriving on the plate. Ironically, the obesity victim is really starving for nutrients found only in fresh vegan foods.

Animal foods contain cholesterol which clogs blood vessels. Fruits and vegetables are 100% cholesterol-free—our livers make all we need. There is no dietary requirement for cholesterol. Animal fat is solid at body temperature, whereas fruit and vegetable fat is liquid. Unfortunately, obese children are clogging their arteries, building the cause for future diseases unknown in countries where people are, fortunately, too poor to eat animals and their byproducts.

Even vegan children become obese when white foods are eaten: white flour, refined sugar, salt, white potatoes, starchy, sugary refined cereals, white rice, crackers, breads, rolls, cookies, cakes, etc. Baking and frying require high temperatures. Not only are the heated oils and shortening toxic to the point of becoming carcinogenic, the resultant acrylamide (a deadly golden brown plastic), albeit crunchy to taste, becomes yet another toxin that gets stored in the fat cells and must be diluted with water held in solution—hence obesity. When the precepts of Creating Healthy Children are lived, obesity will no longer be an epidemic but an impossibility.

27

Questions from Parents Striving to Raise Healthy Children

"When you arise in the morning, think of what a precious privilege it is to be alive—to breathe, to think, to enjoy, to love."

MARCUS AURELIUS

Q: I read on vegetarianbaby.com about your experience raising raw children and was wondering if you had any advice relating to your success. My son is 11 months old, has been fed 100% raw since he started eating solids, and has been breastfed since he was born. We, my wife and I, feed him a variety of mostly fruits, some vegetables, and on occasion a little nut and seed butter. He especially loves the flesh of young coconuts. He seems to be thriving very well except he seems a bit small compared to other babies his age. My personal opinion is that the other kids are overfed and therefore overweight, so he appears to be small compared to them. He has never been sick. Even when around other kids who were sick, he never got anything. He is energetic, playful, sleeps well, and all in all we have no complaints or many concerns. Any feedback or advice you may have on how we can optimize his diet, we'll greatly appreciate.

A: You're doing a great job parenting. I have observed raw vegan children are varying heights and weights and know if fed a variety of whole raw foods, they fall into the normal growth curve, as shown to me by our family pediatrician as well as through research done by Dr. Gabriel Cousens. My children grew more slowly than others, especially those who had been eating animal products all along. Both of my children also had a slower adolescence in growth, and my daughter had her first period later than her peers. They do grow, but they grow

245

at a normal rate. Our local pediatrician assured me, although our children were on the lower end of the growth charts, they were growing normally (If a child is noticeably losing weight each month and his/her weight falls significantly below the growth charts, this should be looked into as there may be a dietary deficiency or other problem that does need to be addressed, and this should not be ignored). Later, my husband became concerned about our son's height because he was one of the smallest on his athletic teams, but I knew children on a more natural diet aren't eating growth hormones from animal products, and may grow at a slower, more natural rate. When he was fourteen, he began to have increased growth spurts, and at seventeen, he became taller than both his parents. Vegan children often gain more muscle mass as they get older. Exercise and playing outdoors in nature are very important. Both of our teen-age children look very fit and have strong muscular bodies. Our son plays tennis and basketball, and our daughter takes volleyball classes, dance classes and goes hiking. Because our children were internally clean while they were growing up, they were always able to be around sick children without "catching" anything. When, on rare occasions, they did become ill, they knew from example to fast and rest, and, now, as older teens, still practice this.

Raw vegan foods are so powerful when prepared simply or eaten as is. At 11 months, most of your son's diet should still be breast milk and any solid foods introduced should be fruits. Nut and seed butters would be too hard on his digestion at this young age and shouldn't be introduced until after three years old. Many babies aren't ready to eat solid foods until closer to age two. Since your child has already been introduced to solid foods, you can provide him with a variety of soft fruits cut into bite-sized pieces to facilitate chewing and to prevent choking. You're already aware that soft ripe bananas, grapes, peaches, pears, and melons are some of the wonderful choices. You can also introduce green juices and green smoothies. These foods and his mom's breast milk will supply him with all the amino acids, vitamins, minerals and enzymes he needs during this period. As he grows into his second year and beyond, you can add many new bite-sized raw fruits and vegetables, and later, nuts and seeds. Some moms who attended my classes have told me their older babies loved avocados and did quite well with them. The avocado, a fruit, has a higher water content than nuts and seeds that have been dried. If your child, after age 3, is eating mostly fruits and vegetables, with some nuts or seeds with the vegetables, he should do amazingly well. As your son grows older and goes through growth spurts, he may crave more food and increased fats from nuts, seeds and avocados for a while and then go back to more fruits and vegetables with smaller amounts of nuts and seeds. You just need to be aware of his needs as he's developing, and have a variety of these foods available. Your son is so fortunate to have you as parents. Congratulations to both of you for being informed parents!

Q: The following is a question from Beata, who experienced a pregnancy while eating raw vegan foods and is raising her daughter Sarah on raw foods. Her article appears later in the book. Beata called me from Israel on 1/21/05 to ask about eating raw foods and socializing. She said people sometimes give her two year old daughter Sarah some pita bread and she starts to love eating it. What should she do as a mother when she knows this is not a healthful choice for her little girl? How can we help children avoid the beginnings of a processed food addiction?

A: Dear Beata,

Following our phone conversation, I thought this over a lot. It's never easy living in a world where we're looked at as different. Your little girl is still very young, and I'm sure you are the center of her life. As she grows, it's important to find others who enjoy your healthful way of eating, and will support the way you're raising her. You said people are offering her pita bread. I know it's very hard to interfere because you want to have good relationships with family, friends and even acquaintances. Until at least age three, children have not yet developed all the enzymes to digest starches, and processed starches are especially toxic and indigestible. Other studies have determined digestive enzymes for starches are not completely developed until age four. Eating starches at her young age can cause problems. There are so many delicious fruits and vegetables a child will easily digest and enjoy.

You told me 99% of her food is your breast milk. That's wonderful! Let her nurse for a long time, and she will be getting the best nutrition and protection possible. Not only does it supply everything she needs, it adapts to her needs as she grows. I think children are definitely curious, but we should not give in to their every whim if it will hurt them physically by significantly increasing their craving for starchy, processed foods.

For your child at age 2, bring her favorite bite-size pieces of fruits and veggies, perhaps some which she doesn't eat routinely, to make her food more interesting. When my children were three and older, I used to make special treats for them to bring to birthday parties: raw cakes, ice creams, and raw candies. This is the time to use fruits, dried fruits and nuts to create some exceptional and beautiful party foods. Sometimes my children cried they wanted to eat the cake and ice cream at the parties. It was sometimes difficult, because it did separate them from others in that respect. But your good friends will want to support you. Over the years we made friends who would also make special healthful treats my children could enjoy at parties. It's a good idea to make an abundance of healthful delights to share at parties and gatherings. Many raw families have received raves for the wonderful desserts they've brought to share on special occasions. Relax and take three breaths if your child should eat something unhealthful at a party or gathering. I got very upset when my children did, but that won't serve you or your child either as I've learned. Just continue to bring tasty raw food preparations your child, and others at the party, will want to try. And you can talk calmly to your child afterwards about how he or she feels physically and emotionally after eating certain nutritionally barren foods. Try not to be judgmental, just state the facts about the imbalances that result, and listen to your child. Today, I don't regret not having given the refined sugary cakes and ice creams to my children, or the sodas, loaded with sugar and caffeine, making the children hyper and leading to all sorts of horrible cravings so difficult to control. Once your child is twelve, you may no longer have the opportunity to create the nutritional foundation for a healthy life, but you now have that opportunity so abundantly with your little girl. Give the best gift of life you can provide for her — to live her life to its fullest potential by starting out early to eat healthful, nutritious, live foods.

Q: On another day, Beata called to ask, "What can I do for my daughter who has a fever?"

A: I asked Beata to review what her daughter had eaten in the past day. Sickness in children is almost always related to something eaten, whether the child has fever or other symptoms, such as vomiting, diarrhea, a rash, cough, etc. Raw food children are exceptionally vital and will react quickly to eliminate ingested toxins. I never gave any medicines to my children. And that includes medicines to reduce fever. Although my children rarely experienced fevers, when they did, they would sleep for the greater part of one to three days, drinking only water or diluted fresh orange juice. If you get very worried should the fever go above 103 degrees, a warm bath may help to relax the child and bring the temperature down. Most often it's best to let the fever run its course.

Q: Dear Karen,

I was recently employed as a midwife by a woman on a raw vegan diet. I know some basic information about raw foods and pregnancy from a few books I've read, but the fear that comes up in the midwifery community is starting to make me feel like I'm taking on someone who is crazy! Anyway, I feel strongly that if the mother feels good, her baby is growing well and everything is fine, why suggest eating something different from what she believes? The push from midwives about protein, protein, protein has gone a bit over the top, in my eyes. Many midwives feel 70-100 grams of protein a day is necessary in pregnancy. Do you have any comments or advice on more information re: the safety of raw foods in pregnancy? I'm not adverse to a raw diet for pregnant women. I'm just observing more and more of my peers questioning its overall safety.

Pamela Hines-Powell, CPM, LDM

Circle of Life Midwifery, Salem, Oregon

http://www.midwifemama.com

A: Dear Pamela,

I began researching raw vegan foods in 1993 when my three year old son was suffering from asthma and chronic allergic rhinitis. After trying many allopathic and alternative physicians to no avail, I turned to nutrition. After eating raw vegan foods for almost a year, my son was healed. Since then, I have spent years reading and studying with some of the top experts in this area of nutrition. I teach a class in the New York, New Jersey, Pennsylvania, and Connecticut area called "Creating Healthy Children," and also lead a raw food support group.

Women who follow a varied diet during a raw vegan pregnancy have absolutely no problem with protein. The only raw foodists who may have problems after the birth of the child are those who nurse for under a year since the baby needs breast milk as a source of digestible fat and protein, and even raw food cannot replace it. I have observed and worked with women during raw food pregnancies. They most often feel wonderful and have much easier childbirths.

I do not recommend that women switch to a 100% raw food diet during pregnancy because the change to this cleansing diet could release toxins into the bloodstream that accumulated from years of eating refined and processed foods, known to build up debris in the cells. If your client is already a raw foodist, my opinion is she will do very well as long as she eats a variety of fruits, leafy greens and vegetables, and small amounts of nuts and seeds several times a week. Please feel free to contact me if you have any other questions.

Best wishes, Karen Ranzi

Q: Miko Nelson emailed me some questions about consuming kefir. I referred her to Dr. Douglas Graham:

Dear Dr. Graham,

Our family of 3 (my husband, 2 1/2 year old child and I) have been on the raw foods diet since February 2, 2003. Recently, a friend introduced me to coconut kefir, and it has caused a slight shakeup in our otherwise established dietary ideals. After finding kefir grains, I learned I would have to cultivate them in milk periodically to enable them to survive in the coconut water medium. This causes me to feel I should revisit our family's lack of dairy to the extent that I would be able to use raw goat milk and be able to create my own probiotic in this way. I read on the Internet, the mucus from kefir is a "good" clear mucus that is favorable in the body. I don't understand what this means. I realize you have never recommended this, nor do I expect you to, however, the "why" part of what we choose and don't choose to eat is the key to sticking to our convictions.

Sincerely, Miko Nelson

A: Miko,

I cannot in good conscience recommend any adult consume the mammary excretions of a goat, I am sorry. I don't really care what you do to the milk, even if you ferment it (basically, this means you have taken a food that was never meant for human consumption and allowed it to go bad). There is no reason to consider the milk of an animal as fit food for humans.

Dr. Graham

In a comment on the intelligence of raw food children, Eric Rivkin writes, "In my observation, I notice in general, raw vegan or vegan mothers give birth to children who are smarter, and of course, they don't get sick like the children of meat/dairy eating mothers. This is due to toxic ketones and acetone built up in the blood from eating animal products that can cause fetal brain damage. The results of one study showed children with meat eating mothers scored 10 points lower in IQ tests than children with vegetarian mothers. Also, we see positive changes in school children's behavior, grades, and attendance, and less violence in schools that banned junk foods from cafeterias.

I also learned most of the great philosophers, scholars, and spiritual leaders in history were vegetarian. The Ancient Greeks knew the secrets of intelligence and longevity were proportional to the amount of flesh eaten, and so did the Essenes as far back as Moses, and the Hindus before him."

Eric Rivkin, raw food instructor and chef

Excelsior, Minnesota, living in Costa Rica since 2007.

Q: Sarah Parker asked about nosebleeds and vomiting that were happening to her children when they started eating mostly raw vegan foods.

A: Dear Sarah,

Regarding your children's nosebleeds or vomiting after eating cooked foods. I discussed this with Dr. Timothy Trader, and we both feel you will eventually have to feed your kids more cooked or more raw foods to avoid these symptoms. Because your children are extremely vital, each time they eat something not natural to their systems, their bodies will try to get rid of it. Dr. Trader pointed out the nosebleeds are a sign of high blood pressure. The blood pressure will rise as a result of the body's attempt to get rid of poisonous substances. If the blood pressure gets high enough, the nosebleed will result. You may want to bring some healthful food with you when you go out, and if you do go to a restaurant, take a list of what they could give you to make a good salad. You can make a delicious dressing and bring some avocados or something else the children love to eat that you can add to the salad. When your children do get sick, it's important to talk with them about the reasons they are not feeling well. Do this calmly, so you don't start a conflict. I can tell you from experience; it needs to be done with much love and tenderness.

*Also note that an excess of salt causes high blood pressure. Most processed foods are loaded with salt.

Q: My 7 month old daughter has lots of energy, gives me normal diapers, nurses on demand, and babbles. She's hitting all of her physical milestones on average, except she can't sit unsupported yet. The only concern about her development is she has some really irritable and cranky days when she is very clingy and screams if I dare put her down. However, when she is in my arms, she is happy, smiling, laughing, babbling...so it's probably a stage, *but* I read one of the symptoms of failure-to-thrive is when a baby is irritable, so I just can't get that out of my head.

A: Young children need to be carried unless they want to be put down. I remember my son cried whenever I put him down, and I thought he was just irritable and cranky, but I learned later through an attachment parenting group I attended, young children need to be carried unless *they want* to be put down. I then carried him very frequently from the ages of 5 to 7 to try to make up for the constant carrying he so needed when he was younger because he seemed to be asking for this. People told me I was crazy and had separation problems when I carried him so much, but I no longer cared what others said. It seemed the more I carried him and was there for his needs, the more independent he became. Be there for your children now. You will be amazed at how fast time goes, and they will no longer want you to carry them or sleep with them. It is so important to fulfill their emotional needs while they're young and not always able to express them verbally.

Q: "I eat what I think are healthy raw foods: raw fruits and vegetables, nuts and seeds. I crave nuts and dehydrated foods, but I don't seem to feel well after eating them. I often get a sinus headache and constipation."

A: Overeating nuts and dehydrated foods is not only hard on the digestion but depletes the body of water. We require nourishment from water-rich foods—fruits and vegetables. Nuts and dehydrated foods are also acid-forming. Dehydrated foods, especially those that are store-bought, often contain excess salt and will create salt cravings. As you will see in the chapter on teeth, excessive nuts and dehydrated foods can cause major dental problems.

Q: Many parents have asked me, "How do we get our children to eat more greens and salads? We know it's important to have greens in the diet, but our children seem repulsed by green salads and vegetables."

A: It often happens that once children are consuming a high percentage of fresh fruits and vegetables, they may automatically acquire a taste for greens as well. (See the Raw Family Journey of Sarah Parker and her family.) I read a chat on a raw food website that focused on the greens dilemma. One parent was wondering if anyone ever stops to think about why "green" is such a turnoff. Some parents felt we pass that on to our children. Another parent suggested making beautiful names for the green food such as "green emerald" or "green jade." I think that is a fantastic idea. As I suggest in my general tips section, my children loved giving names to their dishes, and I gave fun or beautiful names to many of the dishes I served them, which made them seem more enticing. A creative mom, Heather Stewart, told me she makes green smoothies and pours them into colorful cups that hide the green color. Since the green smoothies are sweetened with fruits, her two boys love them and don't see they're green. Tera Warner (www.rawmom.com) suggests something you wouldn't think would make much difference, but really does, "When trying to get children, husbands or strangers to eat smoothies (especially GREEN smoothies) nothing gets it down the hatch faster or more eloquently than a *straw*. Slip in a straw, decorate it with a slice of fruit and a sprig of mint and you'll be smiling as you watch the glass empty and giggle when they ask for seconds."

Q: Yuko Lau asked, "Do you know those 100% organic juices everyone is giving to kids? Can you tell me why they are so bad? They are organic and 100% juice with nothing else added. I can't really think of anything except they're just not that fresh. What do you have to say about them?"

A: Dear Yuko,

Boxed juices are total sugar. The fruits in those boxes are no longer real, and, in actuality, the teeth will be sitting in sugar. The only way the body can assimilate vitamins from fruits, is from real ripe fruits presented whole—the way they are found in Nature. When fruits are pureed or juiced, they must be eaten immediately, or else the nutrients evaporate and oxidize. That's why baby foods sitting on the shelves for many months are totally devoid of nutrients and enzymes; and the baby's body has to work hard to detoxify them. The same is true of boxed juices.

To process juices in boxes, they first have to be cooked to be preserved. Because they've been heated and processed, they no longer retain the ability to become alkaline in the body. Processed juices remain acid and acid forming. Had they been raw and fresh they would be alkaline forming as soon as ingested.

Please only eat fruit when whole, raw, ripe, and organically grown. The fresh, whole fruit contains fiber which slows the uptake of sugars so the blood sugar doesn't spike.

Q: A few nursing mothers have asked:"I don't seem to have enough milk for my baby's needs. Is there anything I can do to increase my milk supply?"

A: Relaxing, drinking enough water during the day, consuming plenty of water-rich fruits and vegetables, and letting baby nurse with an unrestricted time frame should help to increase your milk supply. When my children were young babies, well-meaning friends, doctors and nurses told me not to nurse them more than every 3 hours, stressing how important it was to establish a strict schedule. I found, upon first trying to follow these rules, I had created a tremendous amount of stress for both myself and my baby, who needed my total willingness to give milk for nutrition and emotional bonding whenever desired. When I nursed according to my baby's demands, my milk supply increased and began to flow more freely.

In addition to this scheduling question to the mother, I also ask about diet. Women who eat raw foods call me and have some of the same problems other women experience. It makes sense that women who eat predominantly cooked and processed foods may run the risk of difficult pregnancies and childbirths and problems of adequate milk supply. Women eating predominantly water-rich, high enzyme fresh fruits, leafy greens and other vegetables will have more than enough milk for their children, as do all the vegetarian animals in Nature. I ask these women if they are eating dehydrated foods and salt. When these are consumed regularly, I have seen the mother's milk supply negatively affected because they dehydrate the body.

28

Raw Families—Their Journeys to a Healthful Lifestyle

"It's bizarre that the produce manager is more important to my children's health than the pediatrician."

MERYL STREEP

Throughout this book, I've presented my description of my family's raw vegan journey and transition to a wholesome live food lifestyle. The goal of this book is to provide guidance toward healthful living nutrition. Rather than focusing on the percentages of raw food, it's preferable to move the family in the direction of increasing their raw food nutrition. Initially, my husband wasn't in favor of increasing the raw food in our diet because I had abruptly pushed it on him. It would have been more advantageous to move gradually and less overtly toward raw foods. All of a sudden, not only was he being deprived of his favorite cooked foods at home, but his wife was embarrassing him by bringing avocados and tomatoes to add to salads whenever we went to restaurants. Raw foods made so much sense to me, especially when I saw how they were of great benefit to my son's healing from allergies, chronic ear infections and asthmatic symptoms. It simply seemed realistic to me to dive totally into live foods overnight, but my husband hadn't yet understood the health rewards of the raw food lifestyle.

As time went by, and I tried to become less of a coercer and more of a good example, I was happy to hear my husband giving raw vegan health advice to friends and family. He now accepts and supports the way I chose to eat and has increased his own intake of fresh fruits and vegetables. Whether one eats 30% or 70% or 100% raw vegan foods, everyone is on his own individual path toward learning and growing. Whoever has been exposed to this natural lifestyle stands to benefit from this important life-enhancing information.

In this chapter, I present many other families who discovered the raw food lifestyle provided them with physical, mental, emotional and spiritual benefits above anything else they had ever encountered. Rather than setting up straight interviews with these families, I gave them questions and asked them to write about the most significant aspects of their journey to a healthful raw food life-style. Some of the questions included: When did you become a raw foodist? What inspired you to move toward raw vegan foods? Did you plan a pregnancy on raw foods and how long were you eating raw foods before the pregnancy? What did you eat during your pregnancy? How did you feel during pregnancy? How did you give birth, and were you happy with the outcome? Do you have a supportive spouse? What kind of exercise are you doing? What are your sleep patterns? What are you and baby eating, or is baby solely nursing? How is the nursing experience? Do you have plenty of milk for baby? Describe your daily diet. What success did you have in transitioning older children to raw vegan foods? Explain any difficulties and/or benefits of the raw food lifestyle. Talk about other areas of healthy lifestyle that benefit your child and your family. Give what you feel would be pertinent, truly valuable advice for other families considering the raw food lifestyle for raising healthy children.

To follow are accounts on the subjects of pregnant women on raw vegan foods, homebirths and/or unassisted childbirths, and nursing babies, some about the journey to becoming a raw food family, and some about raw foodist teenagers. This is the search for a simpler more natural life and a better future for the children. Each article emphasizes what is most important to that family, and what has had the most profound effect. There are teens who believe this way of eating leads to excellent health, the end of animal suffering, and the best diet environmentally for the planet. I feel so blessed to be able to pres-ent these wonderful testimonies, and I applaud all of these individuals and families for fulfilling their most basic instincts:

The Boutenko Family

I first heard about the Boutenko family in October 1997 when my children and I were visiting raw food author and lecturer David Wolfe in San Diego, California. It was just after the publishing of his landmark book, *Nature's First Law: The Raw Food Diet*. David told us of a Russian family living in Oregon who switched to raw foods and were completely healed of all kinds of ill-nesses. David saw the Boutenko family before their 1998 hike on the Pacific Crest Trail, 2,600 miles long, from Mexico to Canada. Read about their story in *Raw Family—A Story of Awakening*.

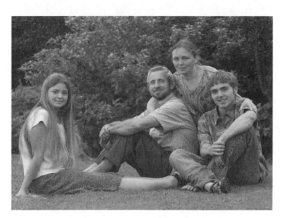

Valya, Igor, Victoria, and Sergei Boutenko

The Boutenko family presented a talk and prepared a raw food dinner at our home in October 2003. Victoria Boutenko spoke with so much passion about the benefits of raw foods, and her listeners were inspired. Her husband Igor and son Sergei prepared raw dishes outside on a long table, and got the children involved in the food preparation. They believe children learn about health from an early age through preparing food together. The Boutenko family stayed at our home for a few days, and their talk was spread over two evenings. They slept outdoors on those chilly and drizzly October nights, using only mats and sleeping bags. The whole family sleeps under the stars all year long unless there is heavy rain. They believe oxygen is very important for healing, and a lack of oxygen could be one cause of normal cells transforming into cancer cells. Some attending Victoria's talks, including myself, joined them in sleeping outdoors.

Sergei Boutenko, now in his early 20s, explains when he first began the raw food diet, he committed to a two week period, this then increased to a month, and then he continued. As a result, his grades in school significantly improved, from D's to A's and B's. Sergei and his sister Valya eventually dropped out of school and began homeschooling and taking courses at their community college. Sergei felt his energy and fitness ability improved from the raw foods. At age 16, he wrote, "Now after seven years staying 100% raw, I am able to run 12 miles uphill in an hour and a half and never get out of breath. I can snowboard for twelve hours, six hours in the day and six hours at night, and still have enough energy to go for a long distance run. My self-esteem has increased to the point where I never feel depressed, but in fact I am happy no matter what happens."

The Boutenko family has published some wonderful books that include many of their favorite raw food recipes. They have traveled extensively, extolling the power of the raw food lifestyle. They are a great example of family support through following what they truly believe. The following contains more information about the Raw Family in their own words from their website, www.rawfamily.com:

We are the Boutenko family, also known as the Raw Family. The four of us embarked on a diet of entirely raw foods in 1994, when we had become seriously ill. Victoria had arrhythmia and edema and was obese and depressed. Igor suffered from painful rheumatoid arthritis and had severe hyperthyroid. Sergei was diagnosed with diabetes and was supposed to go on insulin. Valya had asthma. We also had many other problems, like indigestion, lack of energy, mood swings, and dental problems. Medical doctors considered these illnesses incurable.

However, after we went on a raw diet, we healed all of our health problems. You may read more about our story in our book *Raw Family*.

Today we experience radiant health and constant happiness. We do not have any medical insurance because we feel totally in charge of our health, and we continually experience a high level of energy. Each one of us can run for many miles. In 1998, we hiked the length of the West Coast of the United States on the Pacific Crest Trail. We ate only raw foods, and sixty percent of the food we ate was wild edibles we found on the path.

Having been on raw foods for so many years, we have acquired invaluable experience in living on a raw food diet. Being pioneers, we have made a few mistakes that we've studied and corrected. In our lectures, books and videos, we share our experiences. We are constantly doing research and we communicate our updates and discoveries in a monthly e-newsletter.

In Victoria Boutenko's article "Your Body Never Makes Mistakes," she tells how every effort towards natural living makes a difference: "Eating more fresh fruits and vegetables, sleeping with an open window at night, wearing clothing made of natural fibers, drinking pure water, exercising, getting sunlight regularly, not suppressing sneezing, yawning and stretching, reducing stress, turning off electrical devices when not using them to rest from harmful electric fields, reducing use of soap and chemicals, buying organic produce, and thousands more, including giving your microwave to your enemy."

Valya and Sergei Boutenko presented their own teleconferences respectively on March 12 and 13, 2008. Valya, raised on raw foods from childhood, spoke on helping children to eat more healthfully. She is enthusiastic about the importance of green smoothies in children's diets and recommends getting the children involved in the preparation of the smoothies. Her favorite smoothie contains one mango, one banana, one orange, leafy greens (she loves chard but suggests starting children with Romaine lettuce), and two cups of water.

Valya had healed from asthma and Attention Deficit Disorder (A.D.D.). More than ten years ago, her parents explained to her why it was so important to change to a natural diet. Only two weeks after having begun to eat raw foods, she became aware of her increased ability to concentrate—even for 16 hours a day, and her schoolwork improved dramatically. Instead of watching television, she began reading a book a day simply because she enjoyed it. Valya explains, "Many mediocre students who switched to raw foods went from being poor students to excellent students. A.D.D. is food-related. Many children have been able to reduce or completely eliminate medication through dietary improvements alone." Valya further clarifies, "When junk food is not obstructing your mind, you can become calm and learn anything you want." She also points out she has no need to take medicine of any kind because she doesn't get sick.

Every year in Ashland, Oregon, her hometown, Valya plants 60 fruit trees.

Sergei talks about the benefits of picking wild greens, breathing fresh air, and getting adequate exercise. Since wild edibles haven't had contact with humans, they are even more nutrient-rich than organic or biodynamic produce. Wild plants contain 92 minerals, their roots are three times longer than common plants, they give us the opportunity to eat locally, help to boost our immune systems, and are cost-free except for the knowledge, time, and effort it takes to pick them. Since they have never been hybridized, nor sprayed with pesticides, they are more likely to contain vitamin B12, and they don't even need to be watered. Sergei explains there are only 250 poisonous plants out of the 31,000 plants available to us. He describes Miner's Lettuce as "tender, succulent lettuce, rich in vitamins A and C, and very good for eliminating stomach upsets. Wild edibles, including dandelion, purslane, lambsquarters, sorrel, wild berries and so many others are immune system boosters. Sergei leads hikes and walks, searching for wild edibles, internationally, and can be contacted at www.harmonyhikes.com. Sergei also expresses his love of green smoothies but underlines the importance of alternating the leafy greens they contain since nature makes it possible to eat a variety of foods to avoid toxicity. One of his favorite smoothies contains 4 ripe peaches, 1 banana, 2 handfuls of spinach and 2 cups of water. Sergei says, "I'm not into 100% raw food to be dogmatic, I'm into it for its health benefits."

The Kimmel Family

I met a most amazing raw vegan family, the Kimmels, when I spoke at the Living Now Festival in Western New York in August, 2004. The family sings and plays great music together with their family band, called Ashanan Music. They used to live in New York, but have moved to California. One thing I noticed immediately was how relaxed baby Djembe seemed, how trusting, and how content he was to be held in the sling with mother Yemaya while she was singing with the family band. When I first asked Yemaya to write for the book, she exclaimed it was a timely opportunity as Djembe was thriving on raw foods, but she was getting all sorts of comments from people about how she wasn't giving him enough protein/calcium/B vitamins, etc., only later to hear those same people comment on how healthy and happy he looked. And her new pregnancy was turning into a raw pregnancy after all. Yemaya said it was just where the baby was leading her. She didn't do it intentionally because she was concerned about detoxification, but baby talks, mommy listens. Yemaya Kimmel wrote the following article on her experiences with baby Djembe in 2004. In 2007, she and Mike had another child, Ayla-Sage. See picture of Yemaya nursing her children on page 99.

Mothering Djembe by Yemaya Kimmel, March 2004

Djembe was born at home, after 5 days of labor—actually a wonderful, profound, spiritually transformational experience for me in which I let go of my old maiden self to embrace my new life as Mother. We honored a Lotus Birth with Djembe, which means we did not cut the cord. It remained attached to the placenta until it fell away on its own, exactly one week after his birth. So he came into this world whole, not cut in any way—no circumcision, no blood drawn, no vaccinations, and we knew we wanted to start this precious new soul's life with the purest nutrition possible, nothing but mother's milk, followed by organic raw plant foods.

Djembe was exclusively breastfed for the first nine months of his life. We planned to wait a year, but the return of my menses at eight months signaled my intuition that it was time. We went slowly at first, starting with tastes of avocado until Djembe got hold of a banana and figured out how to poke a hole in the skin with his four teeth. Then again at 11 months, he initiated a new food at a raw gathering in the woods when he discovered wild apples and instinctively bit into one. Now at 18 months, he eats anything organic and raw that he can't choke on, although he's mainly fruitarian, still nursing, and, I must say, is one of the most lively, energetic children I've seen. He's never been to a doctor either. As far as nutritional supplements go, I generally don't believe in supplementing a healthy kid. I believe in extended breastfeeding, so he is getting all the extra nutrients he needs from my milk. Once he weans himself, I'm sure the B12 issue will come up. And we'll deal with it when we get there. As I think about it though, the question that comes to my mind is—How come other vegan animals—all of them raw foodists, and most of them big and strong, don't seem to have a B12 deficiency? I know there are all kinds of scientific views on it, and, of course, with children, we all want to be sure, but I wonder this: For someone who gets mama's milk for as long as he feels he needs it, while eating fresh, raw, unprocessed, organic plant foods, wild and locally grown as much as possible, breathes fresh air in sunshine, eats plenty of seaweed, and as a toddler gets dirty hands in his mouth every so often, does this person really become deficient in anything? We will cross that bridge when we come to it, and like any other aspect of parenting, I will consult my intuition.

Along with breast milk and raw foods, we also believe in the importance of holding or wearing our baby until he lets us know he wants to play on the ground. Contrary to what some may believe, giving ourselves to our children does not mean giving up our lives. If we are their role models and teachers, then it is of utmost importance that we live our dreams fully. In my life as a musician alongside my husband in our family band, this has meant bringing our baby onstage in a sling at every gig. People have been generous enough to offer to hold him while we were onstage, but I enjoy having him with me, and he belongs with his family, performing music of peace and positive change right along with us. We generally play at outdoor festivals and control the stage volume, so his hearing is not affected. He is much happier being with Mommy while being homeschooled in music at the same time. At 18 months, he is quite the drummer, which we believe has everything to do with being involved in the music his parents make.

On the subject of illness in children, I am so fortunate as not to have too much personal experience with that. Djembe has never seen a doctor. He's had the sniffles or a cold maybe twice, and we just nursed lots of mama's milk and let nature take its course. Just a couple weeks ago, he got his first fever. Thankfully it only lasted from three to four hours. I'm glad I didn't have much time to intervene. His body knew how to heal itself.

I'd love to say it's his raw lifestyle and upbringing that makes Djembe so alert and healthy. It certainly does not hurt, but maybe we just got lucky. Either way, I just feel so blessed.

I met Shawn Kimmel, a 17 year old raw foodist teenager, at the Living Now Festival in the summer of 2004, when he was playing excellent music with his family as part of Ashanan Music:

My Raw Food Journey by Shawn Kimmel, April 2005

My name is Shawn Kimmel. My journey to a better self began when I was four years young. My intuition hit me, and from somewhere deep within me, I just knew it was wrong to eat animals. I told my father and sister how I felt, and together we began eating a vegetarian diet. When I was 11 years young, my younger sister Kyla decided to become vegan. On this diet/lifestyle, she felt and was more alive. She believes people are not meant to eat anything that comes from an animal, and shared with me her philosophies and ideas on this subject of human and animal rights. Soon after her, I decided to become vegan too. I stopped eating dairy and eggs and had great success. I continued on, content to be eating cooked vegan food until at age 12, my friend Yemaya introduced me to the concept of the raw food diet. She gave me a book called *Survival into the 21st Century* by author Viktoras Kulvinskas. This book really inspired me, so I got another book by author David Wolfe, *The Sun Food Diet Success System*, which I highly recommend to everyone. I passionately read through these two books, and many other books about the raw food diet, health, science and nature.

While studying in depth about raw foods, I decided I was going to eat all raw. Jumping cold turkey into such an intense diet change was very challenging for me. The detoxifying process was hard. I went back and forth from eating all cleansing raw foods to binging on cooked junk for about a year. During this time, I lost a lot of weight and was looking and feeling good. I could not figure out how much or how little to eat, and it all seemed hopeless, but I had faith and believed I could achieve health through raw foods. I knew I would figure this out no matter what! I started eating lots of green leafy vegetables and some raw plant fats (avocados, olives, nuts and seeds) and lifting weights. I gained 50 pounds. I went from 110 pounds to 160 pounds in one year and felt better than I've ever felt in my life! I transformed from my thin unhealthy body into a vibrant healthy person. It was truly amazing! I strongly believe the raw food diet is the best diet for us and the planet. My dream is to live in total harmony with the planet and everyone on it, and one day I will. I have been eating 100% raw organic vegan food for three years now, from age 14 through 17, and am feeling great! I eat what my body tells me to—fruits, vegetables, nuts and seeds.

I have known Diana Heather and David since 1996. Diana attended my class "Creating Healthy Children" in New York City, and stayed in touch with me during her pregnancy and after the birth of Ben. Here Diana writes about her pregnancy, childbirth and raising baby Benjamin. In 2007, she experienced her second pregnancy on raw foods.

Monkey Baby Ben-obo
by Diana, March 2005

My name is Diana, and I would like to share with you some of my experiences with raw pregnancy, childbirth, breastfeeding and life with a raw baby. Five months before I conceived, I did a three week fast at Dr. Scott's Natural Health Institute in Ohio. I had expected to do a water fast but after three days had a severe crisis, and so I alternated water days with juice days. Having had some concerns about my fertility in the past, I was hoping the fast would help my body welcome a pregnancy. And it seems as if it did! When I got

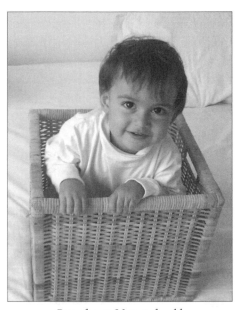

Ben-obo at 30 months old

pregnant, I had been 99.9% raw for nearly four years. I was 38 when my son was born.

Overall, my pregnancy was easy and without complications. For the first four months of my pregnancy, I really didn't have much appetite at all. In the first month I lost seven pounds as I didn't feel like eating much of anything. I never threw up, but I did feel nauseated sometimes. It was a bit frustrating to figure out what I wanted to eat; so many of my old favorites were now un-desirable. Friends and the pregnancy books I read all stressed the importance of eating a lot of protein. For a while, I found myself getting caught up in the conventional fear mode of nutrition, but I finally let that go.

Things got better around the fifth month of my pregnancy when my appetite came back. However, I still couldn't eat as much as I did before getting pregnant. My body would stop me from binging. I didn't really have cravings that everyone usually associates with pregnancy. There were a few weeks when I desired olives, but that was about it. My problem was trying to ascertain exactly what food I wanted; I would walk around the entire Whole Foods store and look to see what might attract me only to be frustrated that nothing called out my name. Fruits went down well, but I sometimes had to force myself to eat salads, nuts and seeds during the first trimester.

My partner, David, had just opened a raw vegan restaurant in New York City, so I was surrounded by delicious raw dishes every day. However, sometimes just looking at all the food turned me off and certain smells would irritate me. It was great not to have to prepare my own food when I felt tired and to have such a wide variety of foods available. I found the agave lemonade to be quite refreshing. In the fifth month, I couldn't get enough of a spicy Moroccan cauliflower dish. In general though, strong flavors like garlic, onions and spices bothered me, especially as my belly got bigger. In my eighth month, I really enjoyed making sandwiches with veggie nut patties and chopped veggies in Napa cabbage leaves. I would usually have fruit or a fruit and coconut smoothie, often with ground flax seeds, for breakfast. For lunch and dinner, I would have salads with either nuts and seeds or patés. I ate one or two avocados per day. Sometimes I would wake up in the middle of the night hungry, and an avocado would satisfy me and put me back to sleep. Snacks would be either fresh fruit or a small portion of dried fruit. Throughout the pregnancy and to this day, I am taking a vitamin B12 supplement since there is no consensus on whether it is necessary. For the first month, I ate some bee pollen, but David was opposed to this so I stopped.

Having read much about natural childbirth, I chose to get prenatal care from midwives instead of from the conventional medical establishment. I had read about unassisted childbirth, but as this was my first pregnancy we felt we needed the reassurance of consulting with a midwife. The only tests I consented to were blood tests to check my iron levels and urine tests to check for protein and sugar. Blood tests in my eighth month indicated my iron levels were very low, so I really tried to eat more iron rich foods like pumpkin seeds, raisins and spinach along with vitamin C rich fruits and vegetables to increase the iron absorption. I was even concerned enough to take a supplement that is widely recommended. It tasted terrible, and David wondered how anything boiled and processed could be beneficial, so I stopped taking it after a couple of weeks.

From the third to the eighth month, I went to prenatal yoga classes two to three times per week. I found them both challenging and relaxing. The classes provided an excellent way to meet other pregnant women and share experiences. All the women had at least one ultrasound, and most knew the sex of their babies. While we had our pregnancies in common, I often felt worlds apart in lifestyle choices. Everyone would comment on how small my belly was, and sometimes their concern would rub off on me, and I would wonder if my baby was all right. Deep down inside, I knew all was well and going as it should, but my fluctuating emotional states would sometimes get the better of me. By the ninth month, I had gained about 17 pounds.

Labor began on a Sunday morning around 11 a.m., when my water broke after breakfast in bed. The initial contractions were very mild and we excitedly began preparing our birthing supplies and being sure our midwife friend was available if needed. The contractions began to get a bit stronger two hours later, and then they were coming every two to three minutes. Around 2:15 p.m., they became so intense that all I could do was close my eyes and stay down on my knees with my arms over the sofa, crying out, "Ow, ow, ow!" David had filled the bathtub but didn't have time to put in the filter bag. So I only got in it briefly, as we didn't want the chlorine in the water to affect the baby. I thought I could try different positions until I found something that was comfortable, but nothing was taking away the powerful energy that was concentrated in my body. I was more or less fighting the flow of the contractions and concentrating on the discomfort. I remembered my midwife had told me to think of the baby and to talk to it. "Come out, baby, I want to meet you!" I said. That seemed to speed things along. At the end, I was totally inside myself and oblivious to anything around me. For the birth, I was kneeling on the floor with my upper body in David's lap. David was sitting on the edge of the bed and was rubbing my back during contractions. A little less than six hours had passed from the water breaking until the baby was born. The baby started crying before it was all the way out. I turned around and saw this tiny person and couldn't believe it had fit inside of me. I picked him up and put him right to my breast; he latched on immediately as he gazed up at me.

The umbilical cord was an amazing sight—it was like a thick, long, radiant braid that was pulsating with energy. The placenta came out about 20 minutes later, and we put it in a bowl next to the baby. I had heard of people eating their placentas as a way to get more nutrients and to supposedly prevent postpartum depression. So I licked a bit of it and found it didn't have any flavor for me. I had no desire to take a bite and eat it. We wrapped the placenta in towels and it remained attached to the baby until 48 hours later. By then, the cord had become very thin, hard and brittle. We wanted the baby to receive maximum benefit from the placenta and umbilical cord. We had heard about Lotus births (where the umbilical cord falls off on its own accord while still connected to the placenta), and we planned on doing one too. But the hard cord had a kink in it that the baby seemed to be using as an arm rest, and it was pulling at his umbilicus. We felt the cord for any signs of action and found none, so David carefully snipped it off. The placenta was also beginning to smell in the very hot, humid, summer heat. We froze the placenta so that we can plant it under a special tree someday. We also saved the dried cord. After we cut the cord, I was holding Ben at waist level, enjoying the freedom of not having to hold the placenta as well. All of a sudden, he started swinging his arms and legs, and climbed up to my shoulder, and gave me the most amazing look in the eyes. He was definitely a little monkey. I couldn't believe a two day old infant could climb like that. We named our little bonobo (bonobos are a species of primate, similar to chimpanzees) Benjamin, and often call him Ben-obo.

When Ben was born, he weighed just over 6 pounds, and was 19 1/2 inches long. He gained weight very slowly, and for the first five months we believed he was in the 10th percentile on the standard growth charts. Most of the babies I saw around us were much bigger. I began to wonder if he wasn't getting enough breast milk. When I tried pumping, I could only get out an ounce or two of milk. Like so many new mothers, I worried about everything. Suddenly, in his sixth month, he had a growth spurt, and people started commenting on how big he was. His cheeks are very chubby now. I had been too busy to dwell on why he was relatively smaller than other babies his age. I truly think that once I stopped focusing on his growth, nature took over and went on its course as it should. Who was I to question, worry and fret when nature is on auto pilot and knows best? It is something I will remind myself of over and over again as we face other parenting "challenges."

Ben's skin has a wonderful glow to it, and many people comment on how lovely it is. I think it is all the colorful produce we eat that makes him so radiant. We have also put him in the direct sunlight for several minutes a day since he was a few days old. We haven't put any creams, soaps or herbal products on his skin or hair—only filtered water. People have also noticed how alert and aware Ben is. They can sense there is something special about him.

Ben was pretty much constantly held from birth to five months of age. Even with carrying him in a sling frequently, in the first two months my wrists got very sore. Because his body had to adapt to my body's movements, he developed a great sense of balance, and head and neck control early on. He loves standing and taking steps, and he has very strong leg muscles. We still hold him a lot, but now he likes to sit and play with his toys and to walk around and explore as we support him under his arms. We practice "Attachment Parenting"—we are very close to him physically and quick to respond to his needs and wants. He sleeps with us in our bed; we couldn't imagine putting him in a cage in another room. We try to keep him diaper-free and practice "Elimination Communication." In the first few months, there was much more elimination than communication!

At eight months (as I write this), he still only gets breast milk. He loves to suck on carrots and celery stalks; they seem to be good teethers. He doesn't have any teeth yet, so we are in no hurry to give him any solid foods. Ben has always been a frequent nurser, and from about four months of age on, he would usually drink from both breasts at each feeding. When he was a newborn, a feeding could take 30–45 minutes. Now it sometimes takes less than 5 minutes. He has become a very efficient nurser.

After Ben was born, my appetite came back with a vengeance, and I am enjoying my food again. My favorite salad these days is mesclun greens with Udo's oil and dulse flakes. I find breastfeeding makes me quite thirsty, so I am drinking a lot of young coconut water. I have lost all but 4 pounds of my pregnancy weight, which I probably need for breastfeeding. Exercise has always been my weakest link, and especially now that I have so little time with all the demands of motherhood. I have to find ways to fit it into the day. A few minutes of jumping on the rebounder here and there and walking are about the only things I've been doing lately. I definitely need to become more disciplined in this area.

Finally, I would like to mention what an incredible support David has been during my pregnancy, birth and his new fatherhood. His main way of contributing is to prepare my meals with love so as to nourish both the baby and me. That we are both committed raw vegans makes things easier. We both feel so blessed finally to be parents and to have such a super baby like Benjamin.

The Corwin Family

We met Beth, Steve, Spencer and Buddy Corwin in 1996 through home-schooling our children, and we became close friends. Steve brought his son Spencer to a science experiment day at our home. He also brought his vegan lunch. I ate my raw vegan lunch. He was very curious about the way I ate, and began almost immediately to make changes in his own family's nutrition. We saw each other frequently for delicious meals. Our families also got together at Hudson Valley New York EarthSave events, and Steve and I started the "raw table" there. They moved from Westchester County, New York to Montauk in Suffolk County, New York, where Steve and Beth asked me to be a speaker for their East End EarthSave event.

This family has always been driven toward a simpler more natural life, which took them away from Westchester, New York to the beaches of Montauk, New York, and then to beautiful Costa Rica where they've built their hacienda in the mountains about 40 minutes from the Pacific Coast.

Raw Evolution by Steven Corwin, December 2004

Whatever I say here today will most likely change in the future as I am forever evolving. Ten years ago, my wife, one year old son and I, all vegans, were living in Westchester, New York. One day my wife complained about the "normal" conversations the friends in her mommy group were having. I said, "Honey, we are not normal, so all normal stuff will seem boring to us." I immediately got on the Internet and began to search for new, like-minded people in the area.

I found EarthSave, and soon we were at a potluck dinner making new friends and having more meaningful conversations. So there we were, vegan, with our new kin and on top of the world. That is, until we met Karen Ranzi. She spoke of something we had never heard of—a raw food lifestyle. I questioned, "Do you mean there is more to healthy living?" Karen introduced us to a whole new perspective, which right from the very beginning resonated with us and became the focus of our existence for the years to come. For my wife and me, anything we get excited about becomes part of our lives and something we enjoy.

It took us a few years to become totally raw. We experimented, listened to others, read books on the subject and experimented more. We tried all the complicated mixtures in many of the uncook books, but found them too difficult, time consuming and just too rough on the digestive system. I was inspired and determined to invent quick and easy recipes that even pleased non raw food people and nearly wrote a book on the subject. Then, once again presented with a whole new level of thinking at a potluck dinner, we gave up olives, olive oil and salt. All my recipes had to change, and I started all over again.

At many of the potlucks, the topic of discussion was finding the best place for conscious raw foodists to live. It was agreed that it had to be warm enough year round to grow tropical fruits, with fresh air and clean water. We went through every state of the union, none of which could meet the criteria. It seemed no such place existed. That was until we vacationed in Costa Rica. While touring the country, it became obvious this was the place we were looking for.

After going back home to New York, life was just not the same. All we thought about was eating that fresh flavorful fruit. It inspired us to spend the next year researching and planning our subsequent trip to Costa Rica to look for land. Combining intuition and Internet, we honed in on a mountainous area in the South, near the Pacific coast, halfway between the small city of San Isidro and the ocean.

We spent two weeks visiting several regions in Costa Rica before looking for land in our chosen area. It didn't take long to find the right spot. We committed, and soon thereafter became land owners in Central America. It all seemed so dream-like, but it was very real, and we were on our way.

During the next six months we rearranged ourselves and surroundings to prepare for the big move. We were both excited and anxious. So many doubts and questions came to mind, but we just followed our hearts. We stopped thinking of what we were "giving up" and focused solely on what we were to gain.

At that point in our lives, we were living as naturally as possible with our two boys, which meant minimal intervention when it came to health other than treating our bodies to the freshest live food we could find and letting our bodies do the rest. It worked very well for us, and we were quite healthy, making it an ideal time for our transition to living in the tropics.

Moving to Costa Rica with enough clothes, books, some bedding and personal items to fit into a few duffle bags and backpacks, at first, felt like we were on vacation. But after a few months, we were all feeling the pain of adjustment which only lasted a short time, thank God. It was then that we all settled in and began to feel like we were home, even while living in the 30 year old very modest farm house.

It didn't take long before we began building a new home for ourselves, a community/yoga center and developing the farm. This was the place we talked about so much at those potluck dinners. A place where we could find the optimum balance by breathing fresh clean air, eating only natural foods grown on the farm, drinking clean alive water, experiencing pure nature and where our very daily actions would bring joy to our hearts and "exercise" to our bodies.

It became apparent that good nutrition doesn't only come from good food. Sun, water, air and our thoughts are just as important and should be ingested in their natural state. Clean air with plenty of oxygen nourishes our cells. Fresh natural sparkling water excites and hydrates the entire body while the sun feeds us through eyes and skin. Doing fun and meaningful physical activities keeps our blood flowing to our muscles and brains, but the absolute best nutrition we have found for our bodies is thinking thoughts of appreciation.

Looking out into the natural surroundings triggers wonderful healing thoughts that replace any of those musty old unhealthy ones that used to swim around in our minds running us ragged. Thoughts are where life begins and lay the groundwork for everything we experience in a given day. They directly affect the outcome of our existence. If we want to experience freedom and joy, we need to think thoughts that will bring us to that place. Living simply in Costa Rica has helped us to see this and practice it as part of our daily diet.

This sounds so simple, and it really is. Life need not be complicated. It's up to us, and all it takes is a fresh new thought to get it going. By living more simply and being surrounded by nature's bounty, our thoughts shift and slow down as well. Sometimes, it's all that's necessary to begin the liberation. So the only way to change this world is to change what we think, one clean, beautiful thought at a time, and let the new era of purposeful and deliberate evolution begin.

Free as a Bird by Beth Corwin, October 2004

Recently, I examined the phrase "free as a bird." Are birds ever really free? Yes, it is amazing to watch them as they have the gift of flight and can soar overhead so freely, but like all animals they are tied to their environment by the food they eat. If the food they eat in the forest is destroyed by natural or manmade disasters, how do they cope? As I see it, they have two choices. They can remain in their damaged environment and possibly die or travel to another environment where food is abundant, and thrive.

This phenomenon directly relates to me and my family as we thrive on the raw food lifestyle. We eat fresh, raw, organic fruits and vegetables. I began dwelling on this concept when we were living in Montauk, New York. We were part of a coop (8 families) and fortunate enough to be able to transport organic fruits and vegetables from all over the world at all times of the year, for a reasonable price. On one level, it is nice to be involved in world trade, exchanging money for organic sustenance. On the other hand, it started to feel like a waste of the world's energies and resources, and also extremely strange to come in from a snowstorm in December and be eating juicy mangoes in front of a roaring fire. So…what's a bird to do? Or in this case, a family of four guided by the raw food lifestyle.

We realized all the food we were eating and desiring came from warm tropical climates, where sun is plentiful and snow does not exist—a place where people not only live in comfort, but thrive without the use of heat or air conditioning. A place where all that is needed is simple shelter, where water is plentiful, air is fresh, sun envelopes the land, and fruits and vegetables grow abundantly. Our bodies were craving that environment as well. We were being driven by our desires. It was time for a BIG change and Costa Rica was beckoning.

And so in the winter of 2002, we visited Costa Rica to see its offerings, and it offered all we desired and more. We spent the next year realizing what a huge change it would be. My husband and I are in our forties and our two sons were 6 and 8. Would we be able to handle dealing with life so differently? Moving away from family and friends, and our local homeschooling group? Learning a new language? Separating from the American way of life and adopting a whole new methodology? We looked at it seriously, we looked at it lightly, with skepticism, delight, and we all decided YES. The time was right, the opportunity for change NOW. Thanks to my husband's unique talent of combining intuition and Internet, he found the ideal location to relocate. On our second trip to Costa Rica in March, 2003, we purchased land, and in December, 2003, we made the move.

Here it is 11 months later, and our decision to move has surpassed all expectations. All of our needs are being met, and all of our dreams are manifesting rapidly. Our farm has an abundant supply of fruit: avocados, bananas, oranges, coconuts, papaya, mango, manzana de agua, guanabanas, guavas, lemons, mamonchinos and mandarinos acidos. We have planted many other fruits as well since our arrival and look forward to harvesting these too: pineapples, marañon (cashew fruit), sapote, jackfruit, durians, grapefruits, figs and carambola (star fruit). Also available to us are many new types of greens, yuplon, hibiscus, cranberry hibiscus, asinasin and sorillo. These provide a fine balance with all of the fruit sugars we're ingesting.

Our family has also increased in size to 5 horses, 11 chickens, and one playful puppy. For our first five and a half months here, we lived very simply in a modest and rustic Tico (Costa Rican) home. We enjoyed the simplicity. Since June 2004, upon its completion, we have been living in "Pura Vista" which definitely lives up to its name, Pure View. As I'm here writing, I can choose to feast my eyes on the raging waterfall, the distant but visible ocean or the majestic mountains. Our family house constructed of local bamboo and other beautiful wood will be ready for occupancy on December 1, 2004. We will break ground for our community center in January, 2005, a sacred space to hold yoga classes.

One of our greatest desires was to integrate with the local "Tico" (native Costa Rican) families who have been here for generations. We are blessed with Edgar Jimenez, our farm manager, who has lived here in this neighborhood his entire life. Not only is he trustworthy, hardworking, honest, intelligent and knowledgeable, but a real joy to be around. With his passion for life and knowledge of this climate and land, he put together an incredibly talented team of workers. We are enjoying learning their natural ways of farming and caring for animals, and they are respectful and accepting of our organic 'no chemicals' policy and our unusual lifestyle. The sharing of knowledge surpasses farming and animal care—our family has been invited to share their customs for celebrations such as graduations, communions, weddings, Sunday afternoon meals, Good Friday lunch and Christmas and New Years parties. What is truly amazing at these events is that they even honor our lifestyle and diet. While they are eating their rice, beans and meat, they are serving us their fresh fruits and salads. There is a high level of respect on both sides. I think they understand how much we appreciate their land and enjoy the fact that we are its caretakers and only want to add to its abundance.

All four of us have expanded our skills—from learning how to use a machete, caring for and riding horses, planting and harvesting incredibly delicious fruits and vegetables, working with local woods and building useful household items, and mastering a new language. The boys and I are also teaching English at our local school which has 20 students ages 7–12. The children are open and welcoming, and it is such a great way to exchange customs, languages, games, songs and humanity.

And so as I reflect upon this last year, I feel very full, in mind, body and spirit. I am grateful that we had the courage to follow our dreams and listen to our hearts. It has been an incredible year of growth and manifestation. How grateful I am that we chose to move to an environment that contains all of our food. By living with the land and eating its local gifts, a real shift has taken place for our family, as we feel more connected and harmonious to our true desires.

A huge acknowledgment to Karen Ranzi. I was fortunate enough to meet Karen at an EarthSave potluck dinner in 1996. We had never been exposed to the raw foods lifestyle, and at first didn't know if we would be up to the challenge, as living the vegan lifestyle at that time was already a huge commitment. But by realizing there are always many levels of evolvement, and being open-minded had always been a good thing, we decided to pay close attention to the message that was being offered. We listened, we watched and observed, and decided to align our desires according to the raw food principles. For us this meant changing slowly and steadily. We began with fruit meals for breakfast (instead of grain) and gradually having grain-free lunches as well. At first, for us and the children, the grain-free lunches provided a huge challenge, but the more creative we became with our menu and the more we let joy and simplicity in, the easier the process became. We stopped buying certain items and started buying others. As we were liberating ourselves, shedding appliances and processed foods, living with fewer things started to become very enjoyable. We were more connected to the journey than the destination of a 100% raw food diet.

After some time, I also made the choice to be a relaxed raw foodist instead of a righteous one. I had been around too many righteous people in my life and had been righteous about things before, and realized that type of energy just seemed to push people away instead of creating connection. The relaxed way just felt so much better, and it is a real gift to allow others to choose. Being a powerful example in the raw food movement and holding the torch instead of the sword seems to have incredible effects. Thank you, Karen, for being the messenger who delivered this incredibly powerful message. My life has never been so rich and rewarding.

You can explore their website at: www.vidanatural.info.

I met briefly with Erika and Ofek and their baby daughter Momo when I was presenting on "Raw Parenting and the Continuum Lifestyle" at the Portland International Raw Food Festival in Oregon, August 2003. I looked up their website, www.economads.com to find so much valuable information about natural parenting, green intentional communities around the world, and much more. Erika, Ofek and Momo left Israel in search of egalitarian, green intentional communities in January 2001. I was very excited to have Erika write about their experiences:

Erika, Ofek and Momo
September 2003

When I met my partner, Ofek, back in August, 1999, he had been vegetarian all his life (fourth generation), vegan for five years, and was interested in going raw. I, on the other hand, had just gone back to eating meat after a few years of being vegetarian and was not at all interested in raw vegan food. We soon got pregnant, and then it was very important to him that I eat an all-vegan diet for the health of our unborn child, so I did. Over the next couple of years, he often commented that we should eat all raw, but I wanted some time to get used to the vegan diet, and I really enjoyed cooking new vegan dishes.

When Momo was 5 months old, we took off backpacking around Europe (and eventually the U.S.) in search for community (see our website www. economads.com). In December 2001, we finally made it to Spain to visit the raw foods community, Ecoforest. We prepared ourselves for the fact that we would be eating all raw for the first time. We stayed there for a month and a half eating 100% raw vegan foods, and then we did some sightseeing for a month in Granada, and then visited two more communities for two weeks each, and then back to Ecoforest for two more weeks, all while keeping on an almost 100% raw diet. Then we went to Morocco and we fell off the wagon because we really wanted to try the cooked Moroccan specialties, and for the next nine months, we were visiting communities and relatives, but it was very hard to keep raw when there was always cooked food around. So depending on the place, we were on and off—it was easy to be raw when there were other raw foodists at the place we were visiting. Momo was always a great eater, eating lots of fresh fruits and veggies. However, we found that with time, if she saw one cooked dish on the table, she would push aside the greens and stuff herself with whatever else was there, leaving little to no room for the live food.

In January 2003, we went to visit my partner's uncle (who is a raw vegan M.D./Naturopath) in Minneapolis, and we lived there for three months, in the same building as his 100% organic raw vegan restaurant Ecopolitan. There we had our own kitchen and access to plenty of good food. We were a block away from the largest food co-op in the U.S., which every day at 6 p.m. would give away their produce that hadn't sold. Not only was more than 75% of our food free, we were surrounded by raw foodists and raw food talk—the restaurant carried every book written on raw foods.

In May, we moved here to Portland where we have our own place again. Our stove has never been turned on, and we continue to maintain a close-to 100% raw vegan diet. Momo, now three, is a raw food lover, though she hasn't lost her addiction to cooked food yet and still has cravings. We are trying to deal with different strategies. On a typical day, she'll have some melon when we first wake up, followed by her favorite—a sliced apple with a thin layer of tahini, and we usually snack on fruit here and there. I get veggies from the farm I work for at the farmer's market, and every day around 4 p.m., we will have a large salad made of some lettuce, dark greens, and whatever other veggies I got, plus a dressing of olive oil and lemon juice and occasionally crushed sesame seeds. These days she prefers her tomatoes out of her salad, and likes her salads just green with dressing. Sometimes I accommodate her wishes, but we don't always like her to be picky like that. Around 7 p.m. or so, we might have another piece of fruit or she'll have whole carrots and a dressing/dip. My next move is to try to get us to eat less fruit and more greens. In the past week, we have tried to have two salads a day, but it's hard to fit them in, especially in fig and plum season. This morning she ate all the cherry tomatoes off our plant, and when she asked for more, Ofek satiated her with a few collard leaves off the plant, which she immediately stuffed in her mouth, making her raw food parents beam with pride.

What I have learned from watching Momo (and ourselves) with food is: If we want her to eat raw, we can't have any non-raw foods around, and we have to be raw too.

Compared with two years ago, I feel I have been totally liberated from the kitchen. I used to spend at least three hours a day planning meals, cooking and washing dishes. Now I only spend a total of a half hour ripping leaves and chopping veggies, and I don't have any pots or pans to scrub.

Still, being raw can be isolating, and the ideal would be to co-live with other raw foodists in an extended family situation. We try not to make any commitments until a core group is formed.

—Erika

[As of 2009, Ofek is guiding 100% foraging trips in Israel: www.lakatim. tvuna.org]

I met Kathy Raine and her family when she and her two children came to my annual Thanks Living Party on the third Sunday of November, in which we celebrate the life of the turkey instead of the cruel slaughter of millions of turkeys at that time of year. We celebrate with a gourmet raw food potluck meal and a gratitude circle where the guests stand in a circle and express their gratitude for so many blessings.

The Raine/Wright family, formerly of Ithaca, New York, moved to Montreal, Canada.

The Raine/Wright Family
April 2005

Kathy Raine wrote:

My husband, my daughter (born 1989), my son (born 1994) and myself started our raw food journey around 1997 in Michigan, where a Hallelujah Acres health minister told me about a way of eating that would cure my chronic jaw pain. Absolutely nothing else had worked for this pain, and after a few more health problems piled up on me, I decided to try raw foods. After two weeks of carrot/apple juice and salads, I was off my codeine pills. I knew I was on to something, and since I was the family chef, so were we all onto something. I

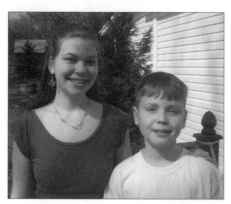

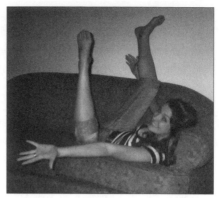

Alexa and Leland Raine/Wright   *Relaxed and radiant Alexa Raine/Wright*

didn't have much information except a few "un-cookbooks," and so I started to explore. Soon I noticed everyone's health was dramatically improving and we weren't getting sick any more.

We moved to upstate New York in 2000, and our raw diet sort of fell apart. Eventually my pain came back, and I knew what I had to commit to. At the same time, one of my children was having intense emotional problems. I knew this child might "outgrow" this "stage," but I might not get through it. It dawned on me that while I myself was eating 100% raw, I still had some reservations about it for my children and husband, who weren't 100%. So now it was full steam ahead with their food plans (with their agreement, of course). I made raw granolas out of buckwheat, fruit smoothies, and raw veggie burgers, raw pizza, raw lasagna, raw vegan sushi, etc. in my dehydrator. The health benefits for my children were many: no longer did we have to run a vaporizer in every room during the winter flu season; my husband wasn't falling asleep all the time while reading, driving, etc; my one overweight child was now at a healthy weight; and my other child, the "ADHD candidate," quit talking about suicide and was enjoying life again.

After about two years on our 100% raw vegan diet, I felt my family's health wasn't as excellent as it should be. Our dental health was starting to deteriorate; we were getting cavities again, and this didn't seem right. My son developed eczema, and my energy level wasn't what it was when I first went raw in 1997. I started taking supplements sold by many of the top raw food experts, and put my son on an herbal cleanse. These measures didn't produce a noticeable change, and I was starting to wonder if I was on the right track with my diet. Luckily I had a few raw friends who were eating simpler. Through their example, I took a long hard look at how I had tried to copy the standard American diet with raw foods. Our raw diet had become dehydrated, dense and high-fat.

So, I cleaned out the pantry again, and soon we were mostly eating just fruit—what a difference! We are now what I call "juicy-fruitarians," by which I mean we try to eat only raw, whole, organic, fresh fruits and vegetables, getting about 80% of our calories from fresh whole fruits, 10% from fats, and 10% protein. While I think this may be the biggest change for us yet, it's also been the best. I get a lot of good ideas from Dr. Doug Graham's research and work.

On a daily basis, we usually start the day mid or late morning with a mono fruit meal, such as melons or grapefruits, usually something juicy. Then when we're hungry again, we usually make a smoothie—no frozen fruit, but we do add ice at the end. We usually toss in lots of greens and eat it with a spoon because using straws would prevent us from insalivating the mixture. We eat when we're hungry, and we take fruit along on trips. At some point in the day, we might make a big simple green salad. I run a small co-operative produce buying club, and I get discount prices on cases of organic produce. I also buy extra special fruits every few days to keep things interesting. Generally, we eat what and when we want, according to what we need.

Besides diet, we also try to work on our health through exercise, sunshine, spiritual connection, and many other ways. We use little trampolines indoors and a big one outside in good weather; we do daily yoga, take long walks, jump rope, etc. We just spent five weeks camping outside in Florida in January and February, and now a family goal is to be south and sunny for the winter. I couldn't believe how wonderful it was to feel the sun every day. Another big challenge is to slow down and try to concentrate on what we think are the most important things in our lives. Sometimes the way we eat and live feels difficult because family and friends are eating differently, but we keep in mind what we know is true and have fun with life.

—Kathy Raine

I met SueAnn James when I presented "Raw Parenting and the Continnum Lifestyle" at the Portland International Raw Food Festival in Oregon, August 2003. SueAnn was pregnant at the time, looking radiant on raw foods. She wrote:

SueAnn James
September 2003

I would love to be a part of this wonderful and progressive project, and to be a divine and living example to women who have the courage and wisdom to take on the basics of a holistic living lifestyle by eating live food, the food created for us.

Before pregnancy, I was eating raw foods for 7 months. I am currently in my sixth month of pregnancy, eating fresh fruits, vegetables, soaked seeds and nuts, sprouted grains, fresh herbs and spices. Here are my typical daily meals in the order they occur:

16 oz. kale and freshly made apple juice
Water

Breakfast ball with sesame seed milk:
Ball—sunflower seeds, dates, one apple, raisins, one banana, and
    sometimes blackberries
Milk—sesame seeds, raisin soak water, flaxseeds, maca root powder,
    vanilla, cardamom seed pod

Snacks—raisins, tomatoes, blackberries, grapes, or nectarines

16 oz. kale and apple juice

Nori rolls:
Lettuce, tomato, green onion, bell pepper,
Seed paté: sunflower seeds, pumpkin seeds, fresh thyme, oregano, and basil

Snack—raisins
Water

I am privileged to have a very motivated and supportive spouse who is also 100% raw. He helps with the preparation of juices and foods, food shopping, cleaning up, does all the heavy compost work, and always has a positive attitude.

My exercise includes walking and dance. I usually sleep 8 to 9 hours a night with rare naps during the day.

I would like to stress the importance of the kale and apple juice in my diet. Before I started drinking 32 oz. of green drink per day, I was bed ridden with nausea, dizziness and fatigue. Within days of regular apple juice with greens, I was on my feet again with vigor. We knew I needed green juice for basic nutritional requirements; however, the taste of dark leafy greens juiced with carrots was more nauseating than no juice at all. I would literally throw it up. Then thankfully, taking the High Priest Kwatamani's advice, we started juicing the kale with apples, and the rest is history. The apple amazingly covers up any "green taste" and it's actually pretty yummy.

In the spirit of supreme love,
SueAnn Maria James

I met Francesca Repass at the Portland International Raw Food Festival in August 2003.

She was very excited to be experiencing her pregnancy on raw foods, and looking forward to having her first child. In September 2003, we began emailing back and forth and continued throughout her pregnancy. Later, she wrote about the horrific ordeal of her baby daughter's sequestration soon after birth. She pointed out the lack of knowledge on the part of the medical establishment and government agencies regarding the truth about health:

Francesca and Elizabeth Repass
September 2003, December 2003, July 2004, February 2005

In September 2003, Fran wrote: I am two and a half months pregnant and haven't had a stitch of morning sickness. Not once. I attribute it all to the raw food diet. I am very hungry. I do crave fish, so I occasionally eat it raw…sushi. I eat all sorts of other things. For breakfast, I used the juicer to make raw yam juice. I have been making almond milk as well and eating everything I have cravings for, except of course, cooked food. I don't have a husband. At age 39, I decided it was high time to have a baby. I met the most gorgeous 30 year old you would ever want to meet, and asked him if he would get me pregnant. He said sure, as long as he would not have to be responsible. It took me five years to get pregnant. After I went on raw foods and cleansed, I was able to conceive. During the five year period before that with real boyfriends, there was no pregnancy. Finally, I believe the almond milk helped, and the 30 year old. I got pregnant!

I love kale and canteloupe, and I do take a prenatal multivitamin.

In December 2003, Fran wrote: I have absolutely no side effects from this pregnancy. No pain, no nausea at all, no aches, no nothing, except for some occasional weepiness and tiredness. That is it though. It's a total breeze. I hardly know she's there.

I replied to Fran: I'm writing to find out what you are eating. Are you still eating raw fish? I know it's a source of B12, but fish is also loaded with mercury and chemicals like PCBs, and is too high in animal protein and saturated fat for human consumption.

Fran answered in December 2003: The baby is due April 21st. I had an ultrasound on Thanksgiving, and I am 4 months pregnant. The baby is totally healthy. The doctor who saw her on the ultrasound was so happy because she is perfect in every way—perfect kidneys, perfect skin, heart perfect…he was just thrilled because I will be 40 when the baby is born. The doctor was worried about Downs Syndrome and spina bifida, but not to worry, because baby is in perfect health, and I owe it all to my raw food diet. And the baby is a girl. I am thrilled. I thought it was a boy, because she is such a demanding, little live wire. No, I'm not eating raw fish now. I went through a craving for it. I am very good, following my cravings, but eating ultra healthy raw vegan.

I am going to the hospital to give birth. They are giving me a midwife also, as well as renting a tub for me in which to give a waterbirth. This is the best hospital in the country, they say. I thought of having just a midwife, but I want absolutely nothing to go wrong, so I will be in the hospital.

In July 2004, Fran wrote: Hi. I am very sad. My baby is extremely healthy, a nine on the Apgar scale. The birth was super easy. A three hour labor and she slid right out. It barely hurt; no complications at all. She is super smart, and started nursing within ten minutes after she was born. The entire hospital was impressed with her perfect skin and perfectly formed head, which didn't lose shape in the birth canal (I think because of all that good calcium from the raw greens I ate).

Anyhow, four days after she was born, Social Services came and took her from me, declaring me an "unfit" mother. I didn't hurt my baby, I love her, and I am not an addict of any drugs as you are all too aware. What happened was when I was pregnant, I sought cheap care at the Peoples' clinic. It's a place for low income people because I had gotten Medicaid. Although I didn't agree with their practices, and argued with them, I stayed with them because it was free. My friends kept urging me to get a midwife, but I didn't want to spend the money. I wanted to save it for my baby girl. Well, I fought with them. They kept wanting me to take this drug and that to prevent this and that rare disease or whatever. I kept saying, "No, she will be fine." They wanted me to take Paxil because I told them I had some mood swings, and I said no. I am pregnant, going through normal hormonal changes, and besides, I am fine. I don't want to contaminate my baby.

Well, the People's Clinic considered me a "bad mother" and called Social Services on me. That's not all; they did an illegal drug test on me which turned out to be negative of course. But in any event, they weren't trying to help me. They were looking for anything they could get on me. So I lost my baby. Only for

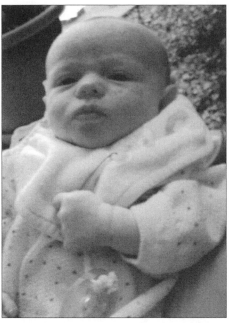

Elizabeth at 2 weeks – Already her face has broken out from the toxic sugar formula, in contrast to her clear skin at birth.

now, I hope. Social Services forced me to vaccinate her (which I didn't want to do), and told me if I refused, they would never give her back. What they did was criminal, but I have no power to fight them. They are the government.

My baby has been in two different foster homes now, and she has gastrointestinal reflux because she is allergic to her formula. She cannot digest it. Due to the stress and fighting this in Court, I have lost all of my breast milk, which I wanted to provide for her as the main source of food.

I am extremely sad. I don't trust the system. They say that I may get her back in six months to a year if I comply with them and do everything they tell me to do. One thing is getting all of her shots, and making sure she sees the doctor at every suggestion of theirs. I also have to do therapy similar to anger management, and yet I am already managing my anger extremely well, considering what they have done to me. They lied to get her taken away. They first said my house didn't have running water and electricity. I have both and proved them wrong. Then they said I had mental problems, and forced me to take a psychiatric exam. Their psychiatrist said I have a borderline personality

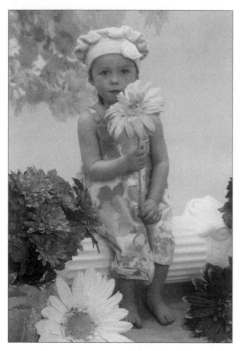

January 2007 – Elizabeth, saddened by her ordeal but recovering and glowing on raw foods.

disorder and a narcissistic personality disorder. I don't think I have either, and so I had my own test done. My psychiatrist said there was nothing wrong with me, and yet I still lost in Court.

It's beyond reason, and insane. A good lawyer wouldn't even help because there are so many lies involved, and the judge believes them every time. I am beyond upset. I just have to do whatever they say and jump through their hoops and pray I get her back. My Court appointed lawyer says I have a 50-50 chance of getting her back. So I pray. You can put this in your book as a warning to all how much the system doesn't believe in raw food "medicine."

I wrote to Fran on February 16, 2005: How are you, and are you making any headway in getting your baby back? I often think of you and pray your little girl will be returned to you soon. How sad it is that the public is so far from understanding healthy lifestyles that children are taken away from good parents.

Fran wrote back on February 17, 2005: I got her back on October 23, 2004, five months after they took her. She was crying daily in the foster home and doctors diagnosed her with "failure to thrive" because she was spitting up the chemical soy-based formula and wasn't gaining much weight. Now, with me 5 months later, she is healthy with rosy cheeks, has gained weight and is a happy baby. And Social Services sees this.

They gave her back because they were destroying her. It almost killed me to see her suffering, and knowing I couldn't help her, but I could if only I had her.

She is a different baby, they say; a happy one now. I am furious and think of suing them, but not now. It's too early, and they aren't out of my life yet.

But I am thrilled to have Elizabeth back, and yes, they immunized her and now they are pushing me to do so as well, although I am saying no. What they did to my daughter was unbelievably ignorant, but at least I have her back and she is thriving in my care, and they see this.

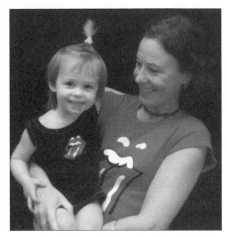

I feed her raw foods, but I also have to feed her (organic only) eggs and meat, and I give her goat yogurt. And, of course, I am giving her plenty of raw veggies and juices and raw fruit and almond milk, etc. What an ordeal I went through! But my daughter is, noted by everyone including the doctors, way advanced for her age, smarter than most babies her age and already crawling and sitting up at five

Elizabeth and Francesca Repass, January 2007

months in spite of "failure to thrive" and gauntness she had when I first got her back from foster care. Even though I feed her proteins like meat because I am supposed to, I have noticed she desires fruit and vegetables much, much more, of which I feed her plenty. Social Services thinks I am a good, loving mother, and I know I am because Elizabeth is such a happy baby. She was emaciated and had a "failure to thrive," and now, how healthy she is looking.

You can put my address in the book, in case mothers in a similar situation with Social Services taking their kids should need my help, or if people would like to send a donation:

Francesca Repass
4640 Greylock Street, Boulder, CO 80301
Phone: (303) 459-0155

Fran and I emailed each other on February 13, 2006. Fran expressed: Elizabeth is healthy and happy, and Social Services closed my case last summer, saying I was an "excellent mom." They couldn't figure that out before taking her away, feeding her only formula, making her sick with a "failure to thrive" diagnosis from doctors during the whole five months they had her in foster care. Now she gets almond milk and mainly raw fruits and vegetables, although I do sometimes give her eggs and some goat milk, for fear they will take her away again.

Author's Note: Rhio and I have founded Health Liberties Network, a not-for-profit organization to protect parents' rights according to their beliefs on how to best care for their children's health. Our vision statement:

Vision Statement of Health Liberties Network

Goals: To gather a coalition of advocates and supporters of freedom of choice in health care, in all fields (medical, legal, research, teachers, social services, legislators, etc.) who will come to the aid and support of individuals, families, and parents being persecuted because of their health care choices, and/or doctors and practitioners guiding those choices, such as:

> *Unless we put medical freedom in the Constitution, the time will come when medicine will organize itself into an undercover dictatorship to restrict the art of healing to one class of men and deny equal privileges to others...*
>
> DR. BENJAMIN RUSH
> PHYSICIAN, EDUCATOR, WRITER, PATRIOT LEADER AND SIGNER OF THE DECLARATION OF INDEPENDENCE
> (1745–1813)

a) Families who have lost custody of their children due to their dietary and health care choices;

b) Families who have lost custody of their children for refusing medical treatments, drugs or mandatory vaccinations;

c) People who have been forced to undergo unwanted medical treatments, drugs or vaccinations;

d) People who have been listed as terrorists because of their health views or choices;

e) People who have been sued for voicing their opinions about products, services, medicines, vaccinations, food products, etc;

f) Doctors and practitioners who are using alternative, complementary, holistic, or comprehensive health treatments and modalities in their practices, or who are following a health care system other than the standard allopathic medical paradigm.

And further, to

g) Protect the privacy of medical records;

h) Prevent substances in natural foods that have healing potential from being designated as "drugs." Substances inherent in natural foods shared freely by Nature belong to everyone—known as "The Commons."

www.healthliberties.org

We would eventually like to see a United States Constitutional Amendment guaranteeing freedom of choice in health care.

Miko Nelson and her family live in Katy, Texas. I met Miko through an email loop called rawbaby@yahoo.com. Miko was so happy to have learned the benefits of raw foods and to give this knowledge to her family. She also realized as time passed, one can get obsessed with food and forget there are many other important aspects to a healthy and happy life.

The Nelson Family
9/14/2003

I am so glad you are writing this book. I was just thinking late last night that I have no raw reference for children, and no support system.

My daughter was vomiting yesterday, and all I had to go by was Morris Krok's advice to drink lots of water and vomit a lot until it runs clear. That was great, and she even enjoyed drinking "to make it all come out." Yet, today, I could not make her go easy on eating, as Krok advises after a good purge. She insisted she really needed bananas, so I gave her one. Now she is out with her dad, enjoying their usual weekend together.

Our family became raw on February 2, 2003. We began the transition on July 6, 2002. Then in February, the day after I read *12 Steps to Raw Foods* by Victoria Boutenko, I got the incentive I needed. Before that, my husband and I agreed our daughter should eat properly, but we did not feel ready to do it ourselves. We realized it was corrupt to continue to sneak our pretzels and breads and the like. We knew we had to be role models and pure in our ways if we wanted to be responsible as her parents. My husband had been vegetarian for some seven years already before meeting me, and his commitment to raw is genuine, though he travels a lot, and many times all meals are served during day-long meetings and cooked fare is his only option. Even when the attempt is made to accommodate him, it seems not all caterers understand the definition of "raw."

My daughter still nurses at two and a half. She is a mono eater, and she eats whatever whole, living foods she likes. We even go to Waldorf classes each week, and she has no interest in the crackers and nut butters everyone else eats with their fruits. It is more stressful for her teacher to deal with our raw diet, as she feels guilty about excluding her. It is a parent-child class designed to guide parents in their relationships with their children. I feel I must homeschool her in the long-run, and I'm already in the mindset that we are homeschooling now. Waldorf ideals have greatly impacted our lives.

We live in Katy, Texas. The raw life is the best thing that ever happened to this family. I feel more honest to the core of my being. I feel clear and bubbling with a sense of centeredness. I want to reach out to God and see His reflection in myself, and I see Him in my daughter, husband and others.

9/30/03

I have been fasting since Sunday, drinking nothing but homemade lemonade. I am juicing in the evenings, as I have felt the need to do this. This is going to be my longest fast and my first juice fast. I consulted with someone about contemplating doing this, and on Saturday, I just felt it was the right thing to do.

My daughter accidentally ate cheese today at the Waldorf School. One of the parents served it, and I forgot to tell my daughter it was not in our diet. Besides, she is only 2 1/2. She wasn't happy about what she ate, and tried to scrape it off her tongue. I'm not sure if this is related, but her nose is really runny.

11/28/03

We enjoyed raw lasagna and sea tangle/carrot/ginger salad wraps for our Thanksgiving feast, which even the extended family thought was tasty. It was too heavy for us compared to our usual fare, but I was impressed by the outcome. I found it on the purejoylivingfoods.com website. I just discovered this vendor, and was encouraged by someone who is raw and has a small child.

[Miko started food logs on www.FitDay.com to record her family's food intake. She sent me two different food logs of family meals for similar dates in December 2003.]

Date	Meal 1	Meal 2	Meal 3
12/19/03	2 apples/2 grapefruits 3 dried apricots soaked and blended	4 cabbage leaves, 12" pc. daikon radish sliced into "crackers" with "chili" mung and lentil sprouts	3 bananas; 7 oz. cabbage juice, head of leaf lettuce, celery, grn onions, broccoli, sweet red bell pepper salad
12/20/03	durian split 3 ways, 2 oranges	2 bananas; strips of butternut, jicama, red pepper, red onion, beets in a salad with red beans	7 oz. mustard greens/ bok choy juice; 1/2 head of tatsoi with light tomato dressing & lentil sprouts on top
12/21/03	durian split 3 ways, 2 oranges	2 bananas, one apple, 10 oz. tatsoi/bok choy juice	red and green leaf lettuce salad with Coco-Yum dressing
12/22/03	young coconut/ grapefruit/ banana blended	2 bananas, 2 finger bananas, one apple, coconut water	live homemade kim-chee with julienned diakon, carrot, cauliflower & green onion salad
12/23/03	2 apples/2 grapefruits, 3 dried apricots soaked and blended	green salad	coleslaw
12/25/03	6 persimmons, a banana	Un-spaghetti, green salad with Coco-Yum dressing, "pumpkin pie"	large green salad with Coco-Yum dressing, daikon salad
12/26/03	8 medium-size persimmons	young coconut, banana	3 apples, coconut water, greens/nori salad with carrots, cashews and red bell pepper
12/27/03	young coconut/banana/ mesquite powder/vanilla blended, 2 apples and 1 persimmon	4 apples, banana	4 persimmons; 10 oz. spinach/cabbage juice

| 12/28/03 | 3 apples, 3 dried apricots soaked | 1 1/2 apples, head of red Romaine, head of escarole, bunch chives 1/2 daikon, 2 sweet peppers | 5 apples, 12 satsuma oranges, cucumber/celery/beet salad, 2 sweet peppers |

Reference for 12/19/03—Mason generally nurses 4 times in 24 hours (Date of Birth: 2/24/2001)

Date	Meal 1	Meal 2	Meal 3
12/21/03	1/3 durian	green salad	one young coconut; tomatoes, cauliflower celery salad
12/23/03	Blended apples, 3 dried soaked apricots	cauliflower/greens/olives/salad	young coconut, 1/4 head of cabbage
12/24/03	4 persimmons	"pumpkin pie," and later, garden "burger"	red radishes, cauliflower, coconut water

Reference—The Garden Burger is a Boutenko Family recipe

Reference—We fed old sprouts to birds in the a.m., and subsequently Mason ate some too.

The Pumpkin Pie recipe consists of 8 to 10 ripe persimmons blended with a teaspoon of extra virgin olive oil and some cinnamon. It is crustless, but Miko pours it into a glass pie dish. Any nut-based crust could be used, but she likes her version as it is healthful and delicious. [Without the nut crust, this recipe is more in keeping with the concept of correct food combining for perfect digestion.] Miko exclaims, "In the refrigerator, the pie solidifies. It is surprising!"
—Miko Nelson

Miko later emailed me to let me know she no longer uses fresh white Thai coconuts in recipes as these young coconuts are treated with formaldehyde and other chemical preservatives before they come into the U.S., and Coco-Yum is a coconut recipe. The coconuts are actually dipped into fungicides.

It's possible to buy untreated domestic organic coconuts at some health food stores and farmers' markets, but they can be quite expensive. Local coconuts, such as the green ones in Florida, California, Costa Rica and other areas, are pesticide-free and absolutely delicious.

My friend Amy Schrift moved from New York to Costa Rica. She bought 17 acres near my friends, the Corwin family. She wrote to tell me of a young couple who were planning an unassisted childbirth there, and the young woman was doing a raw food pregnancy. I was so elated and immediately sent some questions to Amy to ask to the couple about their raw pregnancy and raw food journey. I was so happy to receive this article from Laura Meyer two weeks later:

My Living Food Journey through Adolescence, Pregnancy, Birth and Beyond
by Laura Meyer, October 23, 2005

I was born on August 19, 1987 into a difficult living situation…that I could go on and on about …Just know it was really rough, and I spent my life trying to escape.

I eventually succeeded at the young age of 14. I changed my living situation on my own, and for the first time, I felt brave enough to take control of my life and help myself.

At age 14, I learned not to lie. At age 15, I learned not to drink, smoke, or allow people to use my body, mind and spirit for their own pleasure and unhealthy purpose. I learned to take more and more control of my Being as I grew, and felt stronger and more able. At such a young age, I was forced to tend to myself and take care of my needs because I had no dedicated selfless servant who lived to love me *unconditionally*.

At age 16, I moved out of my mother's home with my lover, Clinton, and began an exciting journey to independence a state away. I felt like I was in a big world full of learning experiences, and I had to stay strong and keep following my heart, even if I was scared or life did something I didn't expect.

I met Clinton when I was eleven, and after three years of a long distance relationship, I started seeing him regularly from age 14 to 15 1/2. Clinton and I were both totally unconscious that cooked food was an addiction that hurt our bodies. We were regularly binging together, not realizing it was unhealthy.

At age 15 1/2, Clinton found an article on the Internet about refined sugar. He had observed the children in his family were craving it in candy, pancake syrup, soda, etc., and he got curious. I used to eat packaged cereal for breakfast every morning at 15 1/2, but the morning after I read that article, I stopped eating cereal because I knew it was true. I could feel it inside me on all levels. So at age 15 1/2, I quit eating refined sugar and white flour. At that point, I already had extremely bad acne for five years, and everyone thought it would leave permanent scars. I wouldn't go anywhere without makeup, and I tried all the chemical products for sale at Wal-Mart and other stores. I was miserable and couldn't look in the mirror without hating myself for being ugly and fat. I was 20 pounds overweight. I weighed two pounds less at full term pregnancy than when I was 12 years old. When I quit eating white sugar, flour and dairy, I shed 10 pounds and a good amount of acne—HAPPILY!

Only a short while after reading the sugar article, I started thinking more about food. I wouldn't eat the chips with the guacamole any more. I would steam veggies, and felt weird about the way my thinking was transformed: "Are they losing vitamins?" It's strange and sad how much I hadn't been aware of. And then Clinton and I were in a Barnes & Noble bookstore with a gift card I received for my 16th birthday, looking for nutrition books. And as I was standing in line ready to pay, miraculously, Clinton came to me with the book, *Nature's First Law: The Raw Food Diet*, saying, "Look how cool, a bunch of naked guys in an avocado tree!" He has always found the coolest information. He plants the seed, and I water it. I was about to move from California to Arizona with Clinton in a couple of weeks, and I didn't open the book until I was on the bus to Arizona. It was just after my 16th birthday, and after reading three chapters, I threw away my lunch (sprouted grain bread with roasted peanut butter and banana) and dedicated my body to health.

Raw foods felt so right. I went into it very hardcore. I was unaware gourmet raw existed, so I ate mono meals (one whole food at a time)—unprocessed whole fruits, leafy greens, seeds, nuts, and herbs as I pleased. No oils, salts, no mixing. I went through extreme withdrawal…Emotions flying—food cravings all the time. Yet, over the course of a month, my skin had no pimples—no more acne, and I lost 20 pounds. I felt beautiful on the outside for the first time since I was 10 years old. After three months, the food cravings calmed down to a manageable level.

For the first seven months of my pregnancy, I ate mono meals—whole living foods, but I got my first job at a gourmet raw foods restaurant. The first time I ate there, I got a bellyache. My stomach was not happy. However, I was quickly addicted to the great taste and full feeling of raw food mixed with olive oil and sea salt. And I began eating gourmet raw from my seventh month of pregnancy. But later, I let go of sea salt and olive oil, and I began to transition back to no packaged or mixed foods, and succeeded by the time my child was born. Because I stopped eating packaged or mixed foods, onions, garlic, and strong spices and herbs, my breast milk was easy for her to digest, and she had no gas. I was highly addicted, and it took a lot of effort to go back to pure living, mono, whole, organic foods after exposure to gourmet, tasty, heavier foods. But, all along, I knew the truth. There were periods at the restaurant and afterwards during which I cleansed for a couple of weeks and ate purely, but I would really have strong cravings and give up, justifying the recipe food because it was "*raw*."

Anyway, my pregnancy went very well. I got pregnant a month after I arrived in Costa Rica, and after two weeks on the beach fasting on the water of wild coconuts. I felt great during the whole pregnancy. I can't remember any discomforts. Did I feel queasy? Certain smells, like onion, would make me queasy. I gained 20 pounds the whole pregnancy, and at the end when I had totally quit salt, I really lost some swelling in my body. You could see my entire body definition with no excess fat, yet my baby was big and so healthy, and I was healthy too. She came out with incredible strength, size and muscle tone.

My body felt better the more pure food I ate, but even though I was eating heavy raw foods for a while, I was always conscious and never overdid it. I felt so energized and joyful. All the way to term, I hiked two miles every day and about one and a half miles at the end of the pregnancy. I danced and felt so capable and strong.

Raw vegan foods gave me something I never knew existed…feeling my body, and feeling good inside of it. I'm so personally thankful to have found this naturally hygienic lifestyle, and I will always follow my higher self on this path. My truth is raw foods. Who knows how high this path will soar, or how it will transcend? For now, I feel great, I feel well, strong, full, able, energized, beautiful. I know how to heal on all levels of my being, and living foods is just one aspect on my healing path.

I love my Mother Earth, and I am thankful for her offerings. I respect her and desire to live in harmony with her.

My daughter, Harmony, came to me in Costa Rica, the place where I came to live in Harmony with Earth. I see my daughter to be a Harmony of me and my lover, one that brings joy: Harmony Joy Meyer/Harvey. Her birth was so beautiful. It was an "unassisted" homebirth. There was no medical personnel, yet I had beautiful angels assisting me, on the physical and spiritual (energetic) levels. Labor is something extremely intense, and has a lot to do with spiritual lessons. However, being in tune with my body and being healthy was certainly a huge help while going through the birth experience.

Harmony is thriving and so am I, on Nature's food and her love.

NATURE FEEDS ME IN EVERY WAY!

EAT FROM THE TREE, NOT THE FACTORY!

I met Sue Nackoney, her partner Jim and baby Persephone when I presented at the Portland International Raw Food Festival in Oregon in August 2003. She was carrying her little girl, Persephone, and they both had a really wonderful, happy energy, and it was easy to feel connected to them. I spoke with Sue quite a bit while I was there. Sue responded to my questions in an interview:

Sue Nackoney and Family
September 2003

Hi Karen!

It was good to hear from you. Wasn't the festival great? I was so happy to make so many contacts. Of course I would be happy to help you with your research; hopefully it will help others in the future. Your questions:

Q: When did you become a raw foodist?

A: Raw and vegan, October 2001 to June 2002; February 2003 to present.

Q: How did you eat during your pregnancy?

A: For the first two months I ate all raw. During the third month I was eating cooked vegetarian food—with dairy and a few eggs included. One time I ate fish, but that was it. By the last trimester, I was eating at least 75% raw again, with some cooked vegetarian food. I also included some raw dairy.

Q: How did you give birth?

A: I gave birth at home with my midwife, partner, and friend present. The baby was 10 days "post date," and I was told I would not be able to have a homebirth if it went another 4 days, so I had my acupuncturist help things along, as it were. We had a water tub, but I didn't use it. Persephone was born into the air of our home…above our toilet.

Q: How did you feel during pregnancy?

A: The first month or so, I didn't know I was pregnant, but I do remember feeling really tired. I kept feeling tired throughout the first trimester, but then my energy was better for the rest of the pregnancy until the last few weeks, which seemed to drag. By the middle of the second month, I had really bad nausea that would last all day, but I wouldn't throw up. Raw food like patés and hummus would not digest well or would give me a stomachache. The nausea got better by the beginning of the second trimester. But even in the second trimester, if I started to eat more raw food, I would notice the nausea returning. By the fifth month, I was getting heartburn. I had to cut out pasteurized dairy, any beans/legumes, baked flour products...By the last trimester, raw food was almost the only thing that wouldn't give me heartburn.

Q: What exercise did you get during pregnancy and after?

A: I got a lot of exercise. I rode my bike up to an hour a day commuting between work and yoga class. I did yoga every day for an hour. By the end of my seventh month, I stopped riding my bike and walked at least an hour a day, and did yoga most days for an hour. My job was active too, on my feet a lot.

Now I walk in the park for an hour carrying 15 pound Persephone at least five days a week. I also carry her and my groceries up to our second floor apartment. I still do some yoga, but less, an hour or two a week.

Q: What were your sleeping patterns during pregnancy and now?

A: I slept well for most of my pregnancy until the last trimester. By then, I wasn't as active and also the baby would be kicking, most often at night. Now I sleep pretty well at night, except when Persephone does a nursing at 2 a.m., I sometimes stay awake for a little while. Generally, I'm so tired I sleep as much as I can.

Q: What is your breastfeeding relationship?

A: I breastfeed Persephone on demand. We sleep in the same bed, and some nights she wakes almost every hour to nurse since a month ago when her teeth started to come in. I used to be careful about what I ate. Now I eat most things, except not much spicy, oniony or cabbage-y foods.

Q: What foods are you giving to the baby and how old is she now?

A: I waited until Persephone was six months old before giving her any foods to eat. She is now seven months old, and she will suck on soft fruit (bananas, mangos, peaches) and gum on hard textures (carrots, celery, cucumbers, apples). She is very interested in leaves of lettuce, spinach, parsley, basil, cilantro, chard and wheatgrass. She will grab them and shove them into her mouth as fast as she can. Then she likes to suck on the pieces of leaves but she doesn't really swallow them.

Q: Do you have support from your spouse?
A: Jim is 100% supportive of feeding Persephone all raw foods. He is also all raw since October 2001.

Q: How do you parent?
A: I'm the one who primarily takes care of Persephone. Jim has to work a lot out of the house. It's really important to me to respond to her needs quickly so she doesn't have to cry, feel abandoned, etc. At the same time, she is as much a part of my day as possible. I wear her in a sling for all outings and around the house while doing chores. We practice sign language, elimination communication, cloth diapering when necessary, and all three of us sleep together in the same bed.

My friends, Nancy Durand-Lanson and Eric Cohen-Solal, came from Paris, France to live in New York. I find them to be awe-inspiring, intuitive parents. Nancy's first child was delivered through Caesarean Section, and her following two children were birthed in a completely natural way after she and her husband had educated themselves on unassisted childbirth. They are very relaxed and trusting parents, and it's wonderful to watch them interact with their children. I have learned so much about positive nurturing parenting from Nancy and Eric. Their children are Lea, Babette, and Armonie.

I met Nancy in 1998 when she called me for a raw food consultation during her pregnancy with her second child, and we have been friends ever since. Nancy has been teaching raw food preparation classes on the Caribbean Islands of Martinique and Guadeloupe since 2003 and in France since 2006. It is her challenge to serve a healthful raw food meal in less than two hours, including instructions, to anyone attending her classes. In 2006, she taught a class of 45 people in Paris.

The Cohen-Solal Durand-Lanson Family
Fall 2004

I still remember the first day I saw Karen Ranzi just after a nature class we had taken with our children. While we were all eating at tables outdoors, I noticed her eating a celery stalk just the way it was. This recalled a documentary on instinctive eating I had viewed on French television fifteen years earlier. At that moment, I knew Karen was eating this way. Later, my friend Laurie told me to speak with Karen at a time when I was experiencing strong detoxification symptoms while eating totally raw foods during my second pregnancy. I feel it was predestined for me to meet Karen since I was ten years old, and all of these coincidences only led to meeting her and having raw foods in my life.

On a Friday night in June 1999 at Caravan of Dreams in New York City, David Klein was speaking about raw food. At that time, Eric and I were looking at ways to reduce the impact of our lifestyle on the environment and had already made some changes in our diet. Everything David said that night made sense. It was the easy way to eat. The next day was the EarthSave Hudson Valley potluck, and there we spent the evening talking with Wilson, who had made the change three months earlier. That same evening on our way back home, we stopped at the store to buy some fruits (because we had no time to eat at the potluck), and we were astonished by how good the fruits were.

The next day I was a raw foodist, and I decided my three and a half year old daughter Lea would also be raw, because I could not make two different meals at home. We decided to finish some of the food we had in our pantry, but we gave away most of the food requiring cooking. I got pregnant two weeks later and stayed raw for the following 14 months before going back to cooked food again. An exception occurred for one month when I ate cooked potatoes in the evening to stop intense detoxification.* Lea was insisting I cook some quinoa pasta for her, and I gave in. I moved back and forth between raw and cooked food for the next eight months. I was frustrated eating only raw foods, and thought I didn't do a good transition. In my mind, had I done the transition properly, I would not have had any cravings. So I decided to wait until raw food would come to me naturally. I was sure it would come. And it came only when I understood I need not stop eating cooked food, but should simply eat raw food. In my mind, it made a big difference.

My first attempt to be raw was hard on Lea because it was not her choice.

---

* At the time of this writing, Nancy had not yet become aware of the superior nutritional value of sweet potatoes compared with white potatoes.

She was miserable each time she was out and around cooked food. It was not the right choice for her. Raw food was my path, not hers. When I understood that clue, it became easier for her to eat raw. We had to have a rule, which was: Our house is a raw house, only raw is bought and eaten here. If one of us wants to eat cooked food, we do it out of the house. We stated it on a general basis so no one would be named. When at first, she would go to birthday parties, I was still preparing her food on the side, but little by little I realized it was useless because she did not want to eat it. I stopped preparing food for her when she was invited somewhere because it would go to waste. Four and a half years later, she was still eating cooked food outside of the house, but at home she was fine eating our raw food. Once in a while, she wanted some cooked food at home, so we would just take her in our arms and remind her of our rules.

We had to state a rule because Babette, born in 2000, had a raw fetal life. Since birth, she has only eaten raw vegan foods. She is still a raw foodist today even when her friends are eating crackers and "funny food" in front of her, but she would like to eat whatever Lea is eating because she wants to be like her older sister. Only last year when she was six did she become aware some people eat food we call "cooked," but she doesn't know how it's done because we don't have a stove. She doesn't ever want to try it. If Babette were to ask me that she wanted to try her friend's food, I would not refuse her. Many times, I have seen her refusing food, saying, "I don't eat that food." I never told her she couldn't have it; she just figured it out for herself. One day at the airport, we went to buy a bottle of water before getting on the plane. She was 2 1/2 at that time. The shop was selling sandwiches, and she asked what they were. I replied, "People call them sandwiches." She stared at them a little longer and responded, "I don't like that kind. I prefer the ones you make at home." It was the first time she was realizing some so-called foods don't look like our food. If Babette would ask me to buy her something processed and cooked, I would give her the same answer I gave Lea, "I can't buy you that because I do not want my money to support an industry that doesn't nourish my children and doesn't provide healthy and environmentally viable options." I came to say that to Lea too because I used to answer, "I can't buy something I know is harmful to you." But soon, I realized I didn't want her to eat cooked food thinking she was harming herself. Whatever we do or don't do, they will eat cooked food, either to try it here and there, or to oppose us. The way we eat our food is often more important than the food itself. If we eat it with happiness, it will digest better.

I had two pregnancies on raw vegan food; the first was not 100% because I became raw so fast, my body started a strong detoxification. Two weeks after I started eating exclusively raw foods, I got pregnant with Babette, so I was detoxifying during that pregnancy. My first three months were terrible. I could barely eat, and even the smell of the forest after the rain made me nauseated. Then one day I had contractions, and that's how I realized I was pregnant. Too much detoxification was going to the fetus, and I had to stop the detoxification to keep the baby. Then I started reading a lot on raw food and pregnancy, and also spoke with Karen Ranzi. For a month, I ate a steamed potato with an avocado in the evening. It did the trick in stopping the heavy detoxification.

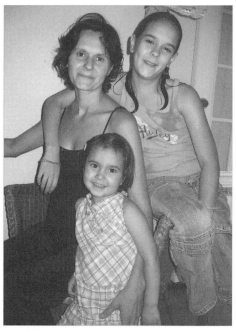

Armonie, age 5, Nancy, and Lea, age 13, in April 2009

Mid pregnancy, we decided to go unassisted. I had a planned C-section with Lea, but the second baby would not make it into the medical world. Eric read a lot on delivering and emergency situations. We also read on happy deliveries, and I knew it would be fine. I decided it would be fine.

I had a very happy and healthy pregnancy. We moved at six months, and I was still skiing at 8 1/2 months, while holding Lea between my legs going downhill. Babette was born after nearly ten months, give or take two or three days. I was not worried, but at one point talking with my family made me worried, so I called a few people to be reassured. I talked with someone who told me in her community, babies were coming when it was their time to come. They would not induce labor because nature does not make mistakes. I was totally fine after that phone call. Babette and I started labor in the middle of the night. I got up that night thinking I was done sleeping and began a puzzle. At six a.m., I went to wake Eric. I told him I thought I was in labor but not sure. He went to work that morning. Lea and I were having our day as usual, and the contractions were still coming far apart and not painfully.

I had read about water birth, and laboring in the water. We decided to take a bath, but the bathtub was clogged. I called Eric at work and asked him to come home. He arrived at two p.m. and took care of Lea, answering her needs. I was laboring in the bathroom, squatting on the toilet because I had the feeling Babette would hurt her head coming out on the floor, the way I was viewing the birth in my mind. Soon I was ready to give birth, but I needed Eric, and he was with Lea, so I waited until she was asleep. When Eric got ready for me, it went fast. I recall asking him when my water was supposed to break. He went to look it up in a book, but I don't remember what he said. Soon I needed to push, so I pushed once and twice, and she was born just like that!

She slid out of my body like an Aries, head and body in one push. The water bag broke at that time. Eric caught her very confidently, even though she was very slippery. I removed the bag from her, and there she was. I had torn. I stepped down from the toilet and sat with her in my arms. Eric went to wake Lea and to get a bowl for the placenta. We had decided to have a lotus birth. I sat in the bathroom for two hours and at one point felt an urge to stand. The placenta came down as soon as I stood up. We washed the placenta with water, but it was too cold and Babette reacted to it, so we finished it in warm water. We dried it as much as we could with towels. We kept in mind that whatever we would do to the placenta, she would feel it. I had made a wooden frame and stapled it onto a piece of voile. We placed the placenta on the voile to let it dry. The next day we washed it again and dried it. Babette was sleeping on me, and the placenta was beside us. It took one week before both of them were detached. The aim of the lotus birth is to give the baby the time needed to transition between uterine and air life. Babette took her time, but in most cases it only takes two to three days.

Babette weighed seven pounds at one week (we didn't have a scale at home to weigh her at birth). She has never had the need to see a doctor so far. She very rarely detoxifies, and when it does happen, she starts a fever and recovers after one or two nights.

Armonie, our third daughter, was born in April 2004. There is nothing to say about the pregnancy. We didn't go to see anybody about it. I knew it would go perfectly right. I kept on living my life, receiving wholesale boxes of raw, organic foods every Thursday, unschooling my kids with all the driving it takes, flying to Guadaloupe every 3 or 4 months to teach raw food preparation classes with my girls, and much, much more. One Thursday, I was restless and very busy—staying up until Friday morning at 3:30 a.m. I slept for three hours and was back on my feet again. Because of the raw food, I don't need to sleep long hours—usually, five or six hours are enough. I was surprised, though, by my high level of energy after a three hour sleep. On Friday, we prepared everything we needed to be out all day and drove an hour north to meet with friends. We had classes in the morning for those who wanted them, and in the afternoon, we went to a little creek where the kids played in the water and the adults conversed with their friends. It was a nice peaceful day for us. I was feeling some contractions, but I didn't know if they were the usual, or if this was *the* day. They were like very mild menstrual cramps, only not painful. I was just feeling the same activity I had already been feel-

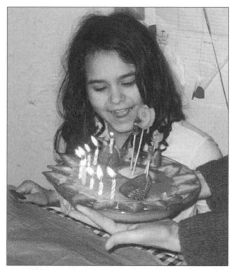

A beautifully prepared "cake" for Babette's 9th birthday, April 7, 2009

ing for two to three months. Anyway, that Friday morning I left home for the day with six towels, just in case. I had no reason to think she would come that day because we were two weeks before what I thought to be the due date. Since Babette was born a month late, I thought Armonie would go beyond her due date too.

We got to the creek around 10:30 a.m. and started to play. I was very happy, and my heart was feeling soon we would see our baby. I was feeling love, and loved. So I asked my friend Heather, "How do we know we are in labor; what tells us?" Heather had five children, so I thought she would be able to tell me. At that time, I had contractions that were there but not painful. I have to say at no time was it painful. I was feeling activity that I knew were contractions. I am reluctant to use the word contraction because of what people know about it, especially birthing women, and I didn't want anybody to worry, thinking I was having the painful kind of contractions.

So we still didn't know if it was happening or not. At 12:00 p.m., I realized I was definitely in labor because when I decided to sit and rest, thinking the contractions would stop, I found out I couldn't sit. My body wanted me to walk. It was very comfortable like that. So I started to cry because it was the most beautiful day since winter. I had planned to be at the creek for five days and could not believe I had to go back home. Here I was, desperate about the situation, trying to accept the moment, when suddenly I understood the "moment." I was going to give birth here. I had no will to go back home. I had been happy all week about the weather on Friday, and all our friends were *here*. I was smiling at the sky because it had been planned all week. At 12:15 p.m., I called Eric to let him know he could come, but I knew he was playing soccer and would get the message only at 1 p.m. At 1:00 p.m., when we finally spoke to each other, I told him my intention was to give birth right here and nowhere else. As soon as my decision was made, things organized fast. In the park was a gazebo. We took it for the day. My towels and some people's cushions made their way there too. We all had towels because the children were playing in the stream.

Each time a contraction was coming, I was closing my eyes to be with it in the moment, and I loved each of them. It was good to be in labor. All the children were playing peacefully and the adults were there, not watching me, just being with me and Armonie. All the children came around to watch, curious to see the new one to come. After Eric arrived, around 4:00 p.m., labor went on faster. I was waiting for him. A few times it slowed down, such as when a police car came to check on the park, and when a high school prom party came and waited for the gazebo to take pictures. A big thank you goes to Heather for organizing a fast, but efficient meditation ceremony to get them to leave. At this point, I needed to wash myself, but I couldn't go anywhere in the stream because the prom teenagers were there also. I asked Eric to drive me back home. Our friend Linda offered to drive us in her van. She lived only ten minutes from the stream, so we accepted since it was all right for me to be naked in the house, as I needed to be.

When we arrived, I went into the bathroom, thinking of taking a bath, and squatted on the toilette facing the tub. I was there for 15 seconds. Eric invited me to go into the empty tub when I felt she was coming out. "Eric, she is coming. Stop everything, she is coming now." So he got into position, I pushed once, and the head came out. Then I remember deciding to take a break. I put one foot down, and then I thought about that poor baby with just the head out, so I pushed again and the body came, the water broke, and Armonie was also born in the bag. We walked back to the room where we set up a bed, enjoying the baby and ourselves, and our friends came to see the baby, still attached to the placenta. After five hours, I got tired of waiting, so I squatted and started to push, but it came out right away. What I think about that birth is, when someone is healthy and has a positive attitude, everything falls into place at the right time. We called our baby Armonie because during the pregnancy and the delivery, everything seemed to flow in harmony.

We are doing the diaper-free method with Armonie. She picked up the idea of my asking her if she needed to go when she was 2 1/2 days, not weeks or months. I was so excited, I offered her to go maybe 15 to 20 times that day, and she did. After the meconium, she pooped only once a week for at least three months. It makes it easier to do for a mom because we can live with a few missed pees on us, but if too many poops were missed, it would soon become hard to do, given our lives outside the house. I think the reason is in our diet, there is very little unassimilated food. Also, she is more aware and faster because her brain and nerves are not clogged with too much mucus. She is light, easy to carry, and

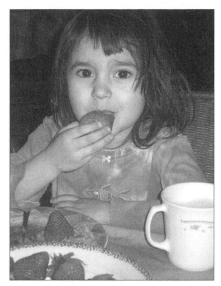

Armonie loves strawberries, April 2009

thin (our family's nature is to be thin). It's such a pleasure to have a baby like Armonie, and the diaper-free method and skin-to-skin contact are easy, simply part of our life together, not something we do, just us.

When we first started eating raw, we all jumped on fruits. They were so good. I remember just how good the fruits were, as if I'd never tasted them before. Now we are still eating a lot of fruits, but a lot of leafy greens also. The girls eat more fruits than vegetables, but when we are with Eric, we eat more greens and sprouts than fruits. We rarely eat our meals together, because we're not hungry at the same times, and we don't want to "push" food down just because it's "time" to eat. We make an exception for holidays and birthdays, but, as we know, on those days we're going to have a meal later, we often hold on to our hunger until that time. We also have a natural tendency to eat whatever is in season. We want more heavy foods in winter than in summer, when we can spend days on juices and light fruits, or light vegetables such as cucumbers, celery or sprouts. We don't say "no" to the girls if they want strawberries in the winter, and I will even buy them non organic if they really want them. I feel their strong bodies can handle the occasional pesticides. It is more important for me that we stay raw. I think we are trying to be like other parents who will go and buy candy, as we have compassion for our kids, and it's hard for them to understand and remember why we live the way we do.

Only now do I find my ten year old daughter Lea is able to understand and remember the meaning of our values. Children understand these principles at the moment we explain them, but then they forget. Between ages eight to ten, they begin to understand and remember.

There is no obsession about the choice we made to eat raw vegan foods. It came as a result of our search. There was no point in telling Lea to eat only raw. First, because she will do what she wants anyway. Secondly, we would be inducing a lot of guilt and pressure. But more importantly, we have already bestowed the gift, the option. Whenever she might feel down in her future life, she will always have the option to return to a healthy, vibrant lifestyle where living food and full acceptance of who she is will be the simplest and most natural principles driving her. We fully realized as a family, we could do a lot for ourselves, and make our life together serene and wonderful.

In Harmony and Serenity,

Eric and Nancy

Beata, brought up in Latvia, was living in Canada when a mutual friend suggested she consult with me regarding her pregnancy on raw foods. When I met her, I found a young woman very excited to learn all she could about a healthy pregnancy for her unborn baby. She has called me from distant parts of the world, including Hawaii and Israel, to further discuss specific questions about raising her precious daughter Sarah, and to get support. I love what Beata writes, and I feel the strength in her maternal instincts.

Beata and Sarah Barinbaum
April 2005

When I became pregnant, I was a student of Osteopathy in Canada. In order to have the pregnancy and the birth the way I wanted, I had to be far away from the people I always thought would be the closest to me; like my family and the father of my child. But that wasn't my reality. I started to move further and further west and away from them, following the necessity to feel safe and create my own nest.

At that time, I was very satisfied living on raw vegan foods for two and a half years. I felt blessed by the simplicity of my diet. I was eating what I enjoyed the most — juicy crunchy stuff. I was starting my day with a watermelon, later had a smoothie, had one big salad per day, created many variations of guaca-moles, enjoyed green juices and raw desserts, nuts and seeds, quite regular wheat grass juice and sunflower greens, lots of celery and cucumbers.

I was swimming and walking a lot, and traveled quite a bit. I was jumping on the trampoline even on my due date, and sitting in a Jacuzzi and dipping into a freezing ocean throughout the winter. In the mornings, I was walking barefoot on the dew, rain or snow, and was practicing Qi Qong. I felt very strong, clear and focused, and filled with energy. Through the entire pregnancy, I felt the best I have felt in my adult life. I didn't take any supplements, but I was adding a raw green powder from Nature's First Law [known as Sunfood Nutrition since 2006] to my smoothies. I didn't do any prenatal exercise, such as breathing or yoga. I did what felt the most joyful for my body and spirit. I was very fortunate, not experiencing nausea or any other symptoms some women have.

I was lucky not to experience cravings for cooked food until the fifth month of pregnancy when I visited Latvia, the country of my childhood. There I was craving potatoes in all their possible shapes and tastes. I ate them and enjoyed them, except the diarrhea part at the end.

At the very beginning, while still not knowing about a new life happening within me, I donated blood on the other side of the globe, in Israel. I had a hemoglobin count of 13 and a good level of vitamin B12. My overall health was very good, although I was quite skinny. By the end of the pregnancy, my hemoglobin was low, but my midwife didn't think there would be a problem because a woman doesn't usually lose more blood than the body will allow during the birth, so she agreed to do a homebirth.

On the miraculous *night of birth*, I was on the magical Island of Maui in Hawaii. To my surprise, the midwife asked us to meet her at the hospital to give birth in the birthing room there. I was already having my contractions so I refused her suggestion. I decided to have the blessed night of birth at the ocean under the stars, embraced by ironwood trees and devoted friends. I was walking in the waves to learn how to open myself for the birth, and running in the water for gravity to help. I sang and danced, and then felt loving hands massaging my belly, feet, head, and legs. Remaining the only one awake for the rest of the night, I journeyed towards opening with each sensation in my belly.

As the new day dawned, we left the beach and drove a short distance to the hospital. The next thing I knew, someone said, "There is a quiet place," and my water broke all over the Bible in the Maui Memorial Hospital Chapel, the quietest place available. I was half standing in the jungle of my own hair, remaining in the power of my instincts, in my own dress, and not connected

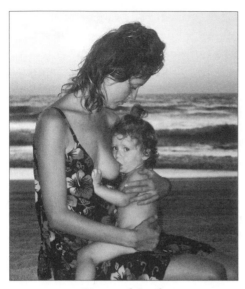

Beata and Sarah

to any equipment. I pushed four times, and a magical red haired girl appeared in my arms. A surprised doctor for the first time received a baby from a standing woman, and gave the just received baby right back to her demanding mother. He was not able to see, touch, weigh, poke, or do whatever doctors are used to doing to babies at birth. I signed that I didn't allow anything to be done to Sarah, and we took the placenta and Sarah and left the hospital.

We were lying in the darkness of the little tent my doula, Robin, made from a big scarf. The most beautiful girl with the eyes of the deep blue ocean was nursing at my breast for the first time in both of our lives. My doula had a cloth scale to weigh the baby so she would remain comfortable and feel as if she were still being held. To everyone's surprise, Sarah's weight was 3.5 kilos (7.10 pounds). When the pediatrician said, "Look at that beautiful baby fat," I said, smiling, "The secret is raw food."

We then left for the jungle house where we lived happily for the next six months. After the birth, we lived in the paradise of Hawaii, surrounded by bamboo forest and the jungle. We were waking up to the songs of tropical birds, and watching the dance of endlessly shaded bamboo and palm trees. This was mesmerizing for the baby, and there was no need for mechanically operated toys above the newborn's head. I was drinking the water of fresh coconuts every morning. Later I would eat some fresh, often newly discovered fruit and a big smoothie with fruits, avocado and blue green algae. Then in our long walks through the forest, climbing mountains, crossing fields and rivers, we were generously fed by varieties of guava fruit, rose apples (the first fruit my Sarah-Manusha was sucking on), pineapples, macadamia nuts, mangos and avocados, all freshly picked.

Coming home, I had a big salad containing spinach, cucumbers, tomatoes, celery, arugula and a pumpkin seed butter or avocado dressing. Manusha curiously fished the green leaves from my bowl and chewed-bit-sucked on celery, her earliest and favorite discovery that lasted a long time, massaging her gums, and continuously getting some juice. I enjoyed miso. In the evenings, I often had miso soup with ginger, seaweed and some of a mashed avocado, or kale salad with miso dressing.

I kept bottles of water in different places, drinking water while nursing Sarah. I always had plenty of milk, and Sarah still chooses to have 99% of her food from mama's milk.

Many women have told me they can't allow themselves to do what I do: not go to work and not send the child to kindergarten. It may not suit everyone, but I can be with my child 24/7 because I really want this. Sometimes I think, "Am I doing the right thing?" I hear lots of questions and doubts, and start having them myself, and then I remember it's up to me. The confusion soon clears and I know again - I want to do it just like this. So, how am I able to do this? Our life is simple, our expenses are minimal. They go toward food, rent, and travel. All of our senses are fed and fully awakened by Nature. We feel different temperatures from the air, sun, rain and the ocean water on our skins; just as Jean Leidloff talks about in her book *The Continuum Concept* (the only book I got to read when Sarah was 18 months)—grass, sand, surf, and earth under our feet; smells of endless blossoms, sounds of live music, stories, and songs of all living creatures. Colors, tastes, touch—all of this is generously and lovingly given to both of us by Nature. I don't need to use money for expensive diapers, wipes, formula, baby food, bottles, a swing, cradles, carriages, pots, soaps, salves, powders, cribs, shampoo, shoulder cloths, etc. I simply don't know how to use all these things. And buying them would surely take a monthly salary, maybe more. I've learned to fold her 12 flannel diapers we have since birth in ten different ways according to the changes. We have learned to spend our time together continuously, discovering each other, and learning about the world and ourselves. I have surrendered to the rhythm of Sarah's instincts, watching the changes in her face and body language, and taking her to the bathroom since she was three months old. Each day of my life since Sarah's birth is filled with the practice of being present, finding answers within me about values, learning about communication, sincere caretaking, independence, and respect, standing behind my words, clarity of my feelings, actions, and thoughts. I listen and see with curiosity. When I skip into something less than honest, my dear mentor reflects it right away, whether it's diarrhea after I ate a bowl of something cooked, or her restlessness when I get into my fears. I stay at home, and I don't have to earn money for all the above things that would require a monthly salary. Many say I am privileged to have the

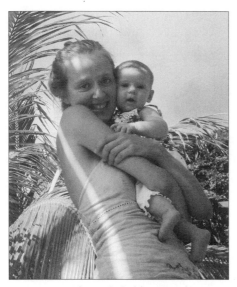

Beata lovingly holding Sarah

opportunity to stay at home, not work, and be with my child, but it's simply my priority. I'm choosing this way over other things at this time of my life. That's how it becomes my opportunity every single day. Some days, I think it could be so much easier to escape this closeness with my daughter and spend time with colleagues at work or school, people my age. I could send my daughter to other people to discover and comfort her, but I can't do it. I want so very much for my little redheaded girl, who is such a big part of my life, to have a mama as much and as close as she wants. I want to do it, and have us be together. I don't have much time for anything because we are always together. I don't have time to read, so I invent, watch, and play it by ear and from the heart in so many different situations. I don't have time to brush my hair, so I cut it. As difficult as this situation might seem, it is a blessing, and I have all of the time and all of me for us.

About our favorite times: Our long walks through rainforests and jungles in Hawaii, climbing for fresh guavas, mangos and rose apples through the forests and bushes; covering sleeping Manusha so she wouldn't get poked or scratched while looking for fresh figs and wild apples in Italy, and searching the ground as I gather hazelnuts and pine nuts generously left by the squirrels. We picked juicy apples, plums, grapes, blackberries, tomatoes, and kale, and gathered fresh seaweed in the Canadian Islands. Now in Israel, we have olives off the trees, Sarah's favorite after figs. She picks them with her tiny fingers with a full smile of the satisfied gatherer. She goes on to pick juicy and colorful grapefruits, pomelas, and fresh carobs. Sarah still plays with most of these, and seriously takes mama's milk as her food. Food for Sarah is always with us as my body is happily producing it, so we can go off far, and for a long time, and travel very lightly: two hats, a bottle of water and a blanket or throw because the ground is always wet with the morning dew. We sing and dance, hide under the huge leaves from the sudden rains, watch rainbows, and play circus in the tall grass. I can do all the silly and fun stuff—often thought of as weird unless a child is nearby. Sarah's playmates are all colors, textures and shapes of flowers, grass, leaves, and rocks, sticks, cones, shells, all the household items, and cats and dogs. A favorite was the telephone cord. There is no need for expensive unreal toys that don't move and smell strange. You always get quite a few of them from friends, and they don't hold Sarah's interest for more than three minutes.

It took me some time to understand why she would want to stay very close to me when I'm doing household chores. That's when she's very interested for a long time. She watches me do everything, often still while riding on my back, whether in the kitchen, garden, market, orchard, store or beach. I wash her diapers in clear, clean water so she can join in and play; and I don't have to worry about her swallowing any chemicals. We are climbing trees, preparing food, planting, cleaning, dancing, exercising, visiting friends, going to concerts, even giving piano lessons together. I've learned all these things are real for her. She demands to play with jars, bottle tops, boxes, pens, telephone cords, bags, tapes, and simply all the things I want to use at the moment—she needs to use them too. I am observing and discovering everything with Sarah; I didn't have my own experience earlier since I was alone a lot without a grandmother to guide me like a mother. I was longing and looking around for a wise grandmother who would teach me everything, and love us like a big Italian mamma, but one didn't appear. So all of the discoveries, diaper tricks, lullabies, and games, we had to teach each other, and they would change from time to time. For some people, this might be all so very easy and natural, but for me it became a huge and beautiful process. I kept choosing people and places to learn these things—I needed support and to be understood. The funny thing is every time I thought I was going to learn something in particular, it would often be completely opposite from what I expected. It is like the anecdote, "Do you know how to make God laugh? ...Tell him about your plans." That's how it was with me, waiting a long time to meet the right person with whom to build a strong family. And it was the same with my plan to give birth at home, and many more examples.

So here we are. Sarah Manusha is a year and six weeks. Ninety-nine percent of her food is mama's breast milk, and the other foods I offer her become her playmates. She does like to bite apples, cucumbers, fennel, celery and carrots. She eats 3/4 of a banana or avocado, a little miso soup and newly discovered sprouted wheat berries and her favorite: sunflower greens.

I've never used shampoos or soaps on her silky skin and copper hair. Her ninth tooth is beginning to emerge. She weighs 10 kilos (22 pounds), and is 72cm (28 1/2 inches) tall. She loves people. She sings loudly and dances very amusingly, extremely animated and interactive. She loves her time by herself too.

In the first year of becoming a mama, I feel the tenderness of discovery in the universe and the joy of learning about love. I trust my instincts, they know it all. I follow them in the food and beyond. I have learned to sleep when tired, to respect people regardless of what they choose to do and how, to offer what I have, to ask for what I want, to be patient, and to enjoy the given. I take time to observe and listen. Our walks in Nature are my favorite—where I receive my true nourishment, where I feel safe and honored—our early mornings when all is so gentle, new and light.

Sarah rides on me during our deeply nurturing walks in Nature. We both get immersed into feelings of gentleness, freshness and wholeness. Here is where I feel the tenderness of discovery in the universe and the joy of finding love. Now I trust my instincts, and I'm devotedly learning to practice, hear, respect and follow them, filled all the while with sacred Gratitude.

—Beata Barinbaum

Rick Philip 2003

I first wanted to meet Rick Philip, a teenager from Florida, when his article, "First Year Journey of a Raw Teen," was emailed to me by a friend from the New York City raw food community who had moved to Florida. Rick was 16 at the time. I contacted Rick by email, and met him in Summer, 2003 at the Living Now Festival in Western New York. Rick made an excellent presentation about his teen raw food journey at the Living Now Festival. After the festival, I invited him to speak to the raw food support group I led in Manhattan. It was inspiring to see this young man who became an animal rights activist and raw foodist through his own research and motivation to be a positive light in the world:

A Teen's First Year Raw Food Journey by Rick Philip

For every raw foodist, there is an experience, and each of ours is unique. As a teenager, trying to find my way in the world, I've encountered resistance and many challenges. Not only have I overcome most of these, but I have used them to my advantage. Raw foods have made me stronger in every way I know. Throughout junior high, I was "the vegan." It was during those years that I first became conscious of the effect one's diet has on the world. I was always interested in health, but I never took it seriously. It was tough being different, but I grew in so many ways because of this. As a vegan, I became angry with the world, and I stored my negative thoughts. I had no idea that later I would be forced to deal with them.

My vegan diet led me to the discovery of raw foods. Three months before my fifteenth birthday, the idea of eating only raw food presented itself to me. I thought it was extreme. I imagined an elderly couple cutting up broccoli and eating it with a fork! After a little research, though, my views changed. This diet made too much sense not to give it a try. Little did I know it was more than a diet; it is an entire way of life. Ready to start a new adventure, I jumped right in…WOW!

Raw foods forced me to analyze all aspects of my lifestyle. My previous diet was anything but healthy, consisting mostly of soy, grains, and condiments. I spent most of my at-home hours in front of the television. I am still adjusting my lifestyle as I grow—an amazing process.

Unlike soy milk, eggless cookies, and meat substitutes, raw foods don't give the impression of denial. No longer am I living solely *without* meat, dairy, and eggs; I am living *with* raw fruits, veggies, nuts and seeds! I was drifting further from the societal norm, but in school, I put up with less resistance. My "diet" was a lot easier to defend. God, nature, and human logic were on my side. Many people who previously were hostile towards me became truly interested. I was becoming a more reasonable, peaceful person, and I didn't even notice.

Transitioning to a raw food diet has been the biggest challenge of my life. I regret not keeping a journal during this pivotal time in my life. A journal would have helped me put everything into perspective. During this time, I ate nuts and seeds by the pound to suppress cravings. My stomach was not used to the light feeling. Occasionally, I'd turn to peanut butter, but I was eating a lot better than before. The change in eating habits was hard, but not the most difficult part for me. I had intense mood swings and emotional releases, which created strain on already weak family bonds.

My parents, avid meat-eaters, mocked my rapid weight loss. "Emaciated" and "anorexic" became frequent words in their vocabulary. For a teenaged male, whose ideal image for himself was one of bulging muscles and gorilla-like strength, these words really hurt. My family bonds were further weakened by money situations. I was constantly asking my mother to buy me bananas and raw seeds. My parents told me I was "fading away," but when I ate, they made me feel guilty about it. I wasn't getting enough food.

The problems I faced left me doubting my new lifestyle. The night of Halloween that year, cravings hit hard. I went to a party and gave into social pressure. A few pieces of candy sent me on a downward spiral like nothing I've experienced. The next two months, I felt like hell. Detox, cravings, emotions, toxins…everything was blurred. I felt like a failure, and I was embarrassed by this. I suffered through intense junk food cravings, but I had no one to tell. I wouldn't even ask for help online, the only place I had raw support. I was too embarrassed.

Towards my family, I used a "raw façade," pretending to be raw, but inside I was fighting myself. I searched for the bottles and packages with the highest calorie and fat content. I ate jars of salsa and drank salad dressing until my taste buds burned. I devoured whole boxes of crackers when no one was looking. As I binged, I might as well have been a cocaine addict, shooting up in an alley. I lived for those releases, the artificial satisfaction brought about by these foods, crushed by an overwhelming sense of defeat and sickness but a few moments later. I cried frequently, and I felt crazy. I confronted my emotions and my tough childhood, not by choice, but because it needed to be done. Despite my setbacks, I persevered. I used my backyard as my getaway, a place to go, free of guilt and pressuring family members. I kept trying and had some good, raw days. On my first raw Thanksgiving, I was truly thankful. It was around January when the guilt became too much. I didn't want to lie or sneak around anymore. I started telling people I was transitioning, but I was in denial. Now, I could eat as much cooked food as I wanted, and I could do it without secrecy. I ate lots of vegan "nutrition" bars, oils, and hummus. Finally, I admitted to myself that my "transitioning" was nothing more than an excuse to binge and a guilt-free way to feed my addictions. By March, I decided to quit my self-abuse. I went raw, 100%, and I felt great! Over one year later and here I am, writing this article.

A lot has happened this past year. Raw foods revolutionized my life and thinking. Some changes have been physical. A few brief fasts over the summer left me feeling much cleaner. For a few months, I had so much mucus it seemed as if I were spitting every few minutes. Needless to say, that was anything but appealing to my family members. My face has cleared, but light acne proves I am still "cleaning house." Cravings are a rarity now, and my need for high-fat foods continues to wane. I'm doing very well on mostly fruits and vegetables, and I'm getting enough food. I am now more active than I have been in my entire life, and slowly, I am gaining muscle.

Once an atheist, I now have faith. To know there is a higher power is a profound feeling! Raw foods have shown me the magic and mystery of the universe. I have a new kind of confidence in the human race, and I strive for peace, within and around me. I wake up every morning, anticipating the wonders of the day. I am living proof that not every teenager has to be stressed, depressed, and hopeless.

As my family continues to become accustomed to my changes, they are changing too. Both of my sisters are now vegetarians, one who aspires to be raw like her big brother. My lifestyle has created tensions for sure, but I'm overcoming these. Overall, our household is much less toxic.

My senses have sharpened, especially my sense of thought. Food was not a problem in school—I faced the halls with sunflower seeds, apples and carrots in my backpack—but schoolwork became dull and tedious. I made my days bearable by doodling, stretching in my seat, staring out windows, and receiving hall passes *whenever* possible. Last fall, however, after my first raw summer, school was different. It was more than a waste of time; it was prison. After much debate with my mom, I left public school. I concluded there are too many things to learn to wait for someone else to assign them to me. Now, the world is my teacher. When I left school, I was worried I'd become a hermit. The opposite is true. It has only been recently, with raw foods and free time, I have begun to reach out and explore the world. I have discovered many new interests, and I am meeting so many people. For a year, I had no raw support besides online e-groups. Now, I am meeting raw vegan people everywhere but only since I've started looking. I even found an organic buying group very close to my home that has expanded my variety of foods.

Raw vegan foods let me live a real life. The things I'm learning now will help me in the future, but I'm living for the present. Besides tutoring students and volunteering at a forest sanctuary, I have been certified as a raw nutrition specialist, helping others on their way to a better life. I donate a lot of my time to helping children and other teens struggling with vegetarian, vegan, or raw food diets. I'm finding the time to write, and I'm working on an in-depth book about my raw food journey. I am also a full-time activist, fighting for those with little or no voice. I like to think of myself as a strong contributor to the raw food movement and a passionate activist who is changing the world. I believe raw food living will continue to show me the way. What way? I'm not sure, but I am reaching out for the special things the universe has in store for me. I have by no means achieved the perfect lifestyle (whatever that is), but I am learning so much, and I keep moving forward. Challenges present themselves, and I work to overcome them. I adapt my lifestyle to fit the opportunities given to me. No matter what our age, we can embrace our struggles for the betterment of ourselves…and the world.

Raw Food: An Alternative Diet? by Rick Philip

I recently attended an animal rights conference, looking forward to being around so many like-minded people. I was irked, though not surprised, when told my diet was "alternative." This was especially ironic at this conference because it seemed the conference was doing everything it could to be "alternative." The word alternative means a choice between two things or a remaining choice. My diet is not alternative. To say it's alternative would mean we simply had to force ourselves to give up meat and soy substitutes and are left with nothing more than watermelon. This is not the impression I want to give people. For me, there is no choice at all. I admit I'm different from most people, and they will not hesitate to point this out; however, by understanding ourselves, as well as society, we know we are not "alternative" at all. We are *not* eating this way to deny society. We are *not* eating this way to deny cooked food. Eating raw plant foods is instinctive, not a choice at all. By continuing to eat cooked food, society at large is in denial of our natural diet, so readily available today. *They* are the alternative.

Alternative: no better word can be used to describe what was served for food at this conference. "Mock meats," dairy substitutes, egg replacements, and vegan cookies were served all weekend. It was a meat-eaters diet replaced by soy substitutes. Ironically, it would have been easier for me to eat at a steakhouse than it was to eat at this conference. By eating this way, the vegan society is denying itself the unique experience veganism is. Transition foods such as soy should not be meals. Do most vegans forget fruit and salads, too, are vegan? Veganism, and certainly raw foodism, is not a kind way to mimic the rest of the world. We need to abolish this perception, within and outside our movement. Then, why do people think this way? Why do most vegans consider raw foodists "alternative?" To answer this, we need to look seriously at how we present ourselves, what we say, and what our actions imply. The way many of us portray ourselves, it's no wonder others term us this way. Before I went raw, I had been a vegan for two years. During this time, I was constantly asked about my lifestyle. My response was always a long list of what I did *not* eat, could *not* wear, would *not* do, etc. This did more harm than good. Only after becoming a raw foodist, did I discover the importance of acting and speaking positively.

Speaking positively prevents confusion. Anyone who has had trouble explaining exactly what "cooked food" means knows this. Is it a good thing for people first hearing about raw foods to be wondering at exactly what temperature enzymes are killed? Probably not. It's much easier to understand "fruits, vegetables, nuts and seeds" than to be burdened with a long, mostly indecisive definition of the word "cooked."

Speaking negatively makes us appear rebellious. Telling people about the myriad foods you don't eat acknowledges the power of those foods over society. However true this is, acknowledging this makes it seem like you are eating raw for no reason but to deny that power. It also creates the false picture that cooked food is the normal thing to eat. We are not rebels, eating cooked food is not normal, and raw food is not about denial. Most people want to hear we take pride in overcoming society's power. They want to be able to brush us off as people looking for a compliment. Let us not give them excuses to look down on us. Do not be proud; be thankful! By secluding ourselves from society, and by stifling interest, we postpone the re-enlightenment of the entire human race.

Words are powerful—expressions even more so. However much we want to do so, shouting "cooked food is poison" does nothing for our cause. It may be hard to control our anger sometimes, but a smile and a happy attitude make all the difference in how someone perceives us. Only by smiling, laughing, and acting as if our lives are truly the gifts they are, will we attract people to our movement. The raw food diet is not a joke, a big experiment, or a fad diet, so be sincere, but positive, in how you present yourself. Even positive speaking won't cover up an attitude no one wants to relate to.

So when do we talk about *why* we eat the way we do? Surely, we have to mention enzymes and toxic caloronutrients. The answer is simple: when they ask. Asking *what* and *why* are different questions. Most people won't be interested in the reason behind the raw food lifestyle if you are negative and depressing. No one wants to live an angry or obsessive life, and few people want to be considered "alternative." By using positive speech and attitudes, you will almost always create interest. When asked, we can explain why eating raw vegan food is so important to our quality of life. Our personal experiences add to this and make conversations more human. After all, we are not the demigods some make us out to be. I don't mean we should never talk about cooked food. We can't ignore the issues, but we have a responsibility to inform and inspire. Don't be afraid to mention how tough it was for you, but focus on what good has come of it. If you're still struggling, explain what you know in your heart will occur.

To go raw is to take a step in the quest for life, and it's a very personal issue. Despite our desires to bring everyone we meet away from that boring, "alternative" lifestyle, we can't pressure other people. It's important never to make people feel guilty about what they do. We are all on a path. Let's open doors—not shut them! Try to make those you speak with so incredibly amazed by what you say they won't want to choose cooked food anymore.

When speaking out about our lifestyles, we should use the real definition of ourselves. We are people who eat with respect for all life, our own included. The word vegetarian was not derived from "vegetable" but from the Latin word "vegetus" to mean *full of life*, or *enlightened one*. So let's strive to be enlightened beings—the true meaning of vegetarian. Smile, laugh, watch your words, and be positive! Let's show the world what wonders we can achieve…without an alternative lifestyle!

The Teenage Product of a Raw Food Lifestyle
(Update for Karen) 2005 by Rick Philip, age 18

Raw is not the best thing that ever happened in my life…because it all got better from there. Two years after writing my article that swept the Internet about my personal journey as a raw foodist, food doesn't seem to matter as much anymore. I have reached the point where my life has little to do with food. My focus is on my life and my purpose: to bring happiness to people and make the world a better place. I live my life to the fullest. This means powering it with raw fruits, vegetables, nuts and seeds, the best human fuel on the planet.

After more than three years of eating nothing but 100% raw foods, eating raw food is still a choice. I even allow myself to eat cooked food; I just choose not to do it. In fact, eating good foods has become such a habit for me, sometimes I forget not *everyone* eats this way, and I have to remind myself why I chose to do so.

Despite not focusing my life on food, the fact still remains—and Karen knows this—I *love* to eat. I try to choose the raw vegan foods that are healthiest for me, knowing not all of them are, but I don't worry too much about my health. If I don't feel great after eating something, I try to eat it infrequently. My favorite foods are many and depend on the season. Some favorites this year are watermelon, young coconuts, banana "ice cream" (frozen bananas in a blender or through a juicer), green veggies with my favorite sunflower seed dip, hummus made with soaked chickpeas, cream of tomato soup (got to love avocados!), durian, and a whole assortment of apples and citrus. Yum!

I do more than the average teenager because I feed my body what it needs. I've been called an overachiever, yet I've come to see that label as an oxymoron. I have so much energy it only seems natural for me to take on so many projects. I have a passion for learning that has me conquering my fourth and fifth languages (French and Russian) as well as steadily working toward two degrees at the university. Raw foods continue to keep my life exciting and allow me the time and energy to pursue my goals and live with passion. Ten pages of goals and priorities, constantly updated, keep me on my toes. In between studying for classes, watching great movies and videos, and teaching Spanish (I *do* have to make money), I regularly find myself writing essays, comedies, and even a novel, planning demonstrations, singing in different languages, cracking people up on stage as an actor or moving them to action as a public speaker. I now speak nationally at animal rights conferences, continue to write for www.vegetarianteen.com, and travel regularly. In November of 2004, I flew to Brazil as the youngest foreign attendee to the World Vegetarian Congress where I got the chance to try delectable—and really inexpensive—tropical fruits, experience an incredible culture, and connect with people in all of my first three languages: Spanish, English, and Portuguese. In summer 2005, I stood in front of 1000 people in Los Angeles to accept an award for my work on behalf of the animals and shortly after hit the streets of Mexico City where I lived it up while trying to make a difference in the lives of the people I met. Regardless of what I do now, though, be sure I will be having a blast, living my life to the fullest, and praising God for letting me experience it!

The most important thing I can say to anyone going raw is not to place too much emphasis on food. We should enjoy our food, and healthful food matters a lot, but life is not about food. After being a raw foodist for so long, I have tried cooked food and find it not very appealing at all. Some people—both young and old—may be at a point in their lives when they need to focus on overcoming a food addiction and correcting that aspect of their lives, but I pray they will rapidly realize what I now know to be the real reason for eating raw: living our lives.

Just a few years ago, not a vegan much less a raw foodist, I commonly occupied my couch, downed up to ten sodas per day, stuffed my face full of chips, and lived for the momentary pleasures I called meals. I tried hard not to fall asleep in class, and I could only dream of doing something great, something important, even anything that mattered. I hold nothing but gratitude for that time in my life. It was a vital step in reaching the life I live now: I am working toward who I want to be, having fun, and making the world a better place every day I live, raw fuel and all. What more could I want?

Rick's words to live by: "Life's an adventure…what have *you* done today?"

I began to communicate with Jenny Silliman when I saw her writings for rawbaby@yahoo.com

Jenny and her husband Cliff have eight children. Her children are not being raised on raw foods, but she is nursing the youngest child while she eats 100% raw vegan foods. They live in Sequim, Washington. At the time of this writing, 2003, Jenny, at age 45, has 8 children ranging from ages twenty-four to one. She and the one year old were both having yeast problems. Out of desperation, she went to the International Raw Foods Festival in Oregon and began eating 100% raw vegan foods the next day. She was very overweight, and lost over 25 pounds in the first five weeks, and an additional 15 pounds doing a master cleanse the month before. Jenny was thrilled to be able to go to her favorite department store to buy a new outfit in a size 16—a far cry from the size 26 she had been wearing. When she wrote to me again later, she had lost 71 pounds, and weighed 149 pounds after having eaten raw vegan foods for a year. Peter, her youngest, at 15 months, was enjoying fruits and veggies and eating primarily raw foods, but his brothers gave him bits of whatever other foods they were eating. Jenny answered my questions in interview style:

Raw Mama
by Jenny Silliman September 26, 2003

Q: When did you start to eat raw foods?

A: I began to eat an all raw vegan diet on July 10, 2003 when our 8th child was almost 4 months old.

Q: Can you talk about nursing and raw food nutrition?

A: First let me backtrack about how this began. On July 10, 2003 at 4 months postpartum, I began to eat all raw vegan foods. I had 60 pounds to lose at that time. We have eight children, seven of whom are sons, and I was tired of being tired and fed up with being fat. I want to be able to go hiking and biking with my sons and be able to keep up and enjoy the recreation. I also want to live a long life and be a spunky, healthy old grandma some day. I read an inspiring recipe book, loaded with information, called *Rejuvenate Your Life!* by Serene Allison. www.rejuvenation.org. My husband encouraged me to try it for 3 days. I immediately went into detoxing and had headaches and diarrhea, but I knew it was time to "clean house." After 3 days, I lost 5 pounds and I felt an energy surge along with crystal clear thinking. It was like the fog had cleared out of my brain. I decided to keep on eating 100% raw veggies, fruits, nuts and seeds, also known as the "ideal diet." I looked up raw food on the web and found over three dozen sites and joined an e-mail loop, rawfood@yahoogroups.com. I asked them all my questions. I was directed to books on the web on Natural Hygiene. I had read about it several times, and about the seven principles of health (which include sunshine, rest, pure water, exercise, emotional poise, fresh air and the ideal diet)—but now I was *doing* it! When I did a search on Google on the phrase "Natural Hygiene," I was shocked to discover 17,000 found! I began reading about the history and was surprised again when I learned it had been around since the 1830s. I began to closely follow the principals of Natural Hygiene including eight hours of sleep, fresh air (open the window at night) and sunshine as a part of my daily routine.

The pounds started simply to melt off me at a rate of about half a pound a day for the first sixty days. I had read in *Eat to Live* by Dr. Joel Fuhrman, in the first month you will lose 20 pounds, second month 10 pounds and 5 pounds every month thereafter until you reach your ideal weight. Sure enough, I lost 20 pounds in the first month as a raw foodist and 10 pounds in the second month. Now, in my third month, I have lost a couple more pounds. I feel absolutely great! It is so exciting to think about next spring when I will be called *Slim* and I'll be at my ideal weight. The raw foodists tell me, "If I keep on eating all raw vegan foods, I WILL NEVER BE FAT AGAIN." I have tried many weight loss programs in over twenty-one years of childbearing. I would always have problems with my milk supply drying up. Now that I juice veggies and eat all raw vegan foods, I have plenty of good rich breast milk.

Our baby boy is 100% RAW breast milk fed and chubby. He will be 6 months old tomorrow, September 27, 2003, has big bright blue eyes, rosy cheeks, and wonderfully soft skin and silky hair. He is strong and active and is already crawling all over the house. He's the picture of health. You've never seen a more alert, happy baby than this boy, our sweet Pete.

Q: Will you give a description of your diet?
A: Here's what I do in a day:
6 a.m. Arise and drink water.
7 a.m. Eat an apple, if I'm hungry.
7:15 a.m. Aerobic exercise for 45 minutes—a 3 mile power walk with a video called "Walk Away the Pounds" by Leslie Sansone.
8:00 a.m. I have veggies for breakfast, lunch and dinner. At 8, I have Juice

#1 prepared with a Champion Juicer, a pint of veggie juice which is a green drink. I always juice celery, a sprig of parsley, chard, spinach, an apple and a few carrots, and sometimes a beet, bok choy and other veggies too. I hope to buy a Green Star Juicer someday that will juice wheat grass.

At 12:00 p.m., I have Juice #2, another pint of green juice for lunch. I prepare veggies all at once in the morning so they're ready to juice at lunchtime. After my second juice, I clean the juicer.

At 2 p.m., I have 2 tablespoons of ground flaxseeds ground fresh in a coffee grinder, which I drink stirred into a pint of water. This is for Omega 3 essential fat which has many benefits. One important one I have noticed is for the bowels; it keeps those toxic wastes moving smoothly on out. I read a list of signs of deficiencies of Omega 3 essential fat and one was miscarriage/ premature birth. Before this baby, I had a miscarriage at 20 weeks. I've been taking Omega 3 fat ever since. Raw nuts, seeds and avocados contain Omega 6 fat which is also beneficial. In the afternoon, I will finish the equivalent of a second quart of water.

At 3 to 5 p.m., I will have seasonal fruits of my choice, such as nectarine, cantaloupe, pear, mango—luscious, delicious fruit. My fruit meal is my favorite one of the day!

Sometime later, I have raw nuts when hungry. One thing I have learned is not to eat if I'm not truly hungry. I limit my raw nuts to about 2 to 3 ounces because I am still learning not to overeat.

I sometimes mix up whole almonds, sunflower seeds, pecans and walnuts, and scoop up a handful for an afternoon snack. Occasionally I make "treat balls" with raw nut butter and/or tahini, and I might stir in coconut, mashed banana and/or chopped dates or raisins.

At 6 p.m., I have a large salad for supper with fresh homemade avocado dressing. I mash the avocado, adding a little water and maybe some salsa which I make with lots of cilantro for a Mexican dressing. Sometimes I use grated ginger root, lemon juice, fresh apple juice and sesame seeds to make a Chinese dressing. I use lots of dark green leafy lettuce, red and green cabbage, spinach, green tops of green onions, red, green, yellow and/or orange bell peppers, black olives, cucumbers, grated sweet potatoes, grated squash, alfalfa sprouts, bean sprouts and tomatoes. There is no eating after supper.

In the evening, I will sip on water. Water is important for getting out toxins, for good elimination, for plenty of breast milk and is essential for burning fat stores and losing weight.

Q: Do you have a supportive spouse?

A: Yes! He enjoys bananas for snacks instead of soda pop and candy bars and joins me for supper with a big salad, but besides that and cutting way back on the sweets, he eats fairly conventionally as do our children. I'm praying for some possible changes in the future.

Q: Please share about detoxification and nursing.

A: I have kept a journal of my raw food journey. I have had about one day a week, or at least one day out of every ten, during which I didn't feel well, and I sort of coasted through my day. I have had canker sores, pimples, rashes, heavy arms, shaky flu-like symptoms, headaches, and fatigue due to my detoxification or healing crises. I have noticed I detox right before losing weight, and I think it's because the toxins are layered in the fat stores of the body. After a detox day, I lose a couple pounds and I feel wonderfully healthy—which makes it worthwhile. Though I have done plenty of detoxing, I haven't noticed any detoxification symptoms in baby Peter. I don't know if the toxins get filtered out so he doesn't get them in my milk. I figured eating raw foods is better than dead, devitalized cooked food.

The food cravings were intense during the first three days—giving up bread and sugar was hard, as if somebody died. I'm not kidding. I went through a grieving process at first. Juicing veggies really satisfies me and cured the cravings. I've read it's important to eat or juice a total of a pound of greens each day. This is where a bulk of vital nutrition is found. I've also read, "A fat person is a starving person." Even though the stomach is full, a person may still be hungry because nutritional needs have not been met. A huge discovery for me is satiety. Because all of my nutritional requirements are now being met, I'm often not very hungry. I used to think if I ate this way, I'd be ravenous. Not true! I eat a little, and I'm completely satisfied. I no longer have a problem with emotional overeating. I feel freed from food bondage.

Besides weight loss, good breast milk supply, clear thinking, more energy—waking up alert and ready to hop out of bed—and with victory regarding overeating, I've experienced freedom from depression, softer skin, even on my elbows, some strange spots on my arm are fading, I have more creativity in my writing, my fingers are no longer stiff and crackly, I no longer need to use deodorant, if I get sunburned it's gone in about a day, and I have a new desire to get out and do things and go places. Today, I went on a bike ride with my eleven year old son and kept right up with him.

In Jenny Silliman's e-mail newsletter, Jenny's Journal, she writes about her life, and is delighted to encourage other mothers, and to give practical ideas about the art of homemaking. To subscribe send a blank e-mail to: jennysjournal@associate.com. Jenny's email is: jennysilliman@juno.com. Jenny has written a book called *Raw Victory* about her weight loss and health gain by eating raw vegan and has written an article, "Confessions of an Overeater," for the Spring 2008 issue of Living Nutrition Magazine.

Sarah Parker of Fort Worth, Texas, read an article I wrote for Vegetarian Baby and Child Online Magazine. She contacted me immediately for a telephone consultation. Afterwards, Sarah emailed me when questions arose. She was greatly relieved to have the support, and to have her questions answered related to raising her children on raw vegan foods.

The Parker Family
August 1, 2005

My husband and I switched from a horrible, fast and junk food diet to what we thought was a more healthful vegan diet almost overnight when we had our twin sons. When the boys began eating solids, I started making my own baby food, and it suddenly hit me: nutrition is truly crucial for health, and I barely knew anything about it. So I started reading everything I could on the subject, and our sons have been raised vegan.

I always knew about raw food, but I thought it was a little over the top. Doesn't everybody need cooked grains and beans to be healthy? Weren't they the food staples of all civilizations throughout history? These raw food people must be lacking nutritionally somewhere, somehow. So went my thoughts. Sure, I knew raw fruits and veggies are great for your health, but to eat ONLY live food? I was fascinated with it, but not convinced, and I knew I could never give up cooked food.

In the meantime, our diet gradually shifted more and more into the realm of vegan junk and processed convenience foods. I kept my children's diet relatively clean, but they were starting to eat way too many natural peanut butter sandwiches on 100% whole wheat bread because we were always on the run. I realized with not a little guilt that sometimes they would go a couple of days without eating veggies, and some days they didn't even get fruit if we got too busy. Also, getting pregnant with my daughter, and being on a horrible diet for the duration of the pregnancy, was keeping me tired, sick and unmotivated to prepare healthier meals. But at least they aren't eating Happy Meals and hotdogs…I kept telling myself.

Then a combination of little miracles happened to us. First, I stumbled across an organic produce co-op in our area. We had lived here for almost two years, and I was almost at the point of giving up hope of finding anything healthy in our area. Then, my not very healthy, not even very vegan anymore husband randomly read an article on MSN news about the raw food diet, and showed it to me. We then decided since we had the wonderful organic produce from our co-op, we would eat all of that stuff raw at home, except for a couple of things like corn and potatoes. This way, we would at least be about 60% raw. We did this for a while, and it was a good transition time for us. Meanwhile, I kept reading and reading, when soon after, I stumbled across an e-book that finally convinced me to make a commitment to go 100%, or at least as close as possible. In your lifetime, some truths just reveal themselves when you're ready to accept them, and when truth speaks, I don't ignore. So I pleaded with my husband to read it too. He did, and that was the turning point for us. We have since overhauled our lives, our diet and our pantry.

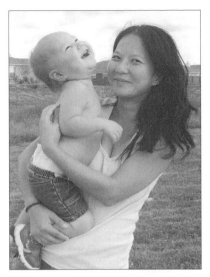

Trinity and Sarah

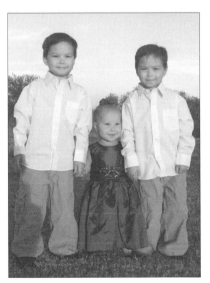

Ethan, Trinity and Elijah

This is definitely a continuing journey. As we keep on with it, so many questions keep coming up, and sometimes the information out there is completely overwhelming. I was especially worried about our kids because we hadn't found a whole lot of good solid information or advice about raw vegan kids. One day, while reading some articles on vegbaby.com, I stumbled across one Karen wrote. It really spoke to me because it was one of *very* few items I'd read about children on raw vegan foods. Thankfully, her email address was listed on the bottom, so I immediately emailed her and pretty much begged her to talk to me about raising kids on raw foods. What do you know…she was actually in the process of writing a book about it! We talked on the phone, and she was so resourceful, answering my endless questions about B12, the issue with grains and beans, getting kids to like greens, social issues, etc. It comforted me to talk to someone who had been a raw foodist for so long and raised her kids that way. I think maybe the best advice she gave me was not to stress out about it, especially where the children were concerned. If we become paranoid or negative about food, our family will be miserable anyway, which defeats the purpose of a happy and healthy life.

We are thankful to have stumbled across the truth of raw foods, and to have the means to live it in our lives. I just want to shout it from the rooftops to all my friends and family, but I know only when truly ready, will one be open to this kind of information. However, through a food blog I started, many friends are already starting to be curious and have been asking me how to improve their diets. My husband lost 20 pounds he really didn't need, and I've gone below my pre-pregnancy weight very easily. My children are happy, healthy and hungry (they eat all day long), and I'm nervous but excited about raising my newborn daughter as a raw vegan. I'm hoping to have a raw pregnancy in the future. For now, we are taking it one step at a time, and every day for us is another precious step to great health.

—Sarah Parker

Sarah had written to me shortly after writing her article, expressing concern her children were eating plenty of fruit, but still weren't interested in green vegetables. I told her the more her children stayed with mostly raw foods, they would eventually enjoy the taste of greens. Two months later, Sarah wrote: "I wanted to let you know things are going well for my family. I told you a couple of times I was having a lot of trouble with my kids not wanting to eat greens. Well, apparently their bodies knew what they needed because, after a couple of months on mostly fruits, my four year olds are *begging* me for a plate of salad every day. And when I serve it to them, they are quiet and eat it with delight. This is crazy amazing for me. No bribery, use of force or torture was employed!"

The Talifero Family

Jingee and Storm Talifero of California have permitted me to quote some of the valuable information they offer in their e-books on *Raw Pregnancy and Childbirth* and *Raising Raw Vegan Children*. Many years ago, soon after she met Storm, Jingee became a raw vegan. Storm has been raw for over 30 years. Jingee quickly lost 45 pounds of unwanted weight, her acne-troubled skin cleared, an undiagnosed lump in her breast dissolved, and she was healed from Candida, hypoglycemia, depression, and chronic fatigue. The following are parts of Jingee's and Storm's story on "Ecstatic Birth: Raw Pregnancy and Childbirth" and "Raising Raw Vegan Children." I recommend purchasing their complete e-books from www.thegardendiet.com. Jingee and Storm have also completed a documentary, *Breakthrough*—a Raw Film Documentary, which is for sale on their website.

Jingee Talifero

I am excited about writing this eBook because my experiences with four pregnancies and births (two cooked food pregnancies and two raw pregnancies) in the last eleven years have led me to believe that staying on a 100% raw vegan diet during pregnancy can lead to a dramatically easier pregnancy with a far easier and quicker childbirth and recovery than usual, while resulting in a healthy and happy baby.

I have spoken with many other raw vegan women who have found the same to be true. I have read the words of raw vegan mothers who described delivering their babies with words like "he slipped into the world like a lamb" (in Dr. Walker's book, *Fresh Vegetable and Fruit Juices*). Hygeia Halfmoon, Ph.D. wrote a book called *Primal Mothering in a Modern World*, in which she describes her raw vegan childbirth as completely pleasurable, orgasmic and ecstatic. She delivered her baby herself with only her two young daughters present. Many women are now delivering their babies on their own. This is called "sovereign birth." I feel a sovereign birth is more natural and easier than a hospital birth because there is no interference and therefore the woman can focus on her labor. However, I believe a husband/wife unassisted homebirth is even more ideal.

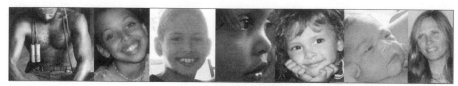

The Talifero Family

My labor with Raven, our first child, with Storm and our friend Oms acting as midwives was 30 hours long. It was complication-free however, a natural homebirth in our living room, and I'll never forget seeing Raven's crown and pushing her out, the most intense and exciting moment of my life thus far. I felt as if I were going to burst wide open. Afterwards, I felt as though I had had a life and death experience and I was just glad to be alive. We were lying down in our loft with the baby nursing and fell asleep exhausted. Raven was a healthy 7 pounds and nursed well, although she was a fussy baby. She would cry every evening at twilight, and the only thing that worked to calm her was flying her around the room, dancing with her, for an hour or two. Maybe there was something in my cooked vegan diet that made my milk disagree with her.

When I took Raven for a "well baby check-up," the doctor was very annoyed with me regarding my vegan diet and my choice not to vaccinate. He said I had a perfect and very beautiful child and I'd be very unhappy if anything happened to her because of my choices. He said very sarcastically, "I'm glad you've decided to take your child's health into your own hands." I think perhaps many doctors really believe we should not take an active part in our own health or not even try to understand anything about our bodies. Fortunately this seems to be changing rapidly for the better. Many doctors now do support people being more active in caring for their own health, and many now do support people in their own choices.

About a year later, I went back to eating 100% raw foods to heal from my Candida which had returned while I was eating a cooked vegan diet. Another year passed and I was pregnant with our son Jome. By this time, I had heard about other raw vegan women who had birthed healthy babies easily, and I was ready to do this pregnancy 100% raw. My health was also so good, I didn't want to give up the diet again. I jogged again during the first five months and walked daily afterwards. I was also involved in singing in a women's music group during the last few months of my pregnancy, and I believe this resulted in the intense musicality Jome has. We were eating out of the Santa Barbara farmer's markets and my diet consisted of big fresh salads, sprouts, lots of green juice and carrot juice, a great variety of different fruits, and plenty of fresh orange juice. I also ate Earthseed bread, a raw "manna" bread. And I ate a lot of tabouli made of parsley, cilantro, green onions, and tomatoes with a dressing of lemons, garlic, olive oil, salt, avocado and honey. I had this at least twice a week. It is a great way to get iron because the parsley is iron-rich while the tomatoes are vitamin C-rich, and iron is more easily absorbed in the presence of vitamin C. I also drank Raspberry Leaf Sun-Tea and lots of water. Raspberry Leaf tea is known to be a great tonic for pregnant women.

My pregnancy was completely easy, and I was very relaxed and happy. I experienced no nausea whatsoever. My childbirth with Jome was also at home, with just Storm and three-year-old Raven attending. My labor was only 45 minutes long with a 10-minute hard labor. It was so easy that right afterwards I said, "Storm, I don't feel like I've given birth." And after nursing Jome and delivering my placenta, I helped to clean up our birthing scene. Jome was a very content baby, just nursing and sleeping. And I feel an unbroken connection of peace and an unbroken stream of energy with him since the day he was born that is still with us today. He also weighed 7 pounds at birth and was totally healthy.

After Jome was born we moved to Vancouver Island, British Columbia, Canada. We had an incredible summer, eating out of our garden and swimming a mile in a pristine lake three times a week. It was the highest level of health I have ever experienced. My body and face rejuvenated to the point where I looked younger than I did in my late teens. I was reaching new levels of creativity in music and business, and I found my emotions were so balanced, I never lost my patience with Raven as I used to sometimes before. This emotional balance, more than anything else, made me want to stay raw for life. I realized when one's colon is stressed from cooked food and the large quantities we have to eat to gain enough nourishment from it, one's whole system is stressed. A stressed colon leads to a stressed body, mind and spirit. I also realized the enormous difference in the level of nutrition in the foods that come straight out of the garden compared with organically grown farm food. On the other hand, most organic farms are on land that was conventionally farmed for 50 years before they became organic. Therefore the farmland soil usually doesn't contain nearly as high a level of nutrients as the virgin garden soil does. This experience of eating out of the garden inspired me to call our raw foods website "TheGardenDiet.com."

During our first winter in Canada, after the gardening season was over, we had trouble finding enough fresh organic raw foods to buy for our family. I once again became a cooked vegan. I knew I wanted to be 100% raw, but

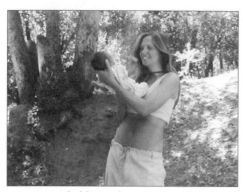

Jingee holding Adagio at 10 months

at the same time I reasoned, now that I was off the path, I might as well eat a little bit of everything not raw first. By the time we conceived Shale in the spring of 2000, I was a total cooked vegan again. I stayed a cooked vegan throughout my pregnancy.

Since Raven's birth was 30 hours and Jome's was 45 minutes, I figured I had better be ready for a 5-minute labor with Shale, if the ratios remained the same. I believed each birth would be easier as my body became more used to childbirth. However, although the pregnancy was as easy as ever, I was in labor with Shale for 40 hours. It was another natural homebirth, but with a painfully hard labor, yet another healthy baby. Two weeks later, it dawned on me, the reason Jome's birth was so easy compared to the others was my pregnancy on 100% raw vegan foods. I suddenly had a vision of the molecules in raw foods spinning fast, going into the body, and becoming bodily tissues made of cells that also spun fast, filled with light, making the tissues elastic, easily expanding to allow a baby's passage into the world. I saw cooked food molecules barely spinning at all, very dense, becoming bodily tissues that were denser and less elastic. This vision explained to me why my labor with Jome had been so easy, as the tissues of my cervix and birth canal could more easily expand to let the baby out. It also explained why the raw vegan diet is so rejuvenating and healing, why raw vegans' skin looks so radiant, youthful, and wrinkle-free, and why Storm's muscles don't seem to notice the influence of 54 years of gravity. This vision was so strong, it made me go back to a 100% raw food diet cold turkey right away. So Shale was nursed by a 100% raw vegan Mother, and has never eaten cooked food in her life. She is three now. Shale was a happy baby from the start and is still a wonderfully healthy and happy little girl. Unlike Raven and Jome who have often been through skinny phases, Shale is a "brick house." This is interesting, considering Raven and Jome have eaten cooked food during my vegan phases, whereas Shale hasn't.

When I found out I was pregnant with Adagio, I ate 100% raw vegan foods, no cheating. Storm totally supported me in my new ideas of non-interference during childbirth, and even when I offered to let him check my dilation he said no. The ideas of no pushing and no interfering with the body made sense to him too. After the birth, Adagio didn't start nursing until hours later, and has been at it ever since. Why did he take longer to start than the others did? Maybe he was so well nourished, he was not hungry at first. Maybe he was more interested in connecting with us and looking around.

I highly recommend you read the chapter on childbirth in *Primal Mothering in a Modern World* by Hygeia Halfmoon, Ph.D. I got this book in my last month of pregnancy and it helped me immensely. If I had gotten it a year earlier, I would have had more time to consciously release all my societal fears about childbirth being a medical emergency. It isn't, although we have been wrongfully led to believe it is. According to Halfmoon's research, hospital births have six times the mortality rate of homebirths. Also, according to Halfmoon's research, mammals have a built in reaction to any interference during labor, and that is to shut down their labor until they find a safe place to deliver. This is why such a high percentage of hospital births result in C-sections, epidurals, induced labors and episiotomies. There is almost no way to have a hospital birth without interference, unless couples specifically request this along with a birthing room. And even then, I'm not sure all hospitals would comply with such a request. Most births are attended by several medical personnel, many of them strangers. Women are examined frequently to determine the dilation of the cervix, the heartbeat of the baby, and the baby's position. There is no way this can be seen as anything but interference. When I was in hard labor, I didn't even want my husband to ask me if I was okay. That's how inward a woman's focus is when in labor.

We still do have our primal instincts. They can't take those away completely. Some women even have them without having to read this kind of information. I talked with a man whose wife had seven children in the hospital. When the doctor told her to push, she told him, "I ain't gonna push, but here you go," and popped the baby out. Then she said, "Let's go on home, hon, we've got laundry to do!" The doctor said she was a baby-making machine. I say she is just one of many women who have survived into the modern world with her primal instincts intact. I found that story very heartening. If this can happen, then people en masse can recognize the truth of the raw vegan diet or find their own way to it even if they don't find a book about it. I think when the evils of the food industry and the medical industry progress so far, they basically hang themselves when things reach a certain level of corruption, and at the same time as people in general are evolving and becoming more intelligent, we are coming full circle, or even better, achieving the next level in an upward spiral, saying, "Hey, something is wrong here with the people and industries in whom I've put my trust. I had better think for myself here, if I want to survive."

I was happy to read in books, such as *Pleasurable Husband/Wife Childbirth* by Marilyn A. Moran and *Unassisted Childbirth, An Act of Love* by Lynn M. Griesemer, both available at http://www.unassistedchildbirth.com, of other women who experienced the sensual touch of their husbands during childbirth, transforming pain to pleasure. The more intense the pain, all the more intense is the welcome pleasurable relief imparted by the sensual touch—painful childbirth is transformed into ecstatic childbirth. As you can see, the father is very much an essential, important and irreplaceable part of the birth of a child. Since the birth of Adagio, Storm and I have fallen in love on a whole new level. We birthed this child completely together, as an act of love. Right after the delivery, the afterglow was incredible and still remains with us in a very strong way. When pleasurable husband/wife childbirth becomes common practice, I believe it will have incredibly powerful changing effects on the world. A bonding hormone called oxytocin is released during childbirth that is like a love potion. The same hormone that bonds mother and baby also bonds father and baby as well as bonding the parents to each other.

Doing well as a raw vegan may have something to do with being 100% raw rather than 99% raw. That 1% makes such a big difference. That 1% cooked food can deplete you. When 99% raw, you become very sensitive to cooked foods, so they can do you more damage than if you were very used to them. This varies with the individual, but I have found it to be true for myself and many others.

I have been nursing and/or pregnant for 11 years straight and have not taken a single supplement, green powder, vitamin, pill, capsule, or medication during this time. Out of the 11 years, I have been 100% raw vegan for half of the time, 50–99% raw vegan for a quarter of that time, and cooked vegan with about 50% raw foods for a quarter of that time.

I tried to get my blood tested for all nutrient levels (calcium, vitamin B12, etc…) during my pregnancy. I had a basic blood test that showed my iron levels were fine. However, I was surprised to find out medical institutions don't have tests for specific nutrient levels. They recommended I find an alternative health practitioner for such tests. They also said good iron levels would indicate you were sufficiently nourished. So, as no medical level testing exists for testing specific nutrient levels, I decided as long as I feel great, I'm going to assume my nutrition is more than adequate.

It is a myth that you need to eat more during pregnancy. I ate very little during my first trimester of this pregnancy because I didn't feel like eating much. I also ate very little during my last trimester as I got full very quickly with the baby taking up more room in my body. During my first and last trimesters, I definitely ate much less than I do when I am not pregnant. During my second trimester, I ate normally, but not noticeably more than usual. I gained 15 pounds during my pregnancy, going from 135 pounds before I got pregnant to 150 the day before my labor. The day after my labor I weighed 140 pounds, due to having delivered a 7 pound baby and burning off the other 3 pounds during labor. A week later, I was back to 135 pounds, even though I was now eating more than usual because I was nursing my new baby, and my appetite was intense.

During my pregnancy, I ate an abundance of fresh organic fruits, about 4 glasses of freshly-squeezed organic orange juice a day, green juice about twice a week (using a variety of one or more of the following ingredients: celery, kale, chard, spinach, broccoli, parsley, carrots, and beets, flavored with either lemon, apple, ginger, onion or garlic), delicious tabouli salad two to four times a week (instead of the traditional cracked or bulghur wheat, we use ground almonds. We take a handful or two of almonds—not soaked—and put them in the blender, grinding them into a fine flour, and then add it into the tabouli salad), a salad of organic lettuce or baby greens with avocado/lemon or tahini/lemon dressing once or twice a week, an avocado/tomato salad sometimes wrapped in a kale leaf which was my staple recipe (once or twice a day), and around every second day on average, I would have some kind of nut or seed milk: either tahini milk, sunflower seed milk, or almond milk. Other foods I would sometimes eat were guacamole, salsa, Earthseed Multigrain (manna) sprouted seed bread, fruit smoothies, blended salads, sunflower seed patés, whole vegetables including celery, bell peppers, carrots, cucumbers, corn, and jicama, whole fruits including durians (the stinky fruit) and young coconuts (durian and young coconuts are both fatty fruits available at Asian markets), berries, apples, bananas, melons, cherimoyas, satsumas, and guava pineapples.

Fruits and vegetables have all the vitamins and minerals you and your baby need. They have all the fats, carbohydrates and protein you and your baby need. Nuts and oils (hemp seed oil, olive oil, and flax oil, all organic and all cold-pressed) have all the omega fatty acids you and your growing baby need. Many raw foodists say nuts and oils aren't even necessary, and fruits and vegetables are enough, even during pregnancy and nursing.

When still eating some cooked food, you will not appreciate the delicacy of raw foods. Whereas if you eat only raw foods, not only do you totally enjoy your food more fully than before, you also lose the cravings for cooked foods. Although this is true for me at all times, it was amplified during pregnancy.

The root of morning sickness is junk food, chemicals in food, and cooked food.

Tahini seems like it brings an abundance of milk. Any leafy greens are great too, in green juices, salads, or on their own. These include lettuce, chard, kale, parsley, cilantro, spinach, and baby greens. Lots of water is good. Freshly-squeezed orange juice is great. Nut milks are wonderful. Tahini milk is fantastic. When nursing, rather than during pregnancy, is when I eat a lot more than usual. It makes more sense for the baby to attain most of its growth after it passes through you.

—Jingee Talifero

Storm Talifero wrote:

The main goal of the raw vegan diet we designed while Jingee was pregnant was to eat just what the body needed. We had to find out what the essential building blocks were, and if it was possible to obtain them from simple raw foods. And if it was possible at the same time to eliminate all the chemicals in processed and non organic foods. The answers we found were amazing. The simplest foods such as oranges and apples contain an abundance of nutrients we need, whereas foods such as dairy and meats contain very little in the way of nutritional building blocks. We had to overcome huge myths such as the need for animal proteins and vitamin B12 from artificial sources and the part they play in the development of newborn babies.

When thinking of nutrition, one must consider the anatomy of a single cell. A cell is surrounded by fluid and receives nutrients and discharges waste through the cell wall. A cell does not care what your food tastes like; it is only concerned with getting the building blocks it needs to function. Heated oils, for instance, don't provide the cell with anything it can use. They are very hard to break down and clog the system, slowing down all of the cellular processes. Trans fatty acids, contained in processed foods, actually surround the cell wall, preventing it from either receiving nutrients or discharging waste. It doesn't matter how much food you eat if in the end the cell cannot use it. If the cell is prevented from operating at its maximum capacity, you are suffering from malnutrition. And nowhere is this more of a paradigm than in our modern diet. So to make up for this, they say we have to take supplements. But when we eat organic fruits and vegetables, even though we don't feel we've eaten a full meal, the cells are fully nourished, and we no longer experience the irony of starving with a full stomach. I believe this to be the main reason Jingee was able to bring forth a perfectly healthy child on exclusively organic fruits and vegetables.

Jingee, Shale and I eat about 80% fruit. We do enjoy salads. Jome and Raven will not eat many salads or drink any green juices, so they are about 95% fruit bats. We all enjoy sprouted nut milks and other nut dishes, and they are rich protein sources for all of us. Jingee and I are the only ones who will drink green juices. Of all the kids, Shale is the most muscular. I attribute this to the fact that she eats a greater percentage of salads and avocados than our other children. She has the best appetite and the most positive spirit. This may have nothing at all to do with the fact that she has never eaten any cooked food while the other two have, it may just be who she is as a person.

On the use of supplements, I feel if the diet is totally balanced, it's possible to obtain all the necessary nutrients to build a strong baby from raw living foods. I feel a lot of the supplements cannot be absorbed by the body, and may even do more harm than good—calcium from a natural source is in an easily absorbed format, but it might not be so readily absorbed by the body from non-food or synthetic sources. Vitamins that may not be absorbed or eliminated are sometimes stored in the body where they can turn into undesirable deposits such as kidney stones or gallstones.

On Raising Raw Vegan Children, Jingee and Storm write: For a long time we kept our older kids on raw oats and sprouted Essene bread against our better judgment, to try to put some weight on them. Ironically, it was when we at last let these foods go that they filled out better. They are at a normal weight now eating a large variety of mostly fruits, some vegetables, and daily nut milks. They eat many times a day, they eat quite a lot of food, and usually they drink many glasses of freshly-squeezed orange juice every day.

Occasional Treats are a Trick: When we allow the indulgence in occasional treats because we don't want to deprive our children of a normal childhood, we can create confusion, food addictions, weight loss and poor health. People will be quick to blame the all-live diet for the illness rather than the candy. Straddling the fence is far more dangerous than being clear and simple about our lifestyle choices.

Lunchbox tips: Pack lots of food. Let the amount make up for the fact that all the so-called "essential" food groups are not there. Include fruit servings, vegetable servings, and nut/seed servings—all live trail mix. When sending apple slices, you can dip them in freshly-squeezed lemon juice and the apples will not turn brown. But whole foods are best anyway—celery and carrot sticks with a tahini dip.

All the vitamins and minerals you need are available in uncooked fruits and vegetables—fresh and organically grown. And recent studies show nuts provide a superior protein to meat.

The following came from Jingee's journal in her Daily Raw Inspiration of August 8, 2008:

> I spoke to a woman today who is looking for a diet to help her lose weight. I tried to tell her about this diet, but could tell she just wasn't receptive. She wouldn't even let herself imagine being able to do it. If people only knew! That they can eat more and still lose weight. That raw vegan foods really have more variety and flavor than cooked foods. That it becomes easy after a while. That you look and feel younger every day. That your children thrive on it. That when you do it, you get help from the Universe. That your whole life changes positively. That it isn't really scary at all but blissful once you are doing it. That you can make mistakes and still be fine if you keep adjusting. That after a while it becomes second nature, like breathing, or any other habit. That you really don't need to eat meat. That you really don't need to eat dairy. That you really don't need to cook your food. That you really don't need to take supplements. That your food really doesn't need to be sprayed with toxic chemicals...
> http://www.thegardendiet.com/articles
> http://www.thegardendiet.com/news

Jaylene presented on raw foods preparation at the 2003 Portland International Raw Food Festival. I later emailed her, and she wrote back the following:

Jaylene Johnson
July 13, 2004

I have a few thoughts to share that may be helpful to others. My youngest is turning 12 next week. During the last 30 years of marriage, I was quite cautious about my diet, but only during the last 2+ years have I eaten totally live food and fresh food. I wish I had known earlier what I now know which would have enabled me to have babies with a cleaner, more pure physical body. We are expecting our fifth grandbaby, and I'm hoping to convince each of these little ones and their moms of the advantages of eating only those foods that will help to enliven their minds, bodies, and spirits. We are making progress as we help to create awareness in each one. I've seen some real changes in my children as we have given them the opportunity to have live juices and wheatgrass juice daily, as well as an abundance of fresh produce. We make it readily available. If we satisfy the "sweet tooth" with natural sugars from fruits, our bodies will no longer crave refined and/or artificial sweeteners. For children, this is especially important. We all need a significant amount of glucose to keep our brains functioning at peak. Our children's tastes truly have begun to change, and their thoughts and actions seem to reach a little higher. I have a very strong belief in the value of this lifestyle, but I still allow people their own choices according to where they are in life. My website: is www. jjvitalityfood.com.

The Graham Family—2006

Dr. Douglas Graham and Professor Rozalind Graham have been teaching health and nutrition for more than 20 years and are both in exemplary health. At the time the following article was written in 2006, Dr. Graham was a raw foodist for 27 years and Professor Graham for 20 years. I have learned much from both of them that I've been able to integrate and benefit from in my own life. I thank them for their in-depth research and passion to share their knowledge. Dr. Graham's website: www.foodnsport.com

Here is Rozalind's loving description of the lifestyle they lead:

For Karen

I was born with an innate love of animals. This love led me to take a vegetarian path at a young age. Awareness of the cruelty involved in the production of dairy products grew within me until I made a vegan choice some years later. Another blessing I was born with was a love of life, which was accompanied by a distinct dislike for feeling ill. I eventually started to ask questions such as, "Will eating this food make me healthier or sicker?" My dear long-suffering mother always did her best to answer my questions and never once complained about my unusual dietary preferences. She toiled in her kitchen preparing me a vast array of vegetarian delights mostly born of her own imaginative creativity. Were it not for her endless support of my health-seeking endeavors, I may have ended up somewhere quite different from where I am today.

For other reasons, however, my childhood was deeply distressing and traumatic. Each of us has a story and mine is certainly no exception. I have shared it with others in the past, but will not do so here. I have come to understand that telling it simply keeps the memory and pain alive. Suffice to say, I had more than sufficient cause to use food as an emotional analgesic throughout the first three decades of my life.

It was the constant struggle with disordered eating that led me to study nutritional science in search of answers to my eating turmoil. So severe were my food addictions, compulsive binges, and weight loss obsessions that I came dangerously close to my demise. I was at my dietary sickest at age 23, a time when I was faced with the choice of giving up the fight altogether or drawing on the little remaining strength I had left and finding a way back to dietary peace. I knew no half-hearted approach would be enough. I also knew I had neither the time nor the energy to hold down a job while at the same time pursuing the answers I sought. After much consideration, I decided to etch out a new career for myself; I decided to make a career of getting well. There is a saying: "Once one is committed, providence moves in." This was certainly true in my case.

What quickly followed was my discovery of Natural Hygiene and the raw food diet, which together literally saved my life. My hunger for food progressively became replaced with a hunger for learning. I accessed every Natural Hygiene resource I could lay my hands on. I became an insatiable student of the science of human health and actively set about creating my own superior level of vibrant wellbeing. Parallel to my nutritional studies, I developed an interest in physical exercise. This was not easy to begin with, as I was obese at the time. What I did have in my favor was a background in dance, something I had cultivated since childhood. Dance is an innate part of who I am, but back then it was hidden beneath layers of pain-drenched fat.

Fuelled by my commitment to become an expert in health creation, I enrolled in a one year-long course to train as an aerobics instructor. This proved to be the first step in what turned out to be an extensive career in the fitness industry.

My studies led me down many interesting and rewarding paths. One of those paths resulted in my becoming a senior lecturer for London Central YMCA's Training and Development Department. For over a decade, I worked for them as a Course Director and Assessor of Teacher Training for fitness professionals throughout the UK. It was during this time that I was involved in the co-creation of the first postgraduate teacher training course on the subject of exercise for older adults. I also played a significant role in the creation and development of many other postgraduate courses, such as Pre and Post Natal Exercise. Most of all, I was interested in encouraging those who were obese to enter into a more active lifestyle, so as to help overcome their problem and increase their self esteem. This passion resulted in my becoming the sole creator of the first postgraduate course for qualified fitness professionals in exercise programming for obese people. Parallel to my career in fitness, I constantly sought out education in nutrition and other aspects of healthy living. Eventually these studies culminated in my receiving a professorship in health science and applied nutrition, subjects I continued to lecture in for many years at London's Middlesex University.

My search for further education led me overseas to various countries, including the U.S.A. At Georgetown University in Washington, D.C., I met the wonderful and brilliant man who is now my beloved husband, Dr. Douglas Graham. Together we travel far and wide teaching people how to take responsibility for the creation of their own health, fitness

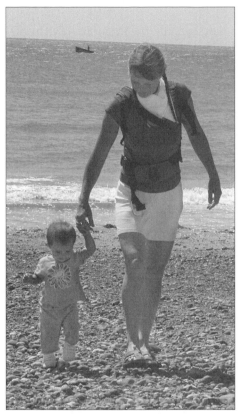

Faychesca and mom, Rozalind Graham

and wellbeing. As private health consultants, international speakers, and writers, we endeavor to bring personal empowerment to the health seekers of the world. The teaching we offer incorporates far more than just individual health. We believe education is meaningless and valueless unless activated by loving-kindness, compassion, nurturing, and awareness. We believe once these inseparable prerequisites of personal, environmental, and global health are integrated, there is nothing that cannot be achieved in the healing of the world. Our mission statement reads:

> *It is our mission to contribute the threads of our teaching to the tapestry of the collective consciousness, to enhance the knowledge and awareness necessary for the evolution of ahimsa as well as global and individual health. It is our mission to do this with professionalism, grace and humility.*

Over the years, the focus of my work has been to help those who suffer the mental and physical agonies of disordered eating by teaching them the science and application of Natural Hygiene and the raw vegan diet. In order to best serve my clients, I have undertaken extensive studies in psychology, counseling, and metaphysics. Education and experience have taught me—only when the diet is corrected in conjunction with the healthful processing of emotional pain can authentic recovery be achieved.

More recently, I have expanded my work to embrace the many diverse aspects of women's health issues. I am constantly honored by the extent to which women allow me into their lives in order to help them, and I am endlessly impressed by the inner strength demonstrated by so many wonderful women around the world.

Last year, at the age of forty-five, I noticed the absence of my usual monthly menses. I sat on my bed captured by the melancholy of realizing I had stepped through the door of menopause, and therefore was never going to be a Mother. In the past, my husband and I had shared the same viewpoint with regard to having a child. We both felt that if we were parents it would be wonderful, but if we were not, it would be equally as wonderful. We thought remaining childless would enable us to continue traveling and teaching, unencumbered by a tiny dependant. I sat on my bed that day, however, and a great sob rose up from inside me. It felt as if the goddess within were bereaving for the child she was never to know. My misery was short-lived, however, for within a couple of days I began to notice a heaviness in my breasts. I had also been feeling nauseous at about 4 pm each day, which I had attributed to the fatigue I had also been experiencing. I awoke one morning to the possibility of being pregnant. I did not dare to believe it. However, if I wasn't, the disappointment would be too great.

I felt somewhat silly going to buy a pregnancy testing kit. The sales clerk seemed to assume I was purchasing the item for a daughter or young friend rather than for myself. I scurried home clutching what felt like my destiny, hidden in a little paper bag. My first reaction, when seeing the test outcome as positive, was to assume I had somehow done the test wrong. I re-read the instructions and performed the test again. Again it came up positive. I stared and stared at the stick with a mixture of disbelief and ecstatic joy surging through my veins. I then put on my coat and shoes, went out of the front door, and walked for several hours in the hills surrounding our home in England.

My husband Doug had just gone overseas at the time, and so I went alone to have a scan to confirm a miracle had truly happened. There she was, a tiny pulsating spirit, nestled in my womb. Tears of wonderment and joy dampened my cheeks as I viewed the monitor. My heart raced to join hers, as its magical beat was made audible to me for the first time. Then suddenly the face of the radiographer changed, as if a cloud had passed across an otherwise blue sky.

"What's wrong?" I asked, aware of the tremble in my own voice. "You have had a bleed" was her matter-of-fact reply. She then went on to tell me, in an equally uncompassionate tone that I needed to see one of her colleagues who would explain the implications of her findings. I walked

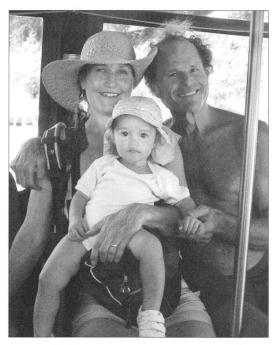

The Graham Family – Faychesca with mom, Rozalind, and dad, Doug

along the corridors, as instructed, following the appropriate signs until I arrived at the correct department. An austere older woman with a masculine appearance took me aside into a small office and viewed the information I had been clutching in my trembling hands. She turned to me with a piteous look on her face and proceeded to tell me how sorry she was. My heart sank like a stone. "At your age, my dear, it is likely this baby will never make it. The bleed from your uterus indicates a problem." I could not catch my breath and at the same time hold back the sea of tears that had suddenly surged into my throat. I swallowed hard. Then it dawned on me—I remembered. Two weeks ago I had fallen while out horseback riding and had ended up in the hospital. I shared this information, almost whispering as I said it for fear the words alone would deprive me of my precious baby. "Well, that probably is the cause of the bleed," she replied, with an expression of almost delight. She then preempted me with what to expect if I miscarried, before sending me out into a cold and bleak world that had seemed so sunny and warm when I had arrived only one hour before. As I walked across the parking lot, the ground came up to hit my feet as if to jolt me into accepting the reality of my nightmare. With every step, the words of the woman pounded in my ears, "At your age…." I heard her condescending voice again and again. I cried so hard on the way home, I turned on the windshield wipers of the car in an irrational effort to see where I was going.

During the days following, I felt as if I were suspended in a state of animation as I waited to discover if this precious baby was to leave my body or remain and grow towards our future together. With every day that passed, I became progressively more certain the spirit inside of me was to be born into the world. I felt a connection, a certainty; I felt the essence of my femininity blossom inside of me. The afternoon nausea was rapidly becoming a reassuring friend telling me of my pregnancy's continuance. It did continue for nine whole months, and so did the nausea (except for the eighth month). Despite many negative predictions and expectations from obstetricians, my baby continued to grow with perfection unmatched by the off-spring of typical mothers half my age. Medics expressed their amazement at my vibrant state of health as my blood pressure hovered steadily around 100/55 and my urine and blood tests gave ideal results.

Throughout my pregnancy, I continued my daily walks in the hills, often lasting for three hours or more at a time. By the time my little one was due to be born, my total weight gain was a modest nineteen pounds. The obstetrician expressed concern it was insufficient weight gain to support a healthy baby, but I thought, and felt, otherwise. Each morning, I would examine my beautiful swollen tummy for signs of stretch marks, but none ever materialized. I attribute this to eating raw fruits and vegetables that so perfectly provide my skin with the nutrients and water it needs to remain soft, moist, and elastic. Were it not for the intense nausea that challenged me twenty-four hours a day, I could honestly report my entire pregnancy was nothing but an entirely blissful physical experience.

As my due date approached, the obstetrician was very eager to induce me two weeks early. The reason I was given for this violent intervention was my age. I refused to entertain the idea despite all efforts to scare me into compliance.

On April 6th 2005, at 1:15 p.m., my little miracle was born to the world just over one week beyond her due date. I birthed her naturally; without any drugs or pain relief of any description. My husband Doug remained with me throughout and, when I was overcome by the exhaustion of having labored for many hours, his loving encouragement brought Faychesca Celeste into the world.

Our little miracle girl was 100% healthy at birth and has remained so ever since. As I type with one hand, she lies sleeping on my lap with her angelic head resting with confidence and trust on my left arm. I look down at her and am reminded of the deep trust we've both had in each other since the beginning—a trust rooted in Mother Nature, the power of the feminine spirit, and love.

Our approach to parenting is different from that usual to families of the industrialized world. It has come about as a result of our extensive research, introspection, thought and insights into the subject. We do not profess to have all the answers, nor do we consider ourselves to be perfect parents. What we do believe is that our approach goes some way towards providing our daughter with a deeply rooted sense of security, self-approval, love and confidence in order for her to thrive in what is becoming a progressively more frightening and soul-destroying planetary and societal environment.

What follows are the key concepts upon which we are approaching our roles as parents along with explanations for our choices. We both know we are going to learn a lot as we go along, and our approaches to parenting will naturally evolve as we gain experience.

Vitamin K

Vitamin K is routinely injected into (or orally administered to) newborn babies in an attempt to assist with clotting of the blood should any type of hemorrhage occur. We have learned the chance of a child developing leukemia resulting from this intervention is greater than that of a hemorrhage. For this reason we did not allow our baby to be given vitamin K—something she created within her own body within a short time after birth, as nature intended.

Vaccinations

The magnitude of information we have accessed regarding this issue is far too extensive to cite here. In summary, it is clear to us from our research into the subject that the risk of long-term, serious and irreversible damage to the body as a result of contaminating it with vaccines is exceptionally high. Attempts by drug manufacturers to prove vaccines in any way help to protect the body from disease appear to be fallacious and are based on the distortion of actual evidence, which clearly indicates vaccines to be health destroying and, in some cases, the cause of immediate fatality. We shall not be subjecting Faychesca to any vaccines or inoculations of any type or description whatsoever. We intend to do everything in our power to assist our child's body to maintain a robust and vibrant state of health to insure maximal natural protection against all manner of microbes.

Attachment

Throughout the natural world there exists great variation in the self-sufficiency of newborn creatures. A baby zebra will be on its feet and able to stand and move unsupported within a matter of hours, and able to keep up with the herd in a matter of days. In contrast, a baby kangaroo is incapable of independent transportation outside of the protective mother's pouch and relies on being carried from place to place for considerable time following birth. Human babies are one of the most defenseless and dependent of all newborns on earth.

They do not have the ability to stand or walk, let alone run, and rely totally on their parents for protection from all manner of environmental and sociological threats. Such vulnerability carries with it an inborn expectation for mother or father to be in very close contact with them at all times. For such a defenseless creature, it is unnatural ever to be out of physical reach of one of its parents, upon whom it depends for its very survival from minute to minute.

Psychologists have discovered that babies up to at least the age of six months have minimal ability to remember. This means each time *mummy* or daddy goes out of view, which in newborns is about 18 inches, the baby does not recall that on previous occasions the parent returned and so assumes they are lost and gone forever. Each time this happens the baby is traumatized. We believe this perceived type of early and repeated abandonment plants the seeds of low self-worth and insecurity demonstrated by the majority of children—a trait commonly carried into adulthood.

In order to provide our daughter with a maximal feeling of self-worth and security so she may grow up feeling confident and secure, we practice what is referred to as "Attachment Parenting." This involves ensuring one of us is always within physical touch or view of our baby at all times until she feels naturally inclined to move away from us. A common reaction from others to this approach to parenting is fear the child will grow up to be too "clingy" and will become overly dependent upon the parents. All evidence we have accessed has proven the opposite to be the case. Children who have been nurtured with attachment parenting show a far greater confidence and boldness than those who have been repeatedly traumatized by the conventional approach, many of whom suffer from bed-wetting, fear of being alone and a reticence for social interaction.

Our application of attachment parenting includes us carrying our baby close to our bodies in a baby sling or baby carrier. We do not use a pram or a stroller, which would render us out of physical touch and sight of our baby given her naturally limited infantile vision. Faychesca has slept skin-to-skin with us in our bed from the day she was born and continues to do so. She has never been relegated to spend the night in a solitary crib, cradle or other receptacle. At no point will we insist she sleep separate from us. We will allow her to lead this transition when she is naturally ready to seek her own space.

Crying

When studying other creatures, it is evident the intensity and frequency of crying demonstrated by the majority of human babies far exceeds that of any other species. Crying is usually a signal of distress of one type or another (including physical discomfort and hunger). In accordance with attachment parenting, we believe a major cause of crying is the trauma that results from perceived abandonment. Psychologists have concluded that the eventual cessation of crying among babies who are left to cry occurs as a result of the baby sinking into a state of hopelessness. We do not subscribe to the common belief that babies who obtain the attention of their parents whenever they cry become overly demanding, selfish and attention-seeking children. We believe such children typically result from a desperate need to be heard and acknowledged. It is our view that babies who are ignored when they cry develop these feelings along with low self-worth and insecurity, and can potentially become limited in their perception of themselves as effective communicators.

Our interpretation of Faychesca's cries is based on the understanding that she is either in some sort of distress or has a need which it is our duty as parents to do our best to meet. It is our intention to always seek out and remove the cause of her distress whenever she cries and never to ignore it or deliberately intend for her to cry herself into silence.

Breastfeeding and Diet

Faychesca is exclusively breastfed and will continue to be until such a time she naturally shows interest in beginning to eat solid food. I shall then continue to breastfeed her as the amount of solid foods gradually increases. I will only discontinue offering her breast milk once she demonstrates a natural desire to fully wean. We believe breastfeeding a baby is neither "dirty," sexual, pornographic, shameful nor immodest but rather a totally natural and beautiful procedure. I therefore do not hide in toilets or any other socially expected places in order to feed her when away from home, nor do we feel the need to disguise the procedure or hide away in our own home when she is hungry.

I have been thriving on raw vegan foods for nearly twenty years, and my husband Doug has done the same for over twenty five years. Our knowledge and experience indicate a low fat (under 10% of total calorie intake) raw vegan diet is the natural diet for fully grown humans, and is totally in accordance with our biological design. We understand any deviation from that diet is therefore detrimental to health. When Faychesca demonstrates she is ready for solid foods, we will introduce her to small quantities of ripe raw organic soft sweet fruits, such as bananas. The variety in her diet will slowly evolve to be the same as ours, and will include a wide range of whole, fresh, ripe, raw organic fruits, vegetables, avocados, nuts and seeds.

Diapers

Diapers are, of course, a human invention and do not exist anywhere in the natural world. While they are very convenient for parents, they do have disadvantages for the baby including causing skin irritation, discomfort, infections, lack of air circulation necessary for healthy skin development and the buildup of unpleasant odors. The bulkiness of a nappy can interfere with the natural movement of a baby's legs and could possibly even cause the legs to grow out of alignment in a bowed manner. While we acknowledge the appropriateness of diaper use at certain times and in certain situations, it is our intention to allow our baby to be diaper-free as often as possible. This has proven challenging in the northern hemisphere where time out of doors is limited by cold weather, but we are attempting to give her every opportunity to move freely.

Cots [Cribs] and Play Pens

Putting a baby behind bars does not resonate with us as being conducive to the healthy psychological development of the infant. We therefore do not use such equipment. As explained above, our baby sleeps with us. We sleep with our baby placed between us so our bodies provide her with a natural protection from falling out of the bed. We have been assured by many advisors (including medical doctors) there is no danger of us rolling onto or squashing our baby in any way when sleeping in this manner. This, apparently, is a tragedy exclusive to the obese or those who sleep with their babies while intoxicated by alcohol or drugs.

Smoking

We strictly take whatever steps necessary to protect our baby from inhaling tobacco smoke. We therefore do not take her into any tobacco smoke filled environments and will immediately remove her from anywhere that becomes contaminated with tobacco smoke during our presence there.

Homeschooling

We are very fortunate in that Faychesca has come to us at a time in our lives when we have the time, resources, and personal and academic development to honor our responsibility of teaching her. In addition, we have no desire for our daughter to spend many hours each day being influenced physically, psychologically, academically and emotionally by strangers whose perspectives, values and morals are extensively opposed to ours.

We intend to provide our child with a carefully structured and comprehensive scholastic pathway based on her developing an authentic interest in subjects that will be of real value throughout her life.

These days both in the U.K. and the U.S.A. there are very extensive support systems and resources for those choosing to homeschool their children, including all manner of syllabus guidelines and approaches to gaining standard qualifications and beyond. We intend to access all such resources we evaluate useful. As Faychesca's academic needs expand, if any subject arises that is beyond the capacity of either one of us to teach, we are open to employing the services of an appropriate independent teacher.

Religion

It is our view there is but one ultimate divine connection available to us all, and one may access that connection via any of a multitude of different pathways—as is demonstrated by the diversity of religions and spiritually oriented practices throughout the world. Rather than deciding on Faychesca's behalf the approach best for her spiritual unfolding, our intention is to educate her in the full spectrum of moral, ethical, virtuous, righteous, and angelic qualities unanimously recognized among all major religions of the world, and in doing so provide her with the framework from which her unique spiritual perspectives can grow.

Violence

We believe children learn by example, and currently in the civilized world, children are taught violence is not only a normal and acceptable aspect of life, but also that it is glamorous.

We do not condone violence in any form and view it as evidence of an immature society, suffering from spiritual depravation. We classify any deliberate word, deed or action that results in the physical, psychological or emotional distress of another, to be an act of violence. It is our intention to teach Faychesca grace by our own example and to demonstrate that all issues can be overcome in a non-violent manner. In addition to our own example, we intend to implement the following:

> Toys will not include imitation guns (or any form of weaponry) or imitation archetypes of violence such as soldiers.
> Toys will not include any imitation of animal abuse including animal farming.
> Television viewing will be monitored and all shows containing violence will be excluded from entering our home.
> We will raise our daughter to maximally practice all aspects of veganism (congruent with our own lifestyle).

Author's Note: I respect and admire Rozalind's views on violence, but I found it difficult, if not impossible, to stick to these guidelines 100% of the time when my children were growing because it would have intervened with their decisions on how to play and with whom. I have friends who moved to a much more isolated environment to get away from many of these influences, but even then, their younger boy began to make knights and swords and play in violent ways, as he showed a desire to learn about this. Both of my children have played with others who exposed them to violent toys, videos or movies, but neither of my children has ever developed any violent tendencies. They have always been extremely social and loving children and teenagers. I believe their resultant behaviors are more related to the non-violent examples we as parents exhibit to our children throughout their growing years that makes the most difference.

Shouting

Currently within the civilized world children are taught shouting is not only acceptable but a normal aspect of life (including family life). We believe the only authentic justification for shouting is when it's necessary in order to be heard, due to distance or over environmental background noise. We recognize all other forms of shouting as an act of violence. We intend to do our utmost to demonstrate to our child that shouting is non-serving, destructive, and unnecessary. Although we realize we will be unable to protect Faychesca from being exposed to the shouting displayed by others, we intend to remove her from such environments whenever possible.

Gender Specific Degradation

While it is common practice for both men and women to seize opportunities to make jokes involving the degradation of the opposite gender, we believe this socially accepted habit contributes to serious social and individual problems, and we intend not to participate in such remarks—be they made in jest or otherwise. We intend to do all we can to ensure Faychesca develops a respectful attitude towards both genders, whereby the natural attributes of both are acknowledged and revered.

Sarcasm

Sarcasm is used when a person is intending to achieve one or more of the following:

Have a negative impact on the self-esteem of the other person;
Communicate they do not want to be honest with the other person;
Show disrespect for the other person;
Insinuate the other person is stupid;
Cause another person embarrassment;
Be perceived as amusing at the expense of the other person's feelings.

We therefore view sarcasm as the most comprehensive form of rudeness and intend to teach Faychesca sarcasm is neither clever nor amusing but rather evidence of poor communication skills and lack of kindness.

Reprimanding in Jest

Young children have not yet developed the intellectual ability to distinguish between authentic reprimanding and that done in jest. We intend to exclude all reprimanding in jest from our communications with our child and replace it, when necessary, with explaining the laws of cause and effect and choice and outcome.

In Conclusion

In our hearts, Doug and I carry the vision of a new world in which peace, harmony, love and respect for all life forms, including Mother Earth herself, predominate. We envision a world where violence, cruelty and abuse in all forms are obsolete. We believe if such a world can be conceived by the intellect, it can be manifested as reality. We believe within each new generation sleeps the seeds of global change, awaiting to be awakened by the intent and sculpting of parents as they teach their offspring about life and right choices. We believe in the same way the health of a person's body depends upon the health of the individual cells—the blossoming of world peace likewise depends upon peace dwelling within the heart of each individual. It is our sincere intent to enable our daughter to fulfill her potential as a single contributor in bringing about the collective shift in human consciousness necessary for our planet's survival.

—Rozalind Graham

Here is Luke Swift's triumphant account of his raw food family path:

The Swift Family

January 2006

My son Adam is almost three years old. His mother gave birth to him naturally, without any drugs or medical interference at a birthing center here in our hometown. She and I trained for the birth by following the Bradley Method, and we hired a birth assistant who assisted in hundreds of natural births. As soon as he was born, he lay on his mother's chest and took in the new world around him with a stunning sense of calm and awareness. No crying, no hysteria and an uncanny expression of real wonder.

We took him home a few hours after the birth, and he has been sleeping in our bed every night. He loves it and we love it. Of course, for the first few months it was hard to get a sound night's sleep, but frankly, I didn't mind so much, as the joy and excitement of having this little being in our bed was really amazing. He now sleeps beautifully and wakes us up with his little charming voice and a priceless smile, "Mommy wake up! Daddy wake up!"

We refused all vaccines and the "normal" medical "treatments," which at the least include antibiotics swabbed in the eyes, a heel prick blood test, circumcision (a barbaric and cruel act), a vitamin K shot and a list of other unnecessary and dangerous medical practices. He has no food other than uncooked, unprocessed organic fresh fruits, vegetables, seeds and nuts. He has been breastfeeding since birth and continues to thrive. He is taller than every boy we have met his age. He is bright, gregarious, receptive, and has an unending amount of energy.

The first food he ate was a bit of organic avocado he reached for on my plate at the age of four months. He liked it and tried a piece of banana not too many days afterwards.

By five or six months, he was eating mashed bananas on a regular basis, a piece of avocado once in a while, and fresh coconut water once or twice a day. He has gained weight and grown in a perfectly healthy manner. He has a fantastic appetite and continually asks for his fruits, vegetables, seeds and nuts. He has been around other children who are eating "normal" food, and much to our surprise, he has never expressed any interest in eating it.

Adam has suffered none of the "normal" childhood diseases. No colic, ear infections, rashes or excessive mucus. His skin tone is remarkable, his hair is full, shiny and thick, his teeth are straight and white, and his eyes are as bright and clear as can be. He has been ill on two or three occasions, most likely brought on by the cold of winter—coughs, sniffles and a fever. Although it is upsetting to see our boy sick, we were confident his body's intelligence was doing its best to correct the situation. No doctors visited, and no drugs taken. The only treatment he received was rest, some fresh juice, and a lot of love and attention. He got better quickly. On two different occasions, there were fevers brought on by teething pain. This was treated with cool cloths to the head, and more love and attention. He breastfed more than ever during this period and always felt relief afterwards. It seems breastfeeding is a great relief to a child in pain. On both of these teething pain occasions, we did apply an herbal remedy to his aching gums. He seemed to think it helped and was happy to have it applied. That was a departure from our philosophy of not treating disease, but we thought the downside (side effects) would be minimal, and fortunately, we were correct.

Both my wife and I are thrilled with the results we have seen raising our little boy according to his natural biological design. We plan on having more children and raising them in the same manner. One of our favorite books on the subject is *A WAY OUT: Dis-ease Deception and the Truth about Health* by Matthew Grace (www.matthewgrace.com). It is quick, to the point, and simply makes a lot of sense. Herbert Shelton's books are also great.

We are both saddened to see so many children suffering unnecessarily and then being drugged to add to their physical turmoil. We live in a very ignorant society that has been completely brainwashed by the pharmaceutical companies and their media. Fortunately, we have created a small community of likeminded parents and children, and it is clear to us there is a distinct difference in the temperament, intelligence, and overall wellbeing of these "natural children."

—Luke Swift

David Klein, author, and publisher of "Vibrance Magazine," sent me a DVD titled *Raising Children Raises Us* by Shannon Leone. I immediately loved the title, and after viewing the lovely story about this Canadian family, depicting homeschooling, attachment parenting and raw food nutrition, I called Shannon to ask her to write a passage for *Creating Healthy Children.*

The Leone Family
March 2006

The Pleasure Principle in Parenting through Food

I love being a Mom and truly believe for some of us it is a Spiritual Calling. For as long as I can remember, all I have ever wanted was to have a family. I always knew with certainty I would have children, nurse them, and devote myself to consciously raising them. When you live in that clear an intention, the Universe conspires to support you no matter what...

Born at a scant four pounds, my survival was precarious. I was always a little frail growing up, but when my beloved single mother died suddenly of a heart attack when I was 16, my immune system crashed. I was diagnosed with severe insomnia, asthma and heart disease in my 20s, and I wondered if I would even make it to my mother's ripe old age of 48...

Well, I have not only survived, I have truly thrived. Becoming a mother is a "Course in Miracles," and feeding my family is a sacred task. This is why I have embraced the living foods lifestyle. Everything about it is in harmony with the pure vibration of a child's potential. I seek only to develop and harness that potential and not to do anything to diminish it.

And so, I have converted my family over to raw foods. It has been so exciting, yet not without its challenges. My husband comes from a strong, well-meaning Italian family—meat, pasta, bread and cheese dominate every family celebration. Being *raw* is tricky—you learn to plan ahead. I fill us up with green smoothies; make the salads, fruit platters and raw desserts. Then I let go and enjoy the party. Tomorrow is another day—we'll all cleanse.

Being flexible and adaptable is a sign of good mental health. For me, family is paramount; and true, overall health is about more than a number. At home, I can be 100% raw, but in social situations with the family, I've learned being rigid is more stressful than allowing occasional compromises, especially when it comes to the kids. I may choose to go to a gathering and be raw, but I do not force the kids; a side dish of homemade pasta lovingly prepared and served is a small sacrifice to keep the peace. However, I draw the line at flesh foods, junk food, soda pop, candy, and anything fried or packaged.

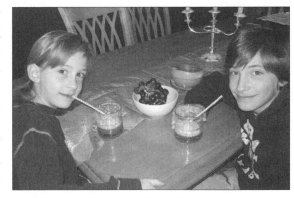

Liam and Landon enjoying their green juices

I've learned the hard way that an overemphasis on food can mar the entire experience and though I am raw and convinced it's the best way to go, I'm more apt to attract people to the benefits if I walk my own path in harmony with others. I feel this food and lifestyle is a very gentle and loving experience for *all*.

In my travels, I was always touched by the loving relationships other cultures had to their foods. Whether in Asia, South America, Australia or Europe, the focus was never on calories or health per se. The central theme seemed to be *pleasure*. Everything about food brought enjoyment: from the beautiful way food was displayed in local markets, artfully prepared and gracefully served and shared—everywhere there was beauty and delight.

This is vastly in contrast to our typical model of fear, guilt, deprivation and binging. We have lost our natural, wholesome relationship to food every bit as much as we have lost these same qualities *in* our food. *How* we eat, our state of being, is as important as *what* we eat, raw or otherwise. When we eat on the run, while driving, watching TV or reading the news, microwave our meals, eat out of plastic containers, while standing up... Where is the sanctity, the nourishment in all that? Sadder still is how everyone here is on a diet—even pre-teens! All the dieting in the world won't guarantee physical, emotional, mental and spiritual health. And no matter how much we binge we still remain hungry and empty on some level. Even raw foodists experience this initially until the internal shift catches up to the external one. So it is not only about what you are eating, but also 'what is eating you.'

Like passionate lovers sensually experiencing each other, is how we may relearn to engage with our food. Only by eating this way, with our senses fully open and awake, will we be truly nurtured and fed. Beautiful, raw food liberates such subtle but powerful distinctions and revelations.

When I fully understood the damage of 'you should' on my family over food, I grew determined to find ways of bringing harmony. I've been creating rituals to reestablish a more balanced, peaceful and 'irresistible' connection with our food. I would like to share some of them with you now:

- I started off by slowing down—my movements, my thoughts, and my pace, centering myself and gaining emotional poise.
- I take the time to think about the atmosphere I can create—a feeling of excitement, or calm, or fun.
- When preparing a meal for myself or the family I light a little candle just for *me*.
- I put on some classical music to enjoy, or I sing, chant or pray. I believe this puts my love into the food. Remember *Babette's Feast* and *Like Water for Chocolate*!
- Then I do what my husband's mother does—I "set a beautiful table" with fresh or wild flowers, or create a centerpiece of golden and crimson leaves, or pinecones, berries and acorns, or seashells and crystals— something lovely to reflect the season, usually gathered by my children on a Nature walk.
- I use the 'good dishes' and beautiful, simple but cared for linens.
- Clearing away any remnants of work, mail, phones or other distractions, I am now ready to ring the dinner bell.
- After all hands are washed and everyone is assembled, my husband lights the dinner candle.
- We all hold hands and sing the blessing. I love to take this moment to see the light in my family's eyes.

Then the feast begins!

I encourage my little tigers to take their time and really *savor* every bite. I really do believe the woman sets the tone in the home, and my husband holds the space for us all. He models good habits by putting his fork down between bites, chewing thoroughly, even closing his eyes and letting out little "Ahhhhhh"s and "Mmmmm"s. He even declares enthusiastically, "Mama sure is the best chef in town!" To which my sons usually chime in, "She sure is!" Having my husband's support makes mealtimes an experience of bonding, laughter, storytelling and true sustenance.

I keep it really simple throughout the day by serving light fare: green smoothies and green juices, fresh fruit, crudités with raw dips or paté, guaca-

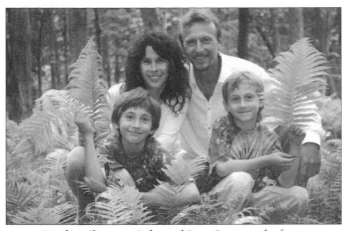

Landon, Shannon, Luke and Liam Leone in the ferns

mole with olives and dehydrated flax crackers, seaweed and veggie salads, or raw soups are some options.

Dinner is a little more elaborate—maybe a main meal salad made with kale, dandelion, parsley and arugula with okra, tomatoes, onion and hemp-seeds topped off with a miso ginger dressing, or perhaps a raw gourmet dish of zucchini pasta with pesto-stuffed mushrooms and raw lemon-raspberry 'un' cheescake; or wild rice 'un' stir-fry with garlic-ginger marinade. If it's Friday, it could be a homemade lentil stew, or curried cauliflower quinoa, or millet-veggie patties with tahini.

Whatever I serve, it will be of the freshest, organic (when possible) ingredients prepared and served with love.

Having a loving and healthy family is the pinnacle of success for me. I am deeply grateful for the exciting works of Dr. Carolyn Dean, Dr. Brian Clement, Victoria Boutenko, David Wolfe and Rudolph Steiner for inspiring me to become empowered to be the mother I've always wanted to be.

Blessings!

—Shannon Leone

Shannon Leone is the author of a beautiful DVD called *Raising Children Raises Us* which looks at homeschooling, raw nutrition, and other facets of conscious parenting. Ms Leone is also the President of The Little Friends Foundation, and can be reached for classes and consultations at (705) 735-4169 or at sjkleone@yahoo.com.

I met Carol Iwaniuk when she was visiting New York City from Australia several years ago. She and one of her sons attended a raw food support meeting I led in Manhattan. She writes of the benefits of a healthy raw food diet:

Carol Iwaniuk and Family
April, 2006

My children and I have thrived on raw vegan food. I started my journey 6 years ago, and the children started theirs 5 years ago. My kids are now 16 and 13, and I must admit, I was a bit skeptical about them being on raw food during their growing years.

But my fears were unfounded, as my eldest, who started his growth spurt late in his fourteenth year, is now nearly six feet tall and very strong. My youngest still hasn't started his growth spurt, but I must say since he's been eating raw foods, he's had no more asthma attacks, dry skin or warts.

After beginning raw foods, my very irregular menstrual cycle was rectified and regular ovulation pain known as Mittleschmerz has healed. After eating raw foods for three months, I started to experience, for the first time in my menstruating life, a normal 28 day cycle, which has continued, as well as the absence of Mittleschmerz. One year prior to starting raw foods, at age 36, when my periods became really erratic, a doctor had told me I was pre-menopausal and should start taking birth control pills to regulate my cycle. Fortunately, I didn't listen and sought other alternatives.

I knew about eating raw foods over twenty years ago from a book called The *Mucusless Diet Healing System* by Professor Arnold Ehret and dabbled in it back then. Even though it felt right and I believed this is how we humans are meant to eat, here in Australia there was no support or further information about it, so I allowed myself to slip back into cooked foods. However, I still kept up my search for the perfect diet, and 15 years later, thanks to Internet technology, I guess I came full circle.

For a good part of the past year, we've been following Victoria Boutenko's idea of green smoothies (green leaves blended with filtered water and fruit) which we usually have for breakfast. We also eat whatever organic fruits are in season, as well as whole fruit smoothies or fruit with creamy fruit sauce (what I call "yogurt"). We make a variety of dips using avocados, tahini or sprouted nuts, which we eat with a large serving of different seasonal non-sweet fruits and vegetables. We snack on nuts and seeds, and we always have a very large salad once a day. The kids' favorite food at the moment is grapes with straw-berry "yogurt" (made by blending a punnet of fresh organic strawberries with a handful of organic pine nuts or cashews). They also love their salads as well as Thai coconuts.

—Carol Iwaniuk, Melbourne, Australia

I met Laura and Brendan Sutton and two of their children, Kai and Junah, when Marco and I visited Costa Rica for the third time in February 2007. They had moved there from Florida and seemed extremely happy with their choice of destination as a raw family. Laura writes with enthusiasm about her family's raw vegan lifestyle. Their daughter, Aria, was born February 2008.

The Sutton Family
March 2007

Hola Karen,

I finally finished my entry for your book…and here it is:

I'm deeply honored to have this opportunity to create an entry in a raw family inspirational book. My story could fill a book I think, but I'll try to be as concise as possible. Since I, Laura, am the one responsible, with God/Goddess blessings, for transitioning my family to the raw diet, it seems appropriate that I tell you how I originally became inspired to go raw: In 1989, at age 19, I decided to go vegan. I found a job in a small health food store which sold many raw food books, such as *Survival into the 21st Century* by Viktoras Kulvinskas and *Recipes for Longer Life* by Ann Wigmore. Upon reading these and many other raw books, it started to make sense to me that not only vegan-ism, but also raw veganism, is the most perfect diet for humans. I used to cry and get chills through my body when I read those books because everything they conveyed resonated very deeply within me; and I wished this information could have come to me much sooner. For the first 19 years of my life, although I was thin and seemingly healthy, I dealt with extreme and embarrassing in-testinal discomfort. As soon as I went vegan I experienced great relief, and began for the first time in my life to have regular bowel movements. Needless to say, I immediately knew I had made the right dietary change. Since then, I've attempted the raw diet several times without success, mostly due to "societal pressure." We definitely live in a "cooked-food-world," making it

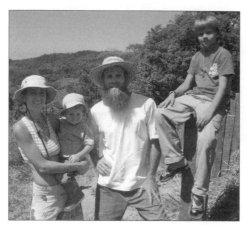

Laura, Junah, Brendan and Kai Sutton in Costa Rica

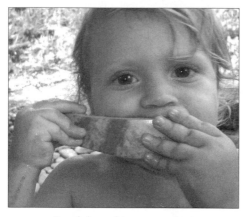

Junah loves his watermelon!

extremely challenging to resist the fragrant temptations of these foods. Developing and strengthening one's willpower, to reach for a banana instead of a slice of pizza for instance, is the crucial key for remaining raw. However, now that I've been 100% raw for the past two years, I've noticed temptations becoming less tempting, and my willpower growing stronger every day. Desiring to be an optimal role model for my husband and children also provides motivation for me to remain raw.

When I met my husband, Brendan, in 1995, he was already vegan and health-minded; so upon imparting the importance and benefits of such a diet to him, going raw was a logical and easy transition. We have two sons, Kai Indigo and Junah Rain. Our first son, Kai, had a natural homebirth in 1996, was breastfed for his first three years and has been vegan since birth. He has always been exceptionally healthy, and is well known wherever we go for his exuberance. After 10 years of eating vegan cooked food, the transition to raw has been difficult for him. He constantly asks to eat at a restaurant whenever we're in town, but at home he's happy with eating 100% raw. We find as long as we always have an abundance of fruits, nuts, seeds, and salad ingredients available, he remains content. He also loves making his own salad each day and experimenting in the kitchen. Junah, who had a natural childbirth at home in 2004, has been mostly raw since birth. He has eaten some cooked food on occasion, but we no longer allow him to share his brother's occasional cooked meal. I believe his body has become very efficient at cleansing any remaining cooked food residue. He has had several intense "colds" accompanied by high fevers since he was 3 months old. I have to wonder though, had I been raw when I was pregnant with him and never fed him cooked food, would he have experienced such intense cleansing episodes? He is still breastfeeding on demand, and still sleeps by my side at night, which I intend to continue as long as he wants.

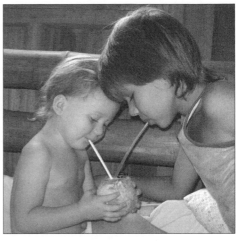

Junah and Kai sipping coconut water (known as pipa in Costa Rica)

When we transitioned to raw two years ago, we had a food processor and a dehydrator. I used to make all kinds of fancy, gourmet foods with those machines: burgers, pizzas, crackers, pies, cakes, cookies, etc., which I believe made the transition much more enjoyable for all of us. However, now that we live in Costa Rica, a tropical fruit lover's paradise, we have simplified our diet even further. We no longer eat any grains, beans, oil, salt, seaweed, or dehydrated foods. My current kitchen tools are a blender for making smoothies and salad dressings, a Spirooli for making cucumber and zucchini pasta, and a mandolin slicer for creating fun salads out of fresh heart-of-palm and carrots. We also have a special tree climbing device now, which Brendan uses to harvest all the coconuts we could ever want. We practice proper food combining, and tuning in, as much as possible, to what our bodies truly need. Moving to a tropical climate has certainly made consuming only raw foods much easier for us due to the abundance of delicious, satiating fruits; and we excitedly look forward to each one coming into season.

After countless attempts to continue on the raw vegan lifestyle path over the past 17 years, I'm thrilled to realize I've finally accomplished my goal, and managed to willingly bring my husband and sons along with me on this beautiful, ever-unfolding journey. My focus is to constantly fine-tune my family's lifestyle, to live the way I believe God/Goddess truly intended humans to live!

In blissful gratefulness,
Laura

I was told about the Schafer Family by my friend, author Paul Nison. I contacted Kristi by email, and she was thrilled to learn of the preparation of this book and was excited about contributing her family's amazing story:

The Schafer Family
May 2007

Our journey on the raw food lifestyle began over two years ago. I had suffered a heart attack at age 28, and six months later, James was in a serious automobile accident and had been told he would never walk again. He had a lot of large wounds to the top of the head, his neck was broken, practically all the ribs on the right side were broken, his liver was ruptured and hemorrhaging, his lung was ruptured, and his hip was pulled out of the socket and the socket was shattered. He was given six blood transfusions to no avail, and when I arrived at the hospital, they sent the chaplain out to break the news to me that he would not make it. Because of what had transpired at the time of my heart attack six months earlier, we had a firm belief in God as a healer and knew He had the perfect diet for curing all of man's diseases. I also firmly believed God would heal my husband in spite of the morbid diagnosis. When I was finally allowed to see him, I immediately put my hands over both of his and started talking to him and sharing my love and energy with him. I was informed he was in a coma, and could hear nothing. I just kept on talking and holding his hands. Very soon, his blood pressure, which had been so low it was hardly there at all, began to come up. Before many minutes, his blood pressure was totally normal and he was responding to me and trying to tell me he wanted the breathing tube out. The next morning he was writing messages on a clip board and visiting with me as normal, only tired. They kept drugging him very heavily in spite of both of our requests not to. The doctors had told me, to begin with, the most critical thing was his broken neck. They were afraid his arms would be paralyzed for life. They told me for sure his arms would be paralyzed for a while. That night I stayed at a friend's house near the hospital, as I had an 8 1/2 month nursing baby. My husband's mother stayed the night by him. That night, I called as many friends as I could think of to pray with me for the healing of James' neck. I had such a peaceful, sure feeling it would be fine. The next morning, upon arriving at the hospital, his mother told me an interesting piece of news. The top neck surgeon had come to his room early, as they were planning to operate on his neck to stabilize it. They said he entered the room and started examining James' neck. He became more puzzled the more he checked, and kept checking the x-ray from the previous day. Finally, he stood up and said there was nothing there…as far as he was concerned, James did not even need a neck brace! They were so puzzled, but I really knew what had happened. My heart was praising God!

The doctors then started pushing for surgery on the shattered hip. We learned if the surgery were to be carried out, he would be required to have hip replacement surgery every five years for the rest of his life…what an outlook for a 30 year old father of five children! They said he probably would be able to walk somewhat, with a bad limp, but kept telling him there was no way he would ever walk again if he didn't do the surgery. James and I decided we would go home and give God's healing way a chance once again.

I had been bringing fresh carrot juice and wheatgrass juice to him every day or several times a day from the time he became conscious. The only foods he was hungry for in the hospital were fruit and melon. Anything else did not sound good to him at all. He had never liked melons prior to that time, so I was surprised to hear him keep asking for melon. We took James home nine days after the accident. He kept on eating fruit and fruit smoothies with a few greens. He was up and walking with his walker about a week after we had returned home. He healed very rapidly and was back to work (he owned his own heating business) laying radiant floor heat six weeks after the accident. This was when we really began to see the importance of eating 100% raw food. James was fine, with no pain or side effects of his accident as long as he was eating raw and vegan. As soon as he would slip and eat something he knew was not good for him, he would feel it in his hip. That truly gives incentive for eating properly. He was doing high jumping again, which he does well, within a few months after the accident. We have truly seen miracles happen when we chose to follow the original diet for humankind instead of the standard American diet (SAD). Our children began to gain weight, and within two months of switching to 100% raw foods, people began to notice and comment about how our children were filling out. They became so much calmer and easier to communicate with. We noted a big change in our oldest son. He had been very difficult to deal with, staring into space when spoken to, and having frequent screaming tantrums. I had been close to despair that I would ever be able to reach my son. Today, he is very loving and responsive…and I am thrilled to say the least!

Why We Love Being a Raw Family

I interviewed every member of our family personally and asked them to share something about why they like being a raw family. Then I asked what each one's favorite foods were.

JAMES: The thing that stands out the most to me is we no longer have to worry about sickness and whether the children are getting what they need the way we used to. When you are totally confident your children are getting the very best nutrition possible, you are no longer afraid any serious illness or disease will strike them. For myself, I like having better energy and clarity of mind. Some of my favorite foods are crushed nettles with a touch of oil and salt. I really like wild edible plants. Greens and grapefruits are probably my favorites.

KRISTI: I enjoy so many foods. Now that I'm breastfeeding, I'm really enjoying an avocado and seeds with lots of greens, and fruits like pears and a pineapple with a few seeds for the evening meal. I feel I now have ten times more energy than I used to before I ate 100% raw foods. With my other babies, I always had trouble having an adequate milk supply. I have never had to worry with this baby, and the more greens I eat, the richer and more abundant is my milk supply. My baby is ten months and very nice and chubby. She absolutely loves avocados, which I allowed her to have once she got her first two teeth. The benefits of eating raw foods are so great they far, far outweigh the social rejection some people may encounter as a result of the change. I would never want to regress to eating dead food. We have a saying at our house: "DEAD FOOD MAKES DEAD PEOPLE, and LIVE FOOD MAKES LIVE PEOPLE."

VANESSA: (age 10) I love being in a raw family because I can create things in the kitchen. I am *soooo* glad my Dad can play with us again. I am *happy* to have a baby sister to play with! (James was told we could have no more children as he had so much nerve damage to the pelvis after his accident.) I am glad I have lots of energy to help my mom. I love to sew and am happy we homeschool. We were not happy when we were sick. I'm so glad Mom and Dad have lots of energy now. I'm glad Mom feels good now so she can do things like playing raw restaurant, making treats, helping me sew, and singing with me. I'm glad we are a happy raw family! I would not want to go back to eating cooked food because it makes me feel so tired and yucky.
My favorite foods are durians and fresh peas.

BRENDON: (age 8) I wouldn't want to go back to eating cooked or baked foods because they seem so dry to me. They just don't have juice like fresh stuff. My favorite foods are avocados, durian fruits, and raw jicama "fries."

NATHAN: (age 6) I would not like to go back to eating cooked food because I don't want mucus in my body, and ticks and mosquitoes bite me when I have mucus. My favorite foods are a jicama "cottage cheese" dish mom makes, and fresh green beans.

DEANNA: (age 5) I would never like to eat cooked food, 'cause raw food is so GOOD! My favorite foods are Brazil nuts and avocados.

DAVID: (age 3) I wouldn't like to eat cooked food 'cause it kills my body. My best food is durian fruit, and I love to do school and write my letters.

RACHEL: When Mommy asked Rachel what she liked, she said "M-m-m, Num!" She was eating a ripe kiwifruit. She loves cucumbers and avocados.

We love to forage for wild edible plants as a family, and our whole family agreed our favorite thing to do is to have a "foraged meal." Each of us takes a plate and scissors or knife (according to age) and gathers whatever looks good for a salad—whatever can be found growing outside. Here are a few examples of what we find: many and varied wild greens such as cockle, wild mustard greens, lambsquarter, crushed nettles, Virginia waterleaf, redroot, wild leeks, Jerusalem artichokes, chives, wild ginseng, chive flowers, dandelion flowers, purple violet flowers, asparagus, wild berries, etc. We have taken a couple of classes on foraging and gathered a lot of knowledge from them. We feel there is so much yet to learn, we have hardly begun.

We then put our "Italian" dressing, made of chia gel or extra virgin olive oil, lemon juice and herbs, on our foraged salad.

We find the raw journey very interesting and exciting. "The true knowledge of a man is what he has when placed alone in the middle of the wilderness." We would all benefit from more of that survival knowledge.

—James and Kristi
Vanessa, Brendon, Nathan, Deanna, David and Rachel

Eric Rivkin had been living in Minnesota but relocated to Costa Rica for cleaner air, purer water, delicious fruits, and beautiful tropical surroundings. His story, unfortunately, is a common one, relating how a spouse with little or no understanding of the benefits of a raw vegan lifestyle can negatively affect the children:

Turning Adversity into Awareness
by Eric Rivkin, July 2004

My two children were taken away from me 9 years ago when they were 12 and 8 by an unsupportive ex-wife who thought I was crazy trying to convert my family to being vegetarian. Even though real research I handed her proved this diet was better than the SAD (standard American diet), she refused to read it or apply common sense, even when I pointed out simple observations like hyperactive behavior after the kids ate a piece of candy, or bladder infections from too many sweets. Raw food veganism was too much for her to handle, although it made perfect sense.

So she divorced me, took physical custody of the kids, and proceeded to feed them SAD junk foods. My daughter gained excess weight, and suffered from sugar addiction, lethargy, extreme bladder infections and acne with a constant stream of antibiotics, and my son experienced extreme acne episodes, constipation, and lethargy. Both endured mild depression, being "down on life," and their performance in school suffered as a result. My ex-wife even fed the children foods to which medical tests showed they were allergic, such as potatoes and milk, and encouraged consumption of sweets at parties and at home, including Halloween junk food every year. I did my best to educate the children and have them experience the raw food magic when they were with me. I could see they were starving for nutrients, so I fed them high nu-trient-rich raw food cuisine which they grew to like. But they came to my house brainwashed, thinking raw food was bad for them because no one else was eating it. Defending raw foods proved futile. I learned I needed a more compassionate and accepting approach.

Lawyers told me no Court at the time would have sided with me, even though there was abundant evidence the SAD diet was tantamount to child abuse and endangerment. Instead of fighting for physical custody, I decided to focus my energy on raw food education. My kids enjoy raw vegan cuisine when they are with me and can absorb my healthful influence. They are slowly ridding themselves of bad eating habits as they see the fantastic improvement in my health and fitness, and my success in teaching raw foods in prestigious places. I see their health and mental abilities slowly improving, as they are doing what they love, and following a good spiritual path toward the higher awareness of truth. I'm happy they have become more enthusiastic about life, and their suc-cesses show it. I am thankful for the examples of other raw food kids, and some of my kids' vegetarian friends in school, who made it easier for my children to understand that what I was saying about raw foods made sense.

In letting go the food controversies between my wife and me, I grew emo-tionally stronger and connected with my children on a deeper level. When she was 18, my daughter's friends influenced her to consider vegetarianism, but lack of her mother's support squashed this awakening. There was a ray of joy when my daughter asked me to provide raw food dishes for her high school graduation party at her mother's house, and my ex provided a fruit platter. I was happy to see this beautiful fruit enjoyed first. Now in college, my daughter has cut down her meat consumption, and is less influenced by harmful SAD propaganda.

Never again do I want anyone to suffer with SAD, as my children and I suffered. So this forms my intense passion for being the best raw food chef I can be, the first to teach a raw food program in public schools under the Five-Fresh-Foods-a-Day Program (now 9 a day, and 13 a day in England) and bringing raw food education into colleges, the American Culinary Federation and Miss U.S.A. Pageants. I will continue to host seminars wherever I am wanted.

I founded the Viva La Raw Project, a nonprofit charity with the mission of raw food education. www.VivaLaRaw.org

—Eric Rivkin

Live-Foods Health Chef and Instructor, Viva La Raw Project Director

emrivkin@gmail.com

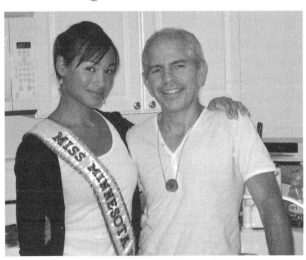

Miss U.S.A. Minnesota, Erica Nego, glowing on raw foods with Chef Eric Rivkin at his raw food preparation class

Dr. Ruza Bogdanovich has been a beloved mentor and friend since I met her at the International Raw Food Festival in Portland, Oregon in 2003, and I asked her to write a foreword to this book. Her family is of Croatian descent, and lives in Croatia, New Zealand and Nevada.

How Jesse Got Well and Stayed Well on All Raw Organic Vegan Foods

A story of triumph over crippling due to polio vaccination

by Dr. Ruza Bogdanovich, N.D., Ph.D.

My husband and I waited nine years to have Jesse. I was very healthy and nutrition conscious. I wanted to have a healthy child. We Europeans are generally very protective and down to earth, but in America there was "pressure" to follow the standard American diet (SAD) that leads to many health troubles.

Jesse was born perfectly healthy. When he was several months old, we reluctantly allowed him to be vaccinated for polio with a few other vaccines all at once. At that time we did not know it was a live polio virus, and dangerous. He reacted with high fever, convulsions and paralysis. His condition degenerated from the medical interventions. A few years later, doctors recommended a ligament surgery to loosen up tightness in his legs, and still later, the removal of his toes and many other procedures.

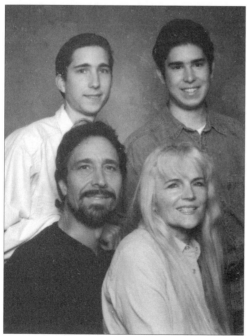

Bottom left to right: Michael and
Dr. Ruza Bogdanovich
Top left to right: Jesse and Sean Bogdanovich
2004

Shocked beyond words, we literally ran from the hospital. No way were we going to allow our child to go under the knife or sit in a wheelchair for the rest of his life. Instead, we set out on a journey in search of the truth. We were told Jesse's situation was serious and would only worsen with time. From one opinion to the next, from America to Europe, from radical to illogical, rational to irrational, natural to supernatural, we could not stop. We felt morally obligated to do everything we possibly could for his wellbeing. We felt guilty, anxious, hoping some new discovery would provide the solution, yet unwilling to subject him, in his fragile state, to any more drastic interventions.

Jesse grew thinner and more fragile. New symptoms surfaced, i.e. juvenile diabetes and stomach problems from medications and the mucus formed from milk and cheese doctors insisted he eat. His feet turned purple. We searched farther out and deeper inward. Besides his inability to walk, Jesse's biggest problem was absorbing nutrients, because he was clogged up with mucus. We were criticized by doctors, parents, neighbors and well-meaning friends for not putting Jesse on steroids, and for refusing to feed him fast foods or milkshakes for weight gain. We were told many times: "If you don't trust your doctor, whom can you trust?" We were learning doctors could be the last people we ought to trust. They are just fallible humans who have been taught to treat symptoms, prescribe drugs, and operate. Many are smart, some are even intelligent, and a few are aware and know the truth of healing. I am grateful we stopped our dependency on doctors and started putting our faith in Mother Nature.

Seeking and Finding Nature's Truth

I read book after book, listened to medical experts, received every health newsletter on the planet and only grew more confused. Everyone seemed to be talking about treating the symptoms with drugs, herbs, surgery, etc. The epiphany came when I knew on a deep inner level, we had to take matters into our own hands. I finally listened to the inner voice of Mother Nature. Unnatural food, pills, drugs, vitamins, etc., were only making Jesse sicker. By this time, my inner voice was whispering to me non-stop, we had to go back to Nature all the way. Then it was shouting louder and louder until it was screaming. Then it clicked, and all the pieces of the puzzle finally fit together.

After a long mind-clearing fast, the answers appeared from all directions. A career change was one of my first steps. But even after receiving my doctorate in Naturopathy, I still had some unanswered questions. I had to look deeper into the law of cause and effect and understand the Hygienic lifestyle because it seemed it was the only thing that worked.

The simple fact is: in order to heal and stay well, we must surrender to Nature's immutable laws. In other words, we must get out of Nature's way, stop our human interventions and totally follow Her path so the body can heal itself. For several reasons, people do not want to believe this truth, especially those in the medical profession. My license and certificate were threatened, but I didn't care. I kept hearing my Papa's words: "Give me the truth and you can have the rest," and, for the first time, I really understood.

Nature's Path to Healing

Jesse instinctively understood the path we chose. The rest just fell into place, although the path itself was not always smooth. Just when he started to feel better on his raw organic diet, healing crises appeared. When we were over the initial shock, he fasted many times, becoming more aware and conscious of his body and of his connection with the Universe. Jesse's heart became pure love and he was listening to it more and more. His mission was clear: he knew firsthand the body can heal itself, and he could help show others the way.

Several years later, when he reached the pinnacle of wellbeing, he told me he could never ever go back to the old way or stray from Nature's path, no matter what! And he has proved the sincerity of those words, through further challenging experiences.

On a 100% raw vegan diet and healthy lifestyle, Jesse's condition improved rapidly. He gained 40 pounds in a few years. This is what happens when the body is freed of mucus—able to absorb the essential nutrients on an enzyme-rich raw vegan diet. He became more peaceful, smiled more, played and was aware of his surroundings. I cried tears of joy when I saw him taking more steps, walking, even running on the beach. He asked me why I was crying. I told him I was glad our problems were now over, I was so sorry he had had to go through all that suffering, and I blamed myself.

I said to him, "Will I ever be able to forgive myself?" He took my hand, pleading with me not to cry, and said: "Mama, I am so glad this happened to me, and if it weren't for all this, how would we know the truth of how to help others? Please, Mama, listen to me now: if we tell parents not to vaccinate their kids, and if we don't charge them, no one will ever be able to stop us from spreading the truth. That is what I want, more than anything in this world, Mama."

I trembled at the words he spoke, the look in his eyes, and the gentleness of his manner, and my tears became a river of relief as I surrendered finally to peace. In that moment I, too, forgave everyone, especially myself.

Natural Health Revelation for Everyone

Everyone can do it; no one has to wait to be a doctor or go to school for 20 years, only to have to unlearn all the brainwashing that starts in kindergarten and continues all the way through college. If you want to become a Hygienic lifestyle coach, you can do it now.

People just don't realize how much we've strayed from Nature and the simple truth of Her Laws. The right natural diet will bring clarity, awareness, healing and peace.

My books, *The Cure is in the Cause* and *Love Your Pet, Let Nature Be the Vet*, were written because of Jesse and his brother Sean—my greatest teachers, my mentors, my angels and the angels of many others.

Today, Jesse and Sean travel the world with us every chance they get and talk to all the kids and parents about how they can heal naturally, without drugs or surgery. It is because of Jesse and what happened to him that we teach Nature's Laws. Jesse is happy, healthy, and remains totally on the vegan Hygienic raw food diet. Jesse and his brother Sean have created a new lifestyle program to show people how they can be close to nature and heal themselves and others by bringing more truth and light. Look up their website: www.thewholelifestyle.com

The Illogic of Vaccinations

It is because of kids like Jesse and thousands of parents like us that pharmaceutical companies must report the side effects of vaccines today. Hopefully, now that the truth is coming out, we can show vaccines are not needed, are totally wrong for health, they do not boost immunity but, rather, are immunity depressors. We are against any manmade interventions, and we are convinced many problems are caused by vaccinations. Their poisons have a cumulative effect, cause many degenerative diseases, and are totally against Nature's Law. The crime that has been committed will have tremendous consequences, and many children will not be able to reach the potential that is their birthright.

I send hundreds of letters every year to parents excusing their children from vaccinations. Society needs to know: although vaccinations are mandated, they are not mandatory. We have nothing to fear in bringing the truth to light. Please join us in this work by bringing this truth to parents and kids.

The conclusion of *The Cure is in the Cause* is: Nature is our ultimate teacher. Get out of Nature's way, but stay on Her path so you can truly heal and help heal others.

Also, we must remember the word "doctor" means "teacher." This is not about treating symptoms with surgery, radiation, etc., but, rather, looking to the cause and eliminating it. There is no better doctor than Mother Nature. There are no rewards or punishments from Her, only consequences.

Nature is wise, so become aware of her immutable laws, and you will be wiser and at peace. When you eat the fruits of her awesome abundance, you will be in tune with your great self-healing gifts. Remember we are here to heal ourselves and then to help heal others. This is true love, freedom, and joy.

Dr. Ruza Bogdanovich is the author of the books *The Cure Is in the Cause, Love Your Pet, Let Nature Be the Vet, Too Much Thinking Not Enough Pooping,* and *Instant, Whole Food Raw Recipes* that she coauthored with her son Sean, available now at: www.thecureisinthecause.com

Contact Dr. Ruza at drruza@gmail.com or call: 775-782-7365. Mail orders: The Cure Is in the Cause Foundation, P.O. Box 1510 Minden, Nevada 89423.

Vaccination Education by Dr. Ruza Bogdanovich

Several years ago, I met Dr. Tim O'Shea and, with Sandi Rizzo, we put on a two-hour public television show that changed many lives and stopped many parents from vaccinating their kids. Please read Dr. O'Shea's book and see the TV show: *The Sanctity of Human Blood: Vaccination I$ Not Immunization.* (The book is available from Living Nutrition and the video from sandina@myexcel. com.) This is what Dr.Tim O'Shea wants us to know:

- Infectious diseases were over 90% resolved by the time vaccines came onto the market.
- There are now 32 + vaccines that are mandated by the time your child is 18 months old, and 58 by age 18.
- Before 1991, there was no system for reporting adverse side effects or vaccine reactions whatsoever.
- Only one country in Europe still has mandated DPT (diphtheria, tetanus, and pertussis) shots, whereas the U.S.A. requires 5 separate shot doses.
- 43% of Gulf War vets suffered side effects from vaccines.
- 80,000 Gulf War vets have permanent medical conditions as a result of vaccinations.
- Vaccination is not immunization.
- Hepatitis B vaccine was outlawed in France after 15,000 citizens filed a class action suit against the government.
- Vaccines do not have to be proven safe or effective in order to be added to the list of shots mandated for American children.
- Hundreds of doctors don't vaccinate their own children but can't talk about it. The same goes for the veterinarians with their pets.
- The mercury in most vaccines is many times in excess of EPA safe levels.
- The vaccine business is the foundation of one of the three biggest cartels in America. They can certainly afford fancy websites, magazines, books and medical journals.

■ It is not so bad most people don't know the information we just learned above. What is unacceptable is so many people don't *want* to know it.

If you want to learn more about this important truth, go to Dr. O'Shea's website: www.thedoctorwithin.com

I learned about Dana Stewart and her family from New Zealand when I subscribed to the San Francisco Living Foods Yahoo Group just before a trip to the West Coast. Dana's family was visiting that area and I was able to contact her through the email loop.

Dana Stewart and Family
July 2008

Understanding living food for us as a family has been our most uplifting and exciting experience ever. It was literally one day I awoke and decided to stop eating cooked food. I had been vegetarian for 12 years and raised my 8 and 5 year old daughters this way. However, I did not truly understand how significant was the effect of the types of food we were eating which limited us in so many ways. The pasta, which I now see as glue, processed cheeses, and products with flour in them were literally gluing us up and stopping the life force from uplifting us in our daily lives. I was waking tired and had a hard time dealing with stress, which I can now see was created by the life-robbing foods I was consuming.

After 11 weeks eating raw, the way I now feel is so incredibly exciting. I have developed muscular strength beyond my wildest dreams which includes a stunning set of abs I thought would never be possible after two children, my skin is glowing, 4 freckles and a growth on my eye have literally fallen off, and I am now able to flow through my day with strength, poise and understanding. My two beautiful daughters are not completely raw. At first, they were annoyed with me, but as the days go by and they increase the amount of living food they eat, the results speak for themselves. Osheana has said she definitely would like to be "raw food" but asked if I could expand my culinary skills to suit her cravings. And my darling Molly-Love has always tended to want lighter, living foods anyway, so I just started buying more of the things she loves, including all fruits and nuts. My partner of 3 years has suffered his entire life

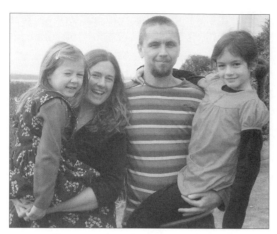

*Molly, Dana (mum), Matty and Osheana
in June 2009*

with ulcerative colitis and is now finally breaking free from this crippling disease. To be able to watch such an extreme transformation in such a short time in someone's mental, emotional, physical and spiritual capacities has been so very encouraging and continually gives me hope for anyone suffering the life depriving effects of eating dead food.

Our connection to the earth has been exciting. We stopped mowing our lawns and now have an ultimate array of grasses, wild herbs and weeds with which to create our decadent salads and green smoothies. Living in an up market, inner city area, it has taken courage to go against the normal lawn mowing lifestyle, but the rewards have been outstanding. I can now create a salad out of more than 30 different types of greens growing naturally here.

I feel like life has just begun!

Thank you for wanting to represent New Zealand in your book... I am so determined to raise the bar here and strive to provide resources for people to take control of their lives again... I have created a first living food forum website for NZ: www.realnraw.com

—Dana Stewart

The following article was written by Andrea Nison, wife of Paul Nison, well-known raw foods author and lecturer. I have known Paul since shortly after I began my own raw food journey in the mid 1990s. Paul was healed of ulcerative colitis by the raw vegan lifestyle: www.rawlife.com

My Amazing Pregnancy and Birth Experience
By Andrea Nison, February 2009

I was very blessed to spend the two years prior to becoming pregnant working at Hippocrates Health Institute (HHI) in West Palm Beach, Florida. This allowed me to prepare my body and enrich it with the nourishment needed for a healthy pregnancy. After having a miscarriage in August 2007, I decided I needed to cleanse and detoxify my body as much as possible before becoming pregnant again. I spent the next year focusing on cleansing, and I really felt it helped my body and mind prepare for a healthy pregnancy. I spent 5 weeks doing the Ejuva intestinal cleanse, and really felt the benefits after that was complete. I also cleansed by using enemas and colonics. Colonics are not recommended while pregnant, so I thought I should take advantage of the time when I could do them.

While working at HHI, I drank green juices three times a day, and ate a delicious, raw salad for lunch every day. The green juices were made using cucumbers, sunflower and pea sprouts, and celery. The salads consisted of numerous sprouts, greens, vegetables, and seaweeds. The Hippocrates Diet does not use any sweeteners or fruits on their salad bar. Although I tried to maintain a mostly raw diet, I was not 100% raw during the entire pregnancy. I ate cooked millet and quinoa in the mornings, and occasionally ate cooked vegetable soups and other vegan foods. I personally do not feel the need to be 100% raw, and find that I am much happier and healthier when I allow myself the freedom to have some items cooked.

When I reached about the 7th–8th week of pregnancy, the hormones started to kick in, and I found myself unable to eat the salads and drink the green juices I was so accustomed to eating every day. Looking at the salads and even smelling them made me feel so sick and uneasy. I didn't have "morning sickness" per se, but I definitely felt nauseated, and the only foods that appealed to me were bland, unseasoned foods, and definitely no salads. I satisfied my hunger by eating sprouted Ezekial Bread and other cooked vegan foods that I had eaten prior to eating more raw foods. I felt I was regressing with my diet, and the foods that appealed to me were the vegan comfort foods I used to eat. No matter what foods I ate, I made sure to take a few digestive enzymes before each meal. I tried not to be too hard on myself at this point, and ate plenty of fruits and other fresh foods that were appetizing.

After the 12th week, I started feeling amazing, and once again, I started to eat the salads and drink the green juices. I actually started to crave them. I looked forward to a delicious, green salad every day for lunch. I supplemented my diet with prenatal vitamins, vitamin B12, probiotics, and E-3 Live. My husband, Paul, made me delicious almond or hemp milks in the mornings. He added maca, chia seeds, green powder and camu powder to the milks and they were delicious. I also did my best not to eat too late at night because I knew I needed to sleep well throughout the night, and late-night eating prevents me from attaining a good night's sleep. I never felt the urge to overeat and I didn't have any weird cravings. It seems that my body was receiving everything it needed.

Before I became pregnant, I took an aerobics class a few days a week. After week 12, I felt that I needed exercises that were less strenuous, so I incorporated stretching in the morning and walks in the evening with Paul. I really felt great throughout my entire pregnancy. I didn't have any swelling or other complications and continued working until 2 weeks before the "due date."

One day after the expectant date, our daughter Noa Raquel was born, weighing 7 lbs. 14 ozs. and 20 1/2 inches long. We delivered her at home with the help of a wonderful midwife. Noa was born completely awake and alert. It was an amazing experience and I feel so blessed we did not have any complications and everything was as natural as possible. Our midwife commented to me that I couldn't have grown a healthier baby. I feel that my diet and lifestyle were the significant factors in my health and our baby's health, and I'm so thankful that I had the knowledge and resources to eat mostly raw, organic foods.

I continued with my prenatal regimen after the birth, and my recovery time was very quick. I was feeling like myself within a few days. I know providing my body with the nutrients and exercise it needed contributed to my amazing pregnancy and birth-giving experience. Free of hindrances, the human body is remarkable and will thrive when allowed the opportunity to do what it is supposed to do.

While Karmyn Malone was living in Costa Rica, she sent me some appealing information about the raw food lifestyle, and I was looking forward to more of her observations. When my daughter and I visited Costa Rica in March 2009, we planned to meet with her, but there wasn't time in our one week trip. Later, with both of us back in New Jersey, I asked her to write for the book:

Karmyn Malone and Family
June 2009

I became vegan back in July 2006. Although I wasn't a 100% raw foodist at the time (I am now),

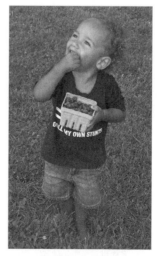

Andrew at age 2

I ate great quantities of locally grown fruits and vegetables available in New Jersey. I felt great eating all those fresh foods! Seven weeks after becoming vegan, I found out I was pregnant with my now two year old son, Andrew.

Once I found out about my pregnancy, I researched parenting philosophies. Attachment parenting made perfect sense to me. I knew I would co-sleep with my baby, wear my baby in my arms and breastfeed my baby.

I'm still nursing Andrew. He's also eating 100% raw foods, no exceptions. He has tried some cooked foods, but he prefers eating raw foods. At a birth-day party about a year ago, he ate a few

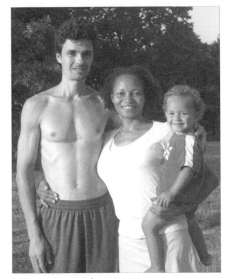

Roger, Karmyn and Andrew, June 2009

bites of a cupcake. Once he saw the fresh fruit platter of watermelon, grapes and apples, he threw the cupcake on the floor and started eating the fruit.

Andrew's favorite foods include watermelon, cantaloupe, grapes, straw-berries, blueberries, peaches, apples, cherries, bananas, grape tomatoes, cu-cumbers, celery, avocados, durians, carrots and salads. While most toddlers scream for candy and cookies at the supermarket, Andrew screams for fruits like watermelon and peaches. He even picks out the best fruits in the store. Once he grabbed an apple and started eating it. After buying it, we tasted it and realized it was the best apple we ever had!

I recently met someone wonderful to share my life, Roger Haeske. Roger has been eating 100% low fat raw vegan foods for the past 8 years. In addi-tion to following the optimal raw diet, he also believes in the importance of exercise as well as other aspects of a healthy lifestyle such as getting enough sleep and minimizing stress. We share so many of the same philosophies on life. Roger is also a great role model for Andrew. It's nice to co-parent with someone on the same page!

Andrew's favorite salad is Roger's Savory Veggie Stew (based on a blended salad). He eats it every day.

Imagine having a child who loves eating only fresh fruits and vegetables.

Imagine having a child who rarely gets sick.

Roger and I do not have to *imagine* as that is *our reality*.

— Karmyn Malone, www.karmynmalone.com

The following speech was presented for Toastmasters in San Diego, August 2, 2006. Instead of a raw family's journey, it's about an individual's path—the wonderful story of a friend, Amy Schrift, who listens very closely to her personal intuition and her connection to Nature. I feel it has great value for all of us who are following a road toward truth in life:

From New York City to Costa Rica, an Inner and Outer Journey
2006

In August of 2003 while living in Manhattan, I underwent a profound transformation. I changed the way I ate. Observing everything that went into my mouth, I decided to eat only foods from Nature, ripened in the sun, thus providing me with life force.

As my body began to cleanse and purify, my thoughts began to change as well, and I started to feel a profound connection with the earth.

With a new sense of calm and focused centeredness, I began to deconstruct conditioned, fear-based thinking patterns and allow for new-found clarity of thought and purpose. My life seemed to take on a momentum of its own.

Besides eating only living foods, I started a daily practice of sun gazing which is gazing at the sun near sunrise or sunset. I soon discontinued the use of corrective lenses—contact lenses I had worn for over 25 years. I began sleeping on the floor, walking barefoot when possible, spending ample time in New York parks—in short, trying to deepen my earth connection in any way possible.

I felt all fear erode away and surrendered to my inner guidance to lead the way.

My internal compass began to point me towards the tropics, where I knew I could always enjoy my five favorite foods: bananas, coconuts, pineapples, papayas and mangos, in a year-round comfortable climate.

The following summer, I planned a month-long trip to Costa Rica where I ended up putting a down payment on a 17.5 acre piece of land I would soon call my home.

As I returned to New York, I understood the profound implications of this decision and felt ready to leave the cement jungles behind for the lush green jungles of Costa Rica. Back in the U.S.A., I was increasingly aware of the toxic environment in which I had lived and desired nothing more than to be in a place with clean air, pure water and fertile land.

By the following summer I had packed my bags, placed some things in storage, said goodbye to my family in San Diego and left for the Promised Land.

I arrived during the rainy season and soon set to work planting hundreds of fruit trees of many varieties which would be my future food source.

When the rains subsided, I built a thatched roof structure with no walls, raised off the ground by a wooden floor in the shape of an octagon. For my personal belongings and food storage, I built a wooden shed with a dirt floor. It has some shelves, and a sink.

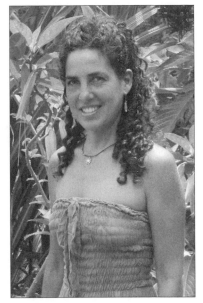

Amy Schrift

I've decided not to use electricity except for recharging a cell phone as a landline is not available. I collect rainwater for bathing, pipe in drinking water from a mountain spring and recycle all my own waste.

Living so simply has allowed me ample time to quietly observe nature both day and night; and never before have I felt so aware of the moon rising and setting and its effects on plant growth and animals.

The monkeys and birds howl and sing in the early morning hours, awakening me from my sleep to begin a daily three hour practice of meditation and yoga. I work and play on the land during the day; sometimes bathing in the river below, hiking to nearby waterfalls or a trip to the beach. I go to bed early, not long after the sun sets and the first stars begin to appear in the night sky.

One of my favorite activities is to lie down on my back and look up at the sky in pure awe and wonder as it is forever changing and impermanent, a true metaphor for our lives.

As I spend days alone in silence interrupted only by weekly trips to town for food and supplies, gatherings with friends or conversations in Spanish with two workers who help me on the farm a few days a week, I find the plants and animals are my teachers and guides. From them, I can learn to live in balance and harmony with my surroundings.

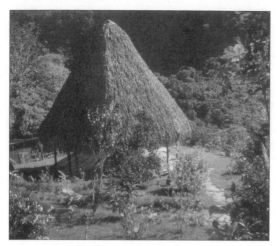

Amy Schrift's tropical farm in Costa Rica

Living in the midst of nature is non-violent, non-judging, always in the moment, honest, peaceful, efficient and sincere.

Life without machines, a car, or pets keeps me endlessly creative in ways that are nurturing and bring me much joy.

By living in the moment, I've released my attachment or fears about what was or what should be, and I'm allowing my life to simply unfold.

The more time I spend alone, the less I fear what was once the unknown— walking in the dark, hiking in the jungle, or sleeping under the open, starry, vast night sky. Rather, I feel embraced and like a child learning new life skills such as building shelter, growing food and living "with" and not just "off" the land.

I guess I would be considered as one of the world's abject poor who are defined as those who build their own homes out of earth or other natural materials and grow or forage for their own food. Our lives don't fit with the corporate model of consumption, and so we are poor in their eyes. We have much to learn from what I call the world's "richest," those who have learned their ways from nature and have lived a peaceful harmonious existence with the earth for many thousands of years.

Ultimately, I'm simply seeking a path of truth, and through my actions hope to inspire others to do the same.

Allowing transformation into your life could be a vehicle for letting go of what isn't or what should be, embracing simply what is, and letting your inner voice guide you to the essence of who you really are.

I believe this life is meant to be a peaceful and gentle journey and consists of nothing more than being fully present and full of gratitude in this moment right now.

Thank you.

—Amy Schrift

[After Amy had relocated to Costa Rica, she sent "GREETINGS FROM THE LAND OF PURE AIR, WATER AND SUNSHINE!" The following are some of her comments showing the happiness, fulfillment and excitement she feels living in such a pure environment]:

As the rainy season begins to wane, ushering in the dry season which goes from December to May, it's an important time to plant trees, so the roots have a chance to become entrenched before the land dries out. So far, I've planted 54 fruit trees of many wonderful tropical varieties and have another 50 to go—zapote, rambutan, papaya, sugar cane, coconut, banana, orange, tangerine, pineapple, starfruit, durian, water apple, jackfruit, jaboticaba (tropical grape), acerola, cashew, macadamia, avocado, sapote, caas, nispero, mangosteen, jocote, noni, sweet lemon, abiut, just to name a few. Each tree has been foliar sprayed with diluted ocean water to give it a full compliment of minerals to choose from. This method has been tried and proven, and my friend Tim had amazing results in Florida.

Yesterday we harvested some hearts of palm and plantains, and the hearts of palm are delicious fresh and raw.

As I spend the days immersed on the farm, planting and watching life unfold, the miracle of a seed transforming itself into a plant is still a marvel to my eyes. The seed opens as life begins to surge through it, and a tiny set of round leaves often appear, followed by a second set that take on the form of the mature leaf. I never throw a seed away, but simply toss it onto the land. I now have hundreds of small papaya plants and other fruits that have simply sprouted where they landed.

Another of the simple pleasures of daily life here is to be able to grab a sweet, delicious banana off a large rack hanging in my home at any time of the day. If I don't have any racks of my own, friends often give them to me. Once you've tasted bananas sun-ripened naturally, there is no turning back!

I find I prefer to eat mono meals or just one thing at a time until I'm full. This allows me to enjoy and appreciate the texture, color, shape and subtleties of flavor of a particular fruit or vegetable, as well as the ease of digestion that follows.

From my observations of nature, I am aware all living beings, except humans, eat mono meals and don't suffer from the myriad of digestive ailments we do. Birds eat insects and seeds and bears consume berries, fish and honey, but never at the same meal. There is no such thing as a "sandwich" or food combining in Nature.

Last week, I took my first rain bath, and stood outside in a downpour, gazing upward, thinking what it must be like to be a tree... Since I've been bathing in rain water anyway, I thought I might as well get it from the source. It felt cool and refreshing, and I never felt cold.

Truly the greatest gift we can give is our presence. Somewhere along the way, we confused "giving presence" with "giving presents."

With a fresh perspective of my new homestead, I am truly grateful for many of the things I have here:

For highly oxygenated air and pure spring water untainted with chloramines and chlorine to render it fit for human consumption.

For the opportunity to grow my own food, allowing it to ripen properly and eating it at the peak of its nutritional value and flavor.

For the experience of swimming and bathing in natural water only: rivers, swimming holes, waterfalls, and the warm ocean.

For the chance to strengthen my body every day, caring for the trees, the garden and many other daily tasks required on the farm.

For the ability to return what I eat back to the earth, allowing microorganisms to create rich composted soil to support new life.

For the chance to work alongside persons who have spent their entire lives planting and harvesting with the lunar cycles, and who humble me with their physical stamina and grace (especially with that machete!).

For the chance to discover new life forms almost daily. Many of them are fascinating insects, each of which plays an integral role in the ecosystem here. I remember asking myself while in the U.S., "Where are all the insects?"

For the possibility of spending days in silence: in quiet observation, reflection and mindfulness.

For experiencing this joy with others who have also come here to work, learn from and live harmoniously in nature.

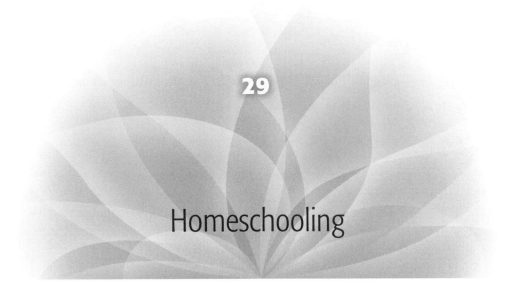

Homeschooling

"No use to shout at them to pay attention. If the situations, the materials, the problems before the child do not interest him, his attention will slip off to what does interest him, and no amount of exhortation of threats will bring it back."

JOHN HOLT

Homeschooling is a continuation of attachment and continuum parenting. How can we nurse and carry our children for years and then force them to separate from us at a very young age by sending them to school? It can sometimes be an environment where they are intimidated and forced into doing work holding no interest for them. When my children were in school, I felt sad to be separated from them, while other mothers seemed thrilled to have the day free without their children. Some of them told me I had separation problems. During all the years spent with my children, I've always loved having them around me. Many years ago, I saw some words that stuck with me, and knew homeschooling was right for us:

> "I do not want to wake up
> some morning
> with an ache in my
> heart, wondering, 'What
> happened? My children
> are gone, all grown, and I
> didn't even know them."
> —anonymous

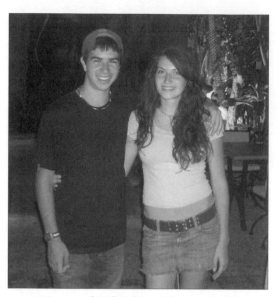

Marco and Gabriela in Colombia, 2006

By the time children reach their junior high years, many of them become so used to being exclusively with their age group, they show little interest in anyone else. One of the main benefits of home-schooling for our family was that our children have grown up together, and have had a close friendship throughout these years.

We also value sleep as being essential for healthy development. I never worried my children were sleep deprived as homeschooling afforded them the sleep time they so needed from early childhood through their teenage years. They could use the bathroom as needed without asking for a pass, and were able to eat when hungry.

Homeschooling is an excellent option, unless a child should desire to go to school. Public schools create conflicting messages about health and nutrition. We do not follow the food pyramid published by the Meat and Dairy Councils, so health and nutrition classes focusing on an animal-food based pyramid would have caused much confusion. Governments use schools as avenues to spread propaganda. Junk food is used as a reward for completion of schoolwork. When our children were in school, I remember pizza parties were held on Fridays for completion of the week's work, and candy was frequently awarded during the week for the completion of papers or tests. According to Alfi Kohn's book, *Punished by Rewards*, rewards can be damaging because they inhibit true motivation.

There is tremendous "peer pressure" to conform in public school. There is also "peer pressure" to conform to other children's eating choices when part of a homeschooling community, but the pressure is less intense than at school. Isolating your family is not the answer either, as it would be harmful for socialization purposes to isolate your children. Children who grow up in strong loving family environments often carry the nutrition and health philosophies of their parents into their daily social interactions.

The main activities of many schools seem to inhibit rather than encourage a child's imagination and creativity. When Gabriela was in second grade, I volunteered frequently at the school. I would sometimes pass her classroom and observe her passively sitting and listening to the teacher during much of her school day. I spoke with the principal and suggested various projects for the teacher, but the situation remained unchanged. My creative, imaginative child had to sit inactively for long periods of time that year. In addition, children at school are most often not involved in decision-making, and this is harmful to their self-confidence and emotional development. When we began to homeschool in 1995, we decided to involve the children in everything we did in our daily lives, from purchasing a car, going to court to challenge a traffic ticket, withdrawing and depositing money at the bank, preparing raw food dishes, planning a trip abroad, etc. The world became our school. We looked for classes with people who were passionate about their work, such as an astronomer who built his own planetarium, a naturalist at a nature center who loved to share outdoor science, wilderness instructors who shared their knowledge of Native American skills, drama coaches who presented improvisation and creative acting workshops, a real life filmmaker to teach a filmmaking class, a permaculture farmer to teach a gardening class, and many more. We also went on field trips often. The children loved all these wonderful, fun classes and trips, and became very involved in the learning experiences because they were so motivating.

People in our town have actually approached me in the past to say I should let my children get out and do things with other children. They think we as homeschoolers completely isolate ourselves, but the truth is exactly the opposite. My children are very well socialized. They have made friends with many school children whom they see after school and on weekends. Marco also often meets his teenage school friends out of school during their lunch periods. Gabriela and Marco have taken part in many area activities, such as community theater and sports. We are part of a large homeschool community that has offered many classes and activities in which our children have participated with other homeschooled children over the years. These events are listed monthly in a homeschooling newsletter. There are also camps for homeschoolers. Our children have attended the "Not-Back-To-School" Camp, organized by the author of *The Teenage Liberation Handbook*, Grace Llewelyn, where they met other homeschooled teens from many states with whom they keep in touch and visit.

My father used to worry my children weren't learning enough academics, but as he observed them growing through adolescence, he realized they were becoming ever more vibrant and dynamic. When they were seventeen and fourteen, he remarked, "I love the way you're raising your children."

The following is an article I wrote in 2002 about homeschooling my children, for the book *Raw Knowledge* by Paul Nison:

Homeschooling: An Option That Makes Sense

After enjoying our lives together during their early years, I sent my two children to public school to sit in classes with many other children of the same age. Something inside me felt great despair and loss at leaving my children in a large, cold building to be raised by someone who is not their mother for a good part of their daily lives. But at the time, I was ignorant of any other options other than expensive, private schools with a smaller teacher/student ratio. I had breastfed each of my children and raised them with the vegan philosophy. It was my natural maternal instinct to remain with my children, but at the time, I neither realized nor understood we could stay together when they reached school age. When Gabriela was in third grade, and Marco was in kindergarten, both in public school, I first learned of homeschooling through some mothers I met at an Attachment Parenting Group, also called a Continuum Group after a book titled *The Continuum Concept*. The belief they held so dear was young children require their mothers to nurture them as they grow and mature through various stages of their lives, and to force separation so prematurely would be harmful to their development.

At the time I began attending this Continuum Parenting Group, my children were still in public school, and I was frequently a volunteer there to be near them. However, once I became more aware there was an alternative, and began reading books about homeschooling, I started to observe incidences in school I felt were detrimental to emotional and educational growth. Gabriela sat at a desk for most of the day listening to her teacher lecture. She was compliant with doing all the work, but she appeared unhappy and unmotivated in the classroom setting. Marco was bored in kindergarten and was reprimanded for trying to leave the room. He was also scolded when he tried to get off of a single file line to hug me when I was volunteering in the library. In addition to these disappointments with the system, I observed junk food being used repeatedly as rewards for completion of schoolwork. This totally upset me because I believe rewards, and food rewards in particular, are obstacles to increasing motivation, and only work temporarily.

I began to feel instinctively public school was a place where my children were not being nurtured, and where commonly held health and nutrition ideas totally conflicted with our values at home.

At this time, in 1995, I had already become a 100% raw vegan, and I knew my children were being confronted with toxic food choices as well as poisonous chemicals in school maintenance products.

Marco was never interested in school, and once he met children who were being homeschooled, he expressed even stronger resistance to attending public school; and so after careful consideration, my husband and I withdrew him that year. Gabriela continued in school for another half year. At a parent-teacher conference with her third grade teacher, I made the decision to take her out of school as well. The teacher explained Gabriela was doing extremely well at school, but she liked writing so much, she didn't want to switch to other subjects. The teacher felt this was preventing her from learning in other areas. I knew Gabriela loved writing and liked to see her projects to completion, but this continued to be a source of conflict between her and the teacher. Gabriela pleaded with us to take her out of school, so after the holidays she did not return to third grade.

We have been homeschooling now for six years. One of the major questions we confront continually concerns socialization with other children. I feel when children are placed into a situation with 20-30 children their own age with only one adult for years on end, socialization is extremely limited. These children most often learn to socialize only with children their own age, and they don't have an adult's individualized loving, caring attention, so necessary as they grow. My children interact with children of all ages and spend a lot of time with loving, nurturing adults as well. My fourteen year old daughter Gabriela has friends as young as five and as old as sixteen. She also considers some of my adult friends to be close friends of hers.

One valuable advantage I've noticed with Gabriela during her home-schooling years is she has maintained her imaginative and playful ways. Girls her age care mostly about popularity at school, while she is still occupied with creative, imaginative play, such as dressing up and acting out a variety of characters she has read or heard about.

If you strongly question the desirability of compulsory schooling, home-schooling is an excellent alternative and is legal in all 50 states. Thousands of people have been homeschooled and have gone on to lead happy, productive lives, and to fulfill their potential.

৶৯

As a homeschooled high school student, Gabriela exclaims she loves her life and loves waking up in the morning and being who she is. Quite amazing considering the pressure on most teenagers, and the depression some of them have to deal with. Each year, Marco says he may like to try high school, but whenever the time comes to make that decision, he decides he likes his life too much with the independence he enjoys.

Award-winning New York State Teacher of the Year, John Taylor Gatto, expressed the following beliefs at a homeschool conference where I heard him speak: "We've built a way of life that depends on people doing what they are told because they don't know how to tell themselves what to do. Homeschooling is a philosophy that locates meaning where meaning is genuinely to be found—in families, in friends, in the passage of seasons, in nature, in simple ceremonies and rituals, in curiosity, generosity, compassion and service to others. School is a fundamental betrayal of the American Revolution. In Benjamin Franklin's autobiography, he said there is 'no time to waste in school.' Students should use their free time to learn something unauthorized from a father or mother, by exploration, or by apprenticing to some wise person in the neighborhood. The trick of learning is to wait until someone asks and then move fast while the mood is on." (www.johntaylorgatto.com).

Today, when young children attend kindergarten, it is no longer the fun, discovery days of play and naps as long ago, but instead involves the beginning of academic subjects, due to more testing which requires students to study earlier and earlier. Many kindergartens now have seven-hour days because there's not enough time for all the required academic subjects. These long days, during which very young children are away from their families for so many hours, create stresses that tear at the emotional bonding and strong value modeling so very much needed by children.

In recent years, there has been much research on the benefits of "play." Much of the imagination and creativity of children is seen in their play. "Play" is children's work, and adults need to respect that children are learning through their play. Who are adults to say only success in academic subjects is the proof of learning. Plenty of "play" may lead to increased skill in problem-solving, confidence in communication, and ability to harness imagination and creativity to solve a variety of life's situations.

Play is fundamental to development. Children's confidence and emotional security are tied in with long-term nurturing relationships with their parents and hours and hours of wonderful time to play. As soon as I realized this, I understood homeschooling was the only option.

A valuable article on play is titled "The Serious Business of Play" by Mary Dixon Lebeau, published in the November 2002 Parent Guide.

One aspect of homeschooling Gabriela and Marco particularly loved was being able to have seemingly endless playdates with their many wonderful

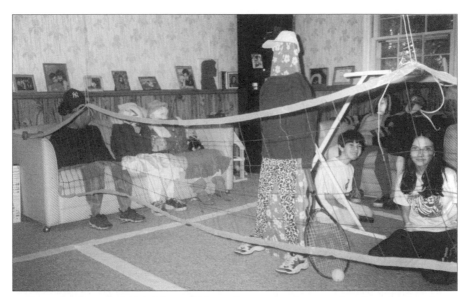

Homeschooling gave Gabriela and Marco the opportunity to explore imaginative play for many hours a day. Here they are creating a simulated tennis match, using dressed brooms, mops and basketballs to comprise the spectators, ironing boards for the tennis players, a volleyball net, masking tape to mark the tennis court, and our furniture.

friends. Often their play would turn into sleepovers and it would be their decision to say how long they wanted to play with their friends, sometimes lasting days at a time. This could not happen with their schooled friends who were unable to take time off school due to their tightly programmed schedules.

It is very important for parents to be playful with their children. Because I had been coerced to perform in a specific way when I was a child, I had lost my ability to be playful. In many areas, I had also lost my creative side. Years of being told my art work was not good by teachers at school had turned me away from artistic desires I might have had. As my children grew, they sometimes told me I wasn't playful. I started to think about it and realized I was missing out on one of the most important aspects of life, especially considering my relationships with my children. Gabriela, Marco and I and some close friends went camping at a nature awareness-survival camp at the Delaware Water Gap. During that experience, the adults were told to put on bathing suits and cover themselves with mud as part of a camouflage activity for the children. I would never have done this before, but I decided to participate and cover myself with mud from face to feet. When the adults jumped out of the woods to surprise the children, my two kids looked extremely surprised, thrilled I had done something so crazy-looking!

Marco and his teenage friends love having poker nights at our house, partly because my husband Harvey enjoys it so much and becomes so playful with all the kids. When the children were younger, he played a chasing game around our living room and kitchen and called it "Sneaky." That was a favorite time for many years for Gabriela and Marco. Attending to children, playing with them and seeing the value in their play can only result in confident happy adults later on.

Homeschooling afforded Gabriela and Marco the time to understand their true interests so they could begin to pursue their individual potentials. During their teen years, Gabriela and Marco engaged in volunteer and internship activities, giving them working knowledge in the areas that motivated them. Progressing logically from the family ideals with which she grew up, Gabriela has decided to make a meaningful contribution toward a cleaner environment. Her successful completion of environmental internships for Clearwater led her to major in Global Environmental Studies at college.

Marco has always loved sports, and homeschooling has provided him with the flexibility and independence to participate in various volunteer programs and internships in the sports broadcasting world. His passion for sports broadcasting has led him to work with some of the top people in that field through internships with Seton Hall University Basketball and Madison Square Garden Sports Network. Both Gabriela and Marco produced remarkable portfolios, illustrating all their rewarding experiences, and both were accepted into top colleges.

Homeschooling can and does lead to acceptance at top universities. Also with astonishing results, many homeschoolers have opted simply to learn from the universe.

Dr. Thomas Armstrong, in his book *Awakening Your Child's Natural Genius: Enhancing Curiosity, Creativity, and Learning Ability*, emphasizes real learning takes place in the context of everyday life:

> In contrast to the old-fashioned dictum that children are to be seen and not heard, kids in positive families are seen and heard doing all sorts of marvelously creative things. They're busy running, playacting, building, drawing, conversing, writing, experimenting, reading, exploring, wondering, laughing, and in many other ways vigorously interacting with the world. The adults in these families are often an integral part of their children's exploratory activities, helping to guide them in practical ways toward a realization of their objectives.

Learning in a positive family climate is not of the look-it-up-in-the-encyclopedia variety where the buck gets passed to a remote and abstract authority. It's a hands-on, everybody-learns-together encounter with the nitty-gritty world of real objects and situations.

At home, children seem to pick up tacit attitudes, beliefs, and behaviors simply by being in the presence of adults who model these learnings in complex and often richly subtle ways. In one sense, elders are like mirrors for a child, reflecting back the child's own developing sense of self.

Children often do their best learning without adult supervision during unstructured playtime. It is often only when they make their own choices about what they wish to learn and how they want to learn it that their motivation and achievement levels go way up. Parents should realize they can usually better help their kids by simply listening to them, respecting their lives, and allowing them the freedom to explore new ideas and subjects on their own, rather than by piling on another French lesson or computer class.

The following is an explanation of "Unschooling" by Nancy and Billy Greer, editors of F.U.N. News:

What Is "Unschooling?"

Everyone has his own definition, but most would agree it involves a more relaxed approach to learning that validates the interests of the child rather than relying on a fixed curriculum. There are many different perceptions of unschooling, and ours is just one view. The unschoolers we know are deeply committed to doing what is best for their children.

We decided the easiest way for us to explain what "unschooling" (also called holistic, organic, child-directed, interest-led, or self-directed learning) means to our family is to print our philosophical beliefs that we place at the beginning of the portfolio we present to our local school district. It is as follows:

Our primary purpose in homeschooling is to keep alive the spark of curiosity and the natural love of learning with which all children are born. We want our children to accept learning as a natural consequence of living, and an ongoing incremental process that continues throughout life. We want their learning to remain an integrated process in which all subjects are interrelated. We also want to allow them the time to pursue a subject as fully as they want, rather than imposing artificial time constraints on them. We believe these aspects of learning are limited by the traditional implementation of a curriculum, and we choose to homeschool as a way to circumvent those limitations.

We have two children who are being "officially" homeschooled, but we believe both are just continuing the lifelong learning process that began at their first moment of awareness. Children spend most of their time learning from us when we are not consciously teaching. A few hours a week of teaching are not as important as the lessons we provide by example for many hours every day. We believe the best way to help our children learn is to live well and to fully include them in our life.

Our confidence in unschooling has grown as we have reviewed our own educational experiences. We have come to realize the skills most important to us are self-taught. We learn best by doing, by having the chance to make mistakes without fear of criticism, and by having the opportunity to concentrate on an idea, or a skill until we have mastered it and made it our own. Now we are trying to provide our children with the same opportunity to make mistakes, to pursue an activity for as long as they want, and to experience that feeling of accomplishment that will pull them on to their next learning experience.

A life worth living and work worth doing—that is what I want for children (and all people), not just . . . something called a better education. —John Holt

For information about F.U.N. News and subscriptions, see http://www. unschooling.org or www.FUN-Books.com., or email FUN@unschooling.org., Nancy and Billy Greer, Editors.

A Feminist View of Homeschooling by Kathi Weiss

I was raised to believe a woman's place was in the home, taking care of her man and children. When I reached adulthood, the feminist movement came into being, and I learned a woman can be and do anything she chooses to do. What I choose to do is stay home and take care of my child and homeschool him. People say this is not a feminist attitude, but I think it is. It's a choice I am making for my child and my family. I work just as much, often more than my husband. He goes to his company and works for 7 hours a day while I stay home with my son and work for 10 to 12 hours per day. I earn every bit of the equivalent of his paycheck just as much as he does. Because I'm taking care of our son, it frees my husband to go to work and earn a living for the family. Yes, this is a feminist value: I am doing what I choose to do. That's what I understood to be the essence of feminism back in the 70s—women choosing what they wanted to do with their lives. In part, I homeschool my son to keep him away from the sexist, racist environment of public schools. Kids are taught to be competitive from kindergarten on. They are pushed to grow up quickly to be ready to join the workforce, but they are not allowed to be children. I want my son to be a child for as long as his childhood lasts. I am a feminist, and I hope to raise my son to respect the feminists he will encounter in his life—to respect all women for their investment in society.

֍

Here is a description of homeschooling made by one parent. These words were exactly how I felt as I had so much time with my children growing up:

> The really great part? Just being with the kids, watching them grow, seeing that "light bulb" go on when they love a topic or just get a concept, whether it be addition or checking out a bug on the grass. Not being rushed most mornings, lingering over breakfast, watching the clouds at 11 a.m. when usually they would be in school, snuggling for two hours on the couch, going for a hike at noon. Doing math at 10 p.m. when my boy is too restless to sleep, reading the *Secret Garden* with my girl at 6:30 a.m., if she gets up early while we lounge in our PJs. Staying up until 2 a.m. to see an eclipse or meteor shower or double feature at the drive-in, knowing they don't have to get up and go off to school. Just knowing you can hug them anytime you want.

My friend Ellen Forman wrote about her children's own personal choices in learning:

> Dylan, age 17, has never attended school, has paved his own path, and will probably sail off to college when he's ready. He loves a lot of random time and space to explore, and thrives on working alone and independently. On the other hand, my daughter Naomi, age 11, decided to try Montessori School this past September and is blossoming in the group environment. A gymnast, she flourishes with routine, structure and consistency. I have always considered myself a facilitator, honoring their interests, needs, abilities, differences,

learning styles, etc; offering and providing the resources that help them follow their hearts, attain their goals and encourage the love of life and learning. We are open minded and embracing how life unfolds: the positive changes and the bumps in the road.

As homeschoolers, I believe we are all aspiring to guide our children toward a path mindful of dear Mother Earth and her residents, perhaps helping to change the fundamentals by supporting them to sculpt a niche as a peaceful warrior rather than just preparing them to survive, collect possessions, or acquire a portfolio, ...teaching them to live in each wonderful moment, with awe and appreciation of the incredible beauty the Earth offers, and contributing in a positive and purposeful manner.

Here is a mother's view of what homeschooling might mean, as she's contemplating on withdrawing her child from school:

Despite fears and uncertainties, I'm reaching out to try to uncover more of what not only homeschooling could mean for my child, but also to glimpse the metamorphosis that would perhaps give birth to a more whole, more calm, more centered, spiritual being…and how this would forever profoundly change me as well.

Exploring Unschooling: Have you heard about unschooling and wondered what it's all about? Would you like to learn more? Here are some places to begin:

Books:

How Children Fail; *How Children Learn*; *Teach Your Own* and other books by John Holt

Parenting A Free Child: An Unschooled Life by Rue Kream. You can find it on-line at www.freechild.info

Dumbing Us Down by John Taylor Gatto

The Homeschooling Book of Answers by Linda Dobson

I Learn Better by Teaching Myself by Agnes Leistico

And the Skylark Sings With Me by David H. Albert

Awakening Your Child's Natural Genius: Enhancing Curiosity, Creativity and Learning Ability by Thomas Armstrong, Ph.D.

The Unschooling Handbook: How to Use the Whole World as Your Child's Classroom by Mary Griffith

Trust the Children: An Activity Guide for Homeschooling and Alternative Learning by Anna Kealoha

For parents and their teenagers:
The Teenage Liberation Handbook: How to Quit School and Get a Real Life and Education by Grace Llewellyn
Real Lives: eleven teenagers who don't go to school by Grace Llewellyn
A Sense of Self: Listening to Homeschooled Adolescent Girls by Susannah Sheffer
The Homeschoolers Guide to Portfolios and Transcripts by Loretta Heuer
And What About College?: How Homeschooling Can Lead to Admissions to the Best Colleges & Universities by Cafi Cohen
The Question Is College: On Finding and Doing Work You Love by Herbert R. Kohl

Websites that are easy and somewhat quick to read:
http://www.holtgws.com/index.html
http://sandradodd.com/
http://learninfreedom.org/
http://www.livingjoyfully.ca/anneo/anne_o.htm

Yahoo groups:
Always Learning- Learning All the Time
    http://groups.yahoo.com/group/AlwaysLearning/
Consensual Living   http://groups.yahoo.com/group/Consensual-living/
Radical Unschoolers List (RUL)
    http://groups.yahoo.com/group/RUL/
Home Education Magazine—Unschooling
    http://groups.yahoo.com/group/HEM-Unschooling/
Unschooling Basics
    http://groups.yahoo.com/group/unschoolingbasics
shinewithunschooling@yahoogroups.com (Anne Ohman)
FamiliesUnschoolinginNY@yahoogroups.com
http://groups.yahoo.com/group/RadicalUNschoolersinNY/
http://groups.google.com/group/UnschoolingDiscussion
http://groups.yahoo.com/group/alwaysunschooled/

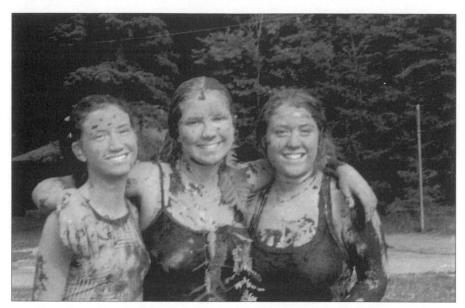

Gabriela and her friends Randi and Stephanie are covered with mud as part of a wilderness survival camp camouflage activity.

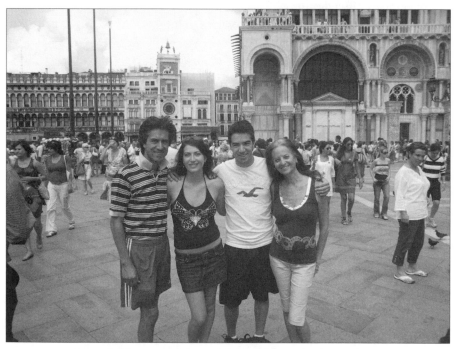

Homeschooling gave us time and flexibility to do what we love—here we are enjoying the wonders of Italy.

30

Nonviolent Communication
with Children

"We are what we repeatedly do. Excellence, then, is not an act, but a habit."
ARISTOTLE

A parenting class on nonviolent interactions with children was offered in New York City with Inbal Kashtan, speaker, teacher and author of articles on nonviolent communication. She explains in an article titled "Compassionate: Nonviolent Communication with Children," in Mothering Magazine, that she wants her son to be "deeply connected to himself and others, to become interdependent as well as independent." She feels by practicing attachment parenting, she and her partner were creating a lifetime of trust and connection with their child. Kashtan believes: "Attachment parenting means nurturing independence and interdependence by prioritizing babies' needs."

Although we may practice skin-to-skin contact with our baby, sleeping together, and holding them, as they get older, it is often more difficult to understand how to respond in respectful ways that create trust. Nonviolent communication deals with these values beyond attachment parenting. NVC has been used worldwide among families, and in prisons, schools and war-torn countries.

Inbal describes NVC's teachings on how a parent can convey three key things to the child: "I want to understand the needs that led to your actions, I want to express to you the feelings and needs that led to mine, and I want to find strategies that will meet both of our needs."

By bringing up children in a compassionate way, without authoritative force, we will be helping to create peaceful people who can solve conflicts in a nonviolent way.

Inbal Kashtan may be contacted by email: nvc@baynvc.org or by phone: (510) 433-0700. BayNVC is administering CNVC's parenting project. Inbal Kashtan is the Director of Peaceful Families, Peaceful World of the Center for Nonviolent Communication.

Marshall Rosenberg is the founder and education director of the Center for Nonviolent Communication. This Center offers nonviolent communication trainings, including parenting workshops worldwide, educational materials and mediation. (CNVC: 818-957-9393; cnvc@cnvc.org; www.cnvc.org).

31

Vaccination and Our Children

"Without basic science research into the biological mechanisms of vaccine injury and death and without methodologically sound, long-term studies which follow groups of highly vaccinated, lesser vaccinated and unvaccinated children over time to measure for all morbidity and mortality outcomes, it is illogical and scientifically irresponsible to assume that there is no connection between the ever increasing numbers of vaccines we mandate for children and the ever increasing rates of chronic disease in our children."

TESTIMONY TO THE CALIFORNIA LEGISLATURE BY BARBARA LOE FISHER, CO-FOUNDER
AND PRESIDENT OF THE NATIONAL VACCINE INFORMATION CENTER

Mass vaccination, accepted without question for more than a century, has recently become a source of great concern. Originally, the word vaccine came from the word "vaca" (cow) in Latin because the first vaccine in 1796 was the smallpox vaccine which was made from cowpox sores. "To vaccinate" means to produce disease in that person. Upon injection, the vaccine goes straight to the DNA.

Acute symptoms, such as high fevers, inflammations, and physical and neurological problems have been reported in many children following the administration of vaccinations. The long-term effects of these vaccines on children's developing bodies are just beginning to be investigated and understood. It's highly possible that immune system dysfunction, chronic fatigue syndrome, allergies, nervous system disorders, cancer, and other illnesses are connected to earlier vaccinations and medications.

After the routine DPT (diphtheria, pertussis-whooping cough, tetanus), MMR (measles, mumps, rubella) and OPV (oral polio) vaccines were administered, thousands of children died or were stricken with debilitating seizure disorders, mental retardation, physical handicaps, learning disabilities, or other chronic illnesses.

After each series of DPT shots, my baby daughter's leg blew up into a "boulder" that was red, swollen and frightening. She screamed for two days each time. The pediatrician told us this was a normal reaction, so we changed pediatricians three times, after each series of vaccines, thinking it was the way the shots were administered instead of the composition of toxins injected. Following the third reaction, I no longer believed the reaction was the doctor's fault. I began to read many books and articles about vaccination. Please see the list of recommended books and websites on vaccination on pages 401 to 402. My husband and I also attended informative seminars put on by Anti-Vac in New York City, and we realized then we were never given information on substances used in vaccines, and reactions and diseases that can result from vaccines. We found out vaccines can contain high levels of mercury and thimerosal, aluminum, and formaldehyde as well as bovine material (mad cow disease?), and monkey kidneys have been used in the polio vaccine.

In the article, "Vaccination: Informed Consent" by Dr. Joe Dzendzel, the dangers of thimerosal are described: "Vaccines are composed of lab-altered live viruses or killed bacteria, along with additives such as aluminum, sodium chloride, gelatin, antibiotics, sorbitol, phenol-xyethanol, formaldehyde, yeast protein, phosphate, glutamine and mercury in the form of thimerosal. Thimerosal, a preservative used to stem fungi and bacterial growth in vaccines, contains ethylmercury, a potent neurotoxin. Dr. Boyd Haley, one of the world's authorities on mercury, said, 'You couldn't even constitute a study that shows thimerosal is safe.' According to internal documents from the 1930s at Eli Lilly, which first developed thimerosal, researchers knew from the beginning it could cause damage—a fact Eli Lilly did not report in its study declaring thimerosal safe. In 1935, researchers at Pittman-Moore, another vaccine manufacturer, warned Eli Lilly its claim about thimerosal safety 'did not check with ours.' They injected dogs with vaccines containing thimerosal and half became sick. Pittman-Moore researchers declared thimerosal 'unsatisfactory as serum intended for use in dogs.' Although not suited for use in dogs, for decades it was routinely used in vaccinations intended for children."

The National Vaccine Information Center (NVIC) in Virginia reported a large U.S. study that found "one in 875 DPT shots produces a convulsion or collapse/shock reaction, which means some 18,000 DPT shots cause American children to suffer one of these neurological reactions every year." The MMR (measles, mumps, rubella) vaccine may cause encephalitis (brain inflammation) and death. The NVIC reported another U.S. government study which found a relationship between rubella vaccine and chronic arthritis, and some nervous system and blood disorders are also believed to be reactions to the rubella vaccine.

In addition to being possible causes of auto-immune disease, cancer, seizures in children, eczema, and sterility, autism is also believed to be a result of vaccinations.

Many parents are sure of the associated time link between the vaccines and autistic symptoms. In summer 1999, Barbara Loe Fisher, President of the National Vaccine Information Center in Virginia, wrote an article for "The Next City" titled "Shots in the Dark: Attempts at Eradicating Infectious Diseases Are Putting Our Children at Risk." She speaks at length on the connection between asthma, diabetes and autism with the vaccinations.

A friend of our family, a researcher interested in autism, found some interesting information regarding a study on mercury detoxification. Hair samples of a control group of children and a group of autistic children were taken. The results found traces of mercury in normally functioning children's hair whereas mercury was not detected in hair samples of the autistic children. From this information, conclusions were drawn that the autistic children demonstrated difficulty detoxifying or were unable to detoxify the mercury from the vaccines, leaving them with no trace of it in their hair. To learn more, read "Autism   New Evidence in Mercury Autism Link." (www.drgreene. com/21_1904.html) A link between certain vaccines and the onset of autism has been presented in numerous publications. Parental reports have pointed out autistic behaviors following the MMR (measles, mumps, and rubella) vaccine and the Hepatitis B vaccine, as well as others. Excellent DVDs on this vaccine connection, produced, written and directed by Gary Null, Ph.D., are *Vaccine Nation* in 2007 and *Autism: Made in the U.S.A.* in 2009.

The following information was presented during April—National Autism Month by Donald Meserlian of Voices of Safety International in North Caldwell, New Jersey:

To All Persons Concerned with Preventing Autism:

April is National Autism Month. According to the Center for Disease Control (CDC), approximately 1 in 150 [1 in 67 in 2008] school age children have Autism Spectrum Disorder (ASD). Many parents of autistic children have stated their child was developing normally until receiving a vaccination which devastated both the child's and the family's lives.

An article by Dr. Paul Offit, et al, "Addressing Parent's concerns: Do Multiple Vaccines Overwhelm or Weaken the Infant's Immune System?" "Pediatrics," Vol 109 No. 1, Jan. 2002, is summarized by Sherri Tenpenny, DO (http://www.mercola.com/2002/mar/27/vaccine infants.htm) as follows:

> One hundred years ago, children received one vaccine (the smallpox vaccine). Forty years ago, children received 5 vaccines routinely (diphtheria, pertussis, tetanus, polio and smallpox vaccines) and as many as 8 shots by 2 years of age. Today children receive 11 vaccines routinely and as many as 20 shots by 2 years of age.

One hundred years ago, autism was unheard of. Forty years ago the rate was probably less than 1 in 10,000. The 1 in 150 present rate [1 in 67 in 2008] can no longer be ignored.

The parents of many vaccine injured autistic children have stated their child was developing normally until a particular vaccine caused their child to become autistic. The pediatricians' response was that the cause of their child's autism was a "coincidence" rather than a "causal factor." This response seems to be supported by both the CDC and FDA based on their failure to address this serious problem.

As both the chairman of "Voices of Safety International" and the father of a 37 year old autistic son, I am providing the following information to all readers as my contribution to "April—National Autism Month": See www.voicesof-safety.com ..."Public Health"...VOSI V50.2 "Standard to Eliminate Mercury from Vaccines, Ban the Triple Vaccines, DPT and MMR, and Permit Freedom of Choice." Click on "View Research Report" and "Review Standard." Note that the research is based on the response from the parents of approximately 1400 children. The children were divided into three groups: those who received "all," "some" or "none" of the American Academy of Pediatrics (AAP) recommended vaccines. The conclusion of the research report was: Children who received all of the AAP recommended vaccinations were 14 times more likely to become learning disabled and 8 times more likely to become autistic compared with children who were never vaccinated. I am asking everyone who reads this message to review both the research and approved standard and send your comments to dmeserlian@msn.com. Those willing to contact the government officials who are responsible for reviewing and utilizing V50.2 should send their names, email addresses and phone numbers (optional) to dmeserlian@ msn.com I will give you the names and email addresses of government officials who must review and utilize applicable private sector standards in accordance with the National Technology Transfer and Advancement Act of 1995. Let's all participate in this effort to make "democracy" a meaningful word!

Donald Meserlian, P.E., VOSI Chairman and ASTM Member
Voices of Safety International
264 Park Ave.
North Caldwell, N.J. 07006
Phone: (973) 228-2258
www.voicesofsafety.com

John Hanchette, in his article, "Mountain Views: Precipitous Increase in Autism Cases May Be Tied to Childhood Vaccines" writes: "Autism is a neurological disorder, first recognized half a century ago, with varying degrees of severity that affects more and more children each year. Classic autism symptoms include lack of speech, repetitive behaviors, little or no social interaction, withdrawal from parental and sibling contact, jerky body motions of specific limbs, head-banging, hand flapping, and strange individual obsessions. The numbers of increased autism cases are shocking. Many parents, doctors, scientists and pediatricians think it's because as the 1990s rolled in and pharmaceutical companies brought new and promising vaccines to market, the number of scheduled shots your baby normally received in the first four or five years of life increased from about 20 to almost 40. And some of these vaccines contained an additive called thimerosol, a preservative that stops contamination of vaccines and preserves shelf-life. Thimerosol contains mercury, a toxic metallic element that attacks neurons. In drinking water, the Environmental Protection Agency (EPA) limit for human consumption is two parts per billion. In landfills, it's 200 parts per billion. Lab tests on some baby teeth have shown a content of more than 3,000 parts per billion. Despite drug company studies from 70 years ago that concluded mercury-containing serum was not fit for cattle or dogs, and with all the huge, expensive federal agencies to protect us from just such a mistake—the Centers for Disease Control, the Food and Drug Administration, the National Institutes of Health, the Institute of Medicine—not one had taken the time to total up how much thimerosal and mercury had been added to the average child's intake with the new increased immunization schedule. In essence, it was a grade-school math problem, but the nation's medical elite hadn't done it. The answer was about 120 times the amount allowed by the EPA for daily mercury exposure."

Jon Rappaport interviews an ex-vaccine researcher at http://www.whale.to/v/rapp.html. Here is a segment of this interview:

Q: Are some vaccines more dangerous than others?

A: Yes. The DPT shot, for example. The MMR. But some lots of a vaccine are more dangerous than other lots of the same vaccine. As far as I'm concerned, all vaccines are dangerous.

Q: Why?

A: Several reasons. They involve the human immune system in a process that tends to compromise immunity. They can actually cause the disease they are supposed to prevent. They can cause other diseases besides those they are supposed to prevent.

Q: What conclusions did you come to in your investigations?

A: The decline of disease is due to improved living conditions: cleaner water, advanced sewage sytems, improved nutrition, fresher foods, and the decrease in poverty. Germs may be everywhere, but when you are healthy, you don't contract the diseases as easily.

Q: Why are statistics quoted which seem to prove vaccines have been tremendously successful at wiping out diseases?

A: Why? To give the illusion these vaccines are useful. If a vaccine suppresses visible symptoms of a disease like measles, everyone assumes the vaccine is a success. But, under the surface, the vaccine can harm the immune system itself. And if it causes other diseases—say meningitis—that fact is masked because no one believes the vaccine can do that. The connection is overlooked.

Q: What contaminants did you find in your many years of work with vaccines?

A: Contamination occurs all the time. You get all sorts of debris introduced into vaccines. The SV40 monkey virus got into the polio vaccine because the vaccine was made by using monkey kidneys. In the Rimavex measles vaccine, we found various chicken viruses. In polio vaccine, we found acanthamoeba, which is a so-called "brain-eating" amoeba, simian cytomegalovirus in the polio vaccine, simian foamy virus in the rotavirus vaccine, bird cancer viruses in the MMR vaccine, and various micro-organisms in the anthrax vaccine. I've found potentially dangerous enzyme inhibitors in several vaccines: duck, dog, and rabbit viruses in the rubella vaccine, avian leucosis virus in the flu vaccine, and pestivirus in the MMR vaccine. These are all contaminants which don't belong in the vaccines, and if you try to calculate what damage these contaminants can cause, well, we don't really know, because no testing has been done, or very little testing. It's a game of roulette. You take your chances. Also, most people don't know some polio vaccines, adenovirus vaccines, rubella and hep A and measles vaccines have been made with aborted human fetal tissue. Remember, this material is going into the bloodstream without passing through some of the ordinary immune defenses.

Q: What was the turning point for you?

A: I had a friend whose baby died after a DPT shot. I found that this baby was completely healthy before the vaccination. There was no reason for his death, except the vaccine. That started my doubts. Of course, I wanted to believe the baby had gotten a bad shot from a bad lot. But as I looked into this further, I found that was not the case in this instance. I was being drawn into a spiral of doubt that increased over time. I continued to investigate. I found, contrary to what I thought, vaccines are not tested in a scientific way. No long-term studies are done on any vaccines.

Dr. Michael Odent has written a letter in the JAMA (1994) where his figures show a five times higher rate of asthma in pertussis immunized children compared to non-immunized children. He is also quoted in the International Vaccination Newsletter (Sept. 1994): "Immunized children have more ear infections and spend more days in the hospital." [See http://www.whale.to/vaccines/baratosy.html]

In Chicago, Homefirst Medical Services treats thousands of never-vaccinated children whose parents received exemptions through Illinois' relatively permissive immunization policy. Homefirst's medical director, Dr. Mayer Eisenstein, reported he is not aware of any cases of autism in never-vaccinated children. "We have a fairly large practice," Eisenstein said. "We have about 30,000 to 35,000 children that we've taken care of over the years, and I don't think we have a single case of autism in children delivered by us who never received vaccines. We do have enough of a sample. The numbers are too large to not see it. We would absolutely know. We're all family doctors." www.homefirst.com

❧

In the 12th edition of *The Sanctity of Human Blood: Vaccination Is Not Immunization,* Dr. Tim O'Shea writes about the following important topics all parents need to know: Learn why they vaccinate your child on the day of birth; Uncover why many physicians boycott school vaccination programs;

Sudden Infant Death; autism; measles; Human Papilloma Virus Vaccine; flu shots and mercury; Why kids can't build immunity anymore; Why American infants are now #39 in infant mortality, worldwide; Even more vaccines are coming soon. Dr. O'Shea continues to provide updated research. His 13th edition of this book is now available.

> A fearsome battle is lining up today in our brave new world. It's as though we're being forced to draw the line to a new threat - an assault on the blood of our children. This is not just a figure of speech. New vaccines are being invented every year, all with the same hope - to be included in the mandated immunization schedule. It's very big money. Today we're up to **68** vaccines mandated for use before a child is eighteen years old. Our infant mortality rate and the health of our children are appalling. The incidence of both infectious and degenerative diseases among adult Americans is skyrocketing. (www.thedoctorwithin.com)

When children become obese, their immunity is severely compromised. There is a pronounced correlation between a high body mass index and suffering from disease. It could be said that obesity itself is a serious disease, curtailing the optimal functioning of the organs as well as locomotion.

Every few years new strains of viruses with their new corresponding disease names develop, and scientists work hard to produce new vaccines in an attempt to impart immunity. But the vaccine can't be manufactured without toxic preservatives and other dangerous chemicals. However, if we keep our bodies clean by eating plenty of green plants rich in phytonutrients, known for building strong immunity, there's no reason to opt for vaccinations. Statistics throughout recent history have shown the obese suffer from diseases in far greater proportions, even after vaccinated. Our choice is to eat commercially processed foods and get the needle, or to strengthen our natural immunity through clean green eating, thereby maintaining a low percentage of body fat and remaining healthy.

You have the right to protect your children, and to interpret God's law in your own way. If you believe God and Nature are one and it's wrong to inject or consume any foreign materials of unhealthy or unnatural composition into the body, you have the right to protect yourself and your family. The first step is to read and acquire as much information as possible, including the websites of organizations such as NVIC in Virginia and Voices of Safety in New Jersey.

Many states have their own vaccination choice organization. Below is a list of the books, websites and DVDs focused on vaccinations:

Resources With Information about Vaccination

Books

The Sanctity of Human Blood: Vaccination Is Not Immunization, 13th Edition by Dr. Tim O'Shea

A Shot in the Dark by Harris L. Coulter and Barbara Loe Fisher

What Every Parent Should Know about Childhood Immunization by Jamie Murphy

Immunization: The Reality behind the Myth by Walene James

Vaccination by Viera Scheibner Ph.D. (100 years of orthodox research shows vaccines represent a medical assault on the immune system)

The Dream and Lie of Louis Pasteur by R. B. Pearson

Evidence of Harm: Mercury in Vaccines and the Autism Epidemic, a Medical Controversy by David Kirby

Vaccination, Social Violence and Criminality, the Assault on the American Brain by Harris Coulter

Vaccines: Are They Really Safe and Effective by Neil Miller

Vaccines, Autism and Childhood Disorders: Crucial Data That Could Save Your Child's Life by Neil Miller

Immunization Theory vs. Reality by Neil Miller

Immunizations: The People Speak by Neil Miller

What You Don't Know About Vaccines Could Hurt Your Child, edited by Jesse Noguera

Dangers of Compulsory Immunizations: How to Avoid Them Legally by Attorney Tom Finn

Vaccinations: Deceptions and Tragedies (Hallelujah Acres)

Websites

http://www.909shot.com (NVIC)
http://www.garynull.com/ Dr. Gary Null
http://www.thedoctorwithin.com Dr. Tim O'Shea
http://www.healthfreedomusa.org Dr. Rima Laibow
www.lifehealthchoices.com Louise Kuo Habakus
www.homefirst.com Dr. Mayer Eisenstein

www.healthliberties.org Rhio and Karen Ranzi
http://www.access1.net/vial (vaccine information and awareness)
http://www.evidenceofharm.com
http://www.generationrescue.org
http://www.mercola.com/townofallopath/index.htm Dr. Joseph Mercola
   You may acquire a copy of your exact state law and a sample
   exemption letter by visiting the following website:
http://www.thinktwice.com/laws.htm
http://vaclib.org   Vaccination Liberation

DVDs

Healing Autism Naturally—a Gary Null production
Vaccine-Nation (www.vaccinenation.net)—produced by Gary Null, Ph.D.
Autism: Made in the U.S.A. (www.AutismMadeinTheUSA.com)—a Gary
   Null production

Organizations

The National Vaccine Information Center (NVIC)
   512 W. Maple Avenue, #206
   Vienna, VA. 22180
   1-800-909-SHOT
   www.nvic.org
   The National Vaccine Information Center (www.nvic.org) has many
   contacts in various states.
Coalition for Informed Choice—Gary Krasner, N.Y. State
   GK-CFIC@juno.com, cfic@nyct.net
Congregation of Universal Wisdom
   www.cuwisdom.org
   Walter P. Schilling, D.C.

Many states in the U.S. and abroad have organizations for choice in vaccination which can be found on the Internet. One of the many is:

New Jersey Alliance for Informed Choice in Vaccination, NJAICV
   www.NJAICV.org
   email: NJAICV@aol.com
   Sue Collins, Co-Founder
   Phone: 1-800-613-9925

32

Your Child's Vision Health

"When one's mind is under a strain one unconsciously tightens the muscles which encircle the eyeball, and consequently squeeze it out of shape and out of focus. But when the mind is at rest these muscles are relaxed and the eyeball is allowed to assume its proper shape and focus."
WILLIAM H. BATES, MD, BETTER EYESIGHT MAGAZINE, MAY 1923

When I was seven, in second grade, unable to read the blackboard, I used to strain my eyes continually by trying so hard to see the small words the teacher wrote. My mother took me to the ophthalmologist who prescribed glasses. Initially, I wore them only at school, but after a very short time, my vision deteriorated and continued to deteriorate. Within two years, I was wearing glasses with a strong prescription—dependent on them during all my waking hours. There is a reason this happens, and as has happened to so many others, glasses became a crutch.

I also believe there is a very strong emotional component to wearing glasses. During my early elementary school years, I was a very depressed and unhappy child. I know this had a great effect on my eyes and vision. My eyes seemed to absorb my emotions.

When my daughter Gabriela began exhibiting vision difficulty in third grade, I had the strong gut feeling it would be wrong to get her glasses. I have always felt my glasses were a "crutch" on my eyes, and I was not going to have my daughter following in my path to weaken her eyes. At that point, there were other problems regarding public school that I felt were interfering with Gabriela's creativity and imagination, and when the vision question also arose, we decided to withdraw her from school. We began to homeschool, and over time Gabriela's vision improved. I recall from a talk given by Victoria Boutenko at my home in 2003 that children in school are usually staring straight ahead, putting strain on their eyes, and they don't use their eyes or turn their heads enough to focus in many different directions.

It is crucial when raising children on healthful foods that we be aware of the whole body, and how it develops naturally. Glasses are unnatural and whoever wears them quickly develops an unnatural dependence. The key to improved vision is relaxation of the eyes. There are natural vision instructors who teach this process.

Robert Lichtman opens his website with an excellent article, "Release, Relax, and Improve Your Vision." www.effortlessvision.com. I asked Robert to write on his experiences with children:

Children and Eyesight

"As for putting glasses upon a child, it is enough to make the angels weep."
WILLIAM H. BATES, M.D.

One of the most deeply held articles of faith modern people cling to is the belief poor eyesight is a genetic flaw exacerbated by the demands of modern life. Although this view implies a measure of hopelessness, it may actually be a relief to those who do not want to confront the facts: Everyone's eyesight is variable to some degree, especially children's eyesight, and only when that variability becomes locked through chronic strain do we experience chronically blurry vision.

The solutions to chronically blurry vision most of us turn to, eyeglasses and contact lenses, actually make our uncorrected vision worse, solving one problem and causing many others, often subtler, ones. For example, children who wear glasses tend to be more nervous and introverted than children with clear vision. They are more prone to headaches and tension. They don't express their emotions as freely, preferring to "keep it inside." To most fully feel the anguish of Dr. Bates' quote above, compare photographs of a child before and after getting acclimated to eyeglasses and note the relative strain in the face and sense of carrying the weight of the world. It is obvious eyeglasses are at best a necessary evil.

To understand why this is so, let's look at how eyeglasses work. Rather than *correct* the blur, eyeglasses merely *compensate* for the blur. If we assume the blur is caused by eyestrain, we can see how lenses actually *require* one to strain in order to see through them. Thus, wearing eyeglasses locks in the strain and encourages more strain. With more strain come stronger lenses and more physical pain until the mind blocks it out. This is what happens when we first put on a pair of glasses and the doctor says, "Don't worry, you'll get used to it."

Dr. Bates, the father of natural vision improvement, attributed much of this strain in a child's life to our educational system. In words surely to be championed by any homeschooler, he wrote:

> In the process of education, civilized children are shut up for hours every day within four walls, in the charge of teachers who are too often nervous and irritable. They are even compelled to remain for long periods in the same position. The things they are required to learn may be presented in such a way as to be excessively uninteresting; and they are under a continual compulsion to think of the gaining of marks and prizes rather than the acquisition of knowledge for its own sake. Some children endure these unnatural conditions better than others. Many cannot stand the strain, and thus the schools become the hotbed, not only of myopia, but of all other errors of refraction.

Nevertheless, in my practice, I work with children who suffer from poor eyesight despite being homeschooled. Typically, poor eyesight can be triggered by the child's inexperience in dealing with emotionally charged situations. Some examples include:

- An intense illness or surgery before age five;
- Death of a loved one before the age we learn how to process grief;
- Moving to a new place;
- Parents' marital strife;
- The changes that occur during adolescence;
- The strain of the first year of college.
- A sense of needing to fulfill expectations the child does not believe him or herself capable of fulfilling.

What do you do if you discover your child is experiencing blurry vision? First, don't panic. Look honestly at your child and yourself and check for stresses and strains that need to be resolved. Are you pushing the child too hard, creating expectations the child despairs of fulfilling? Is there fighting in the house? Is the child eating a lot of junk food and not getting a chance to run around? I once met a very charming six year old girl whose mother had her enrolled in every possible after-school activity. Cutting back her schedule was enough to eliminate her headaches and the first signs of myopia.

One should also be prepared for a trip to the eye doctor. In the very unlikely event your child's blurriness is due to something serious, only an eye doctor is qualified to diagnose and treat it. To be safe, choose an eye doctor who believes in treating eye problems rather than just throwing glasses on a child. And be aware that some of the language the doctors might use sounds worse than it really is. For example, there is a condition called amblyopia where a child does not see through an eye even though there is nothing physically wrong with the eye. If the doctor speaks of this eye being "blind," he does not mean blind as in, get a cane and learn Braille. Through the proper therapy, the eye can be "switched on" again. "Astigmatism" is another minor problem that can unnecessarily scare parents. As a general rule, I'd be very skeptical of performing surgery on a child. Sometimes surgery is only a temporary fix, can make a permanent cure more difficult, and can even cause new problems. In the case of strabismus, it is not uncommon for people to have as many as six surgeries in their lives.

As usual, prevention is the best cure. And the prevention of poor eyesight in children is very easy. First, encourage your child to move. All perception, whether it be sight, touch, smell, taste, or hearing, depends on movement. Encouraging this movement may take the form of dance, sports, rocking back and forth, or just allowing plenty of time for your kid to follow his or her natural, spontaneous attention. Ideally, the child would not watch television. Sugar is best avoided, too.

In his experiments with thousands of schoolchildren, Dr. Bates developed a technique that is as simple as it is effective: The Snellen Test Card (a standard eye chart available at any surgical supply shop) is placed upon the wall of the classroom, and every day the children silently read the smallest letters they can see from their seats with each eye separately, the other being covered with the palm of the hand. Don't worry about the kids memorizing the chart and faking the test; the chart in the doctor's office will be different. What this seems to do is give the children an opportunity to look in the distance, possibly a natural instinct when we experience stress. Also, it turns the eye chart, and the very concept of taking an eye test, into a stress-free, relaxed activity.

—Robert Lichtman

www.effortlessvision.com

⁊ව

Esther van der Werf, located in California, is also a natural vision teacher. I have been to a couple of sessions in which Esther instructed. She talks about daily habits to achieve natural relaxed vision:

Visions of Joy

The three key habits of the Bates method of natural relaxed vision are sketch, breathe and blink. Use these natural vision habits all day long, for improved clarity, color, texture and depth perception.

Sketch – Sketching is Movement plus Centralization. The human eye is designed to see clearly only in the central point of our field of vision. Color and clarity are received by the cones in the fovea centralis. Using that central point, along with movement, good posture and a relaxed neck, will allow for natural clear vision. Peripheral vision picks up movement and the smallest amount of light, but does not provide much color or clarity.

Breathe – Abdominal breathing results in optimum oxygen uptake. Yawn freely.

Blink – Blinking removes dust particles, moistens the eyes, gives the eyes a mini-break, and keeps eyes healthy.

Palming – Palm for further relaxation, and use visualization to train the mind in seeing clearly.

Sunning – The eyes are organs of light, and for health they need the full spectrum of light. Wean yourself off sunglasses by regularly sunning your eyes (with closed eyelids). Use a hat to shade your eyes when necessary.

Reading – Sketch, breathe and blink while reading. Look away regularly; give your eyes variation in focal distance. Pay attention to keeping your neck released. Notice that only one letter at a time is seen clearly.

Massage – Regularly give yourself a relaxing neck massage, and gently massage the area around your eyes with your fingertips.

Glasses – Use reduced prescription glasses, avoid full strength glasses which undo any progress made. Take glasses off as much as possible. Glasses cause tension to be perceived as normal and correct, but the clarity is artificial. Make friends with the blur.

Diet – Educate yourself about a healthful diet. For better health and well-being, get the full spectrum of essential nutrients by including many fresh, ripe, raw, organic fruits and vegetables in your diet. Avoid junk foods, alcohol, coffee, soft drinks, cigarettes, refined sugar, and refined grains. Alcohol has

408 | Creating Healthy Children

adverse effects on almost every vitamin and on many minerals. Particularly vitamins B1, B2, B3, B6, folic acid, calcium, magnesium and zinc are depleted in the body through alcohol consumption. Deficiencies of vitamin A, vitamin B2, vitamin B6, folic acid, vitamin C, vitamin D, vitamin E, chromium, selenium, lutein, zeaxanthin, zinc and essential fatty acids can lead to various vision problems.

Vision improves automatically in better light, when you are relaxed, and are well rested. Age makes no difference if you are following a healthy lifestyle. Your body has amazing capacities to heal itself, once the cause of dis-ease is removed, and when it is allowed sufficient time/rest for healing.

—Esther van der Werf, Natural Vision Specialist,
Joy@VisionsOfJoy.org, www.VisionsOfJoy.org

Here is a list of books on vision health:

Greater Vision, A Comprehensive Program for Physical, Emotional and Spiritual Clarity by Marc Grossman, O.D., L.Ac. and Vinton McCabe, N.V.E. (2001) ISBN 0-658-00643-6

Relearning to See, Improve Your Eyesight—Naturally by Thomas R. Quackenbush. (1997) ISBN 1-55643-341-7

Better Eyesight, The Complete Magazines of William H. Bates edited by Thomas R. Quackenbush. (2001) ISBN 1-55643-351-4

Help Your Child to Perfect Eyesight without Glasses by Janet Goodrich, Ph.D. (1996) ISBN 0-89087-870-6

Natural Vision Improvement by Janet Goodrich, Ph.D., (1985) ISBN 0-89087-471-9

The Art of Seeing by Aldous Huxley, (1942) ISBN 0-916870-48-0

Perfect Sight without Glasses by William H. Bates, M.D., (1920)

In an article titled "The Vision Thing" in the February 2005 Delicious Living Magazine, Phyllis Edgerly Ring points out: "Nutrition plays an active role in eye health, and recent research shows more than a quarter of the nutrients absorbed from food go toward nourishing our sight. Vitamins A and D, abundant in fruits and vegetables, are the most effective antioxidants for the eyes, and may be able to prevent macular degeneration, cataracts and glaucoma, especially prevalent in women over 65. Studies continue to show the importance of lutein (found in dark green leafy vegetables) and zeaxanthin (found in yellow produce) to prevent macular degeneration and possibly to reverse it."

David Wolfe elucidates in *Eating for Beauty*: "Blueberries, bilberries, lychees, and wolfberries (sometimes called goji berries or lyceum) are excellent foods for improving the eyesight, all containing high quantities of antioxidants."

Ingesting excessive fat, even from raw sources, can negatively affect the vision. Dr. Timothy Trader explains: "Overeating on nuts results in less oxygen and thicker blood which affects the eyesight. The blood and lymph are thickened by too much fat in the diet. If there is a lack of oxygen in the blood, nutrients will not be available for the nerves and muscles of the eyes to function properly."

33

Dental Health and Raw Foods

"You don't have to floss all your teeth, just the ones you want to keep."
anonymous

As described earlier, my children and I incurred some serious dental problems during the first few years on raw foods. I remember my children lying in bed in the morning with the dog. When the dog would raise her paw, the children would say, "We all want coconut dates." We did not realize the damage dried fruit, which is quite sticky, could have on the teeth. Neither were we informed of this danger by raw food support group leaders at the time we were transitioning to raw foods. Immediate brushing after eating any dried fruit is necessary. Soaking dried fruits will release some of the sugar into the soak water, so if you do eat some occasionally, it is better to soak it first. Incidentally, complex carbohydrates and refined, simple carbohydrates stick to the teeth in a fashion similar to dried fruits. Most complex carbohydrates, such as potatoes, breads and pasta, are acid-forming, and produce acid waste products that corrode the tooth enamel.

It is important to be aware that many raw foodists eat excessive quantities of nuts and seeds; nuts are acid-forming and cause acid buildup in the blood. The kidneys monitor the blood for pH, and if the blood becomes too acidic, calcium is leached from the bones, teeth and tissues to restore the alkaline balance, but at too great an expense to teeth and bones. A raw foodist can develop many health problems if not focused on keeping his blood pH toward greater alkalinity by not eating acid-forming foods to excess. Dentists who emphasize prevention point to the high potassium and phosphorus content of nuts and seeds. In addition to grains, these acid-forming foods eventually leach calcium, causing cavities and gum problems.

As discussed earlier, most nuts today are heat treated. We may be fortunate enough to get nuts that are sun-dried, but many are chemically dried. According to Dr. Timothy Trader, "Fats begin to break down at temperatures above 110° Fahrenheit. They start to decay, and become carcinogenic and unusable. The acid-forming nature of eating too many nuts can cause significant dental decay." My holistic dentist has expressed the raw foodists who come to him with very severe dental problems are almost always eating excessive quantities of dried fruits and nuts.

Any commercially grown produce would be acid-forming because of the chlorine and fluorine, chemicals used in pesticides and fertilizers, so it is best to eat organically grown ripe fruits and organic leafy greens to achieve correct blood alkalinity.

Some children raised on raw foods have complained of sensitive teeth. Sensitive teeth can often be the result of too much acid in the system—either too great a percentage of nuts, citrus, or dehydrated fruits. For stronger teeth, more alkaline-forming foods are necessary—organically grown vegetables, especially leafy greens. After eating tangerines, grapefruits or other citrus fruits, rinse and/or floss, but don't brush so as not to brush away a layer of enamel that has been temporarily sensitized by the fruit acids.

When one transitions to raw foods, it's crucial to take extra care of the teeth by carefully brushing and flossing after eating. Oral detoxification can result during the transition process. Canker sores and other oral detoxification symptoms that result during a change to more healthful eating practices are signs of a body that was overly acidic, and the mouth needs to be rinsed frequently with water and properly cleansed during this period.

Some raw foodists say eating fresh fruits and vegetables, such as strawberries and celery, naturally cleanse the teeth. I once attended a raw food support group meeting where dental cleaning was discussed. We were told fresh raw fruit would clean the teeth and there was no reason to brush and floss, which could actually be harmful to the dentition. Perhaps this can work for some people who live in chemically-free environments and have been raised on pure raw foods, but I would not recommend it to the majority.

Some claim their damaged teeth were able to remineralize on raw foods, but I have found this to be rare. All areas of a healthy lifestyle, including food, air, sun, emotional poise, sleep, exercise, etc. must be at a high level and in balance. A holistic dentist once told me the only time he had ever seen teeth remineralize was in a patient who switched to a healthful diet, practiced yoga and meditation regularly, left an unsupportive spouse, and significantly in-

creased his rest and sleep—a total lifestyle change, allowing the remineralization of his teeth. This was the only time this holistic dentist had ever observed
a patient to have remineralized dental structure and enamel. Other reports of
remineralization exist.

If your children are away from home and eat decay-causing sweets, such
as dried fruits, but their toothbrushes are not available, have them rinse with
water to wash away debris from their teeth. A good habit to adopt is to swish
the teeth with water frequently after eating. Make sure to have your child
brush at least twice a day, morning and evening, with a soft or extra soft toothbrush. When the child is old enough, buy the dental floss simplest to use and
demonstrate flossing.

For children, make tooth-brushing enjoyable. Try a fun-to-use, colorful
electric toothbrush. And try puppetry. Sometimes a child resisting brushing will love to brush along with a lively, friendly puppet who talks him/her
through the process.

Nontoxic Tooth Soap cleanses and refreshes the teeth and mouth. It
contains no added glycerin, synthetic sweeteners, silicates, fluoride, dyes,
stabilizers or other ingredients that damage the teeth. Raw food author
Frederic Patenaude claims some of his teeth re-enamalized in areas where
erosion had occurred, and this was confirmed by his dentist. Tooth soap is
available through Frederic's website: www.fredericpatenaude.com/toothsoap.
html Aluminum-free baking soda, non-abrasive and alkaline, cleans teeth and
counteracts oral acidity. If you do decide to continue using a fluoride-free,
sodium lauryl sulfate-free toothpaste, cover only one tenth of the length of
the brush with the paste. Fluoride is a dangerous poison. The warning written
on conventional toothpaste brands is associated with toxic ingestion of this
poison. Whatever you choose to use for cleaning your teeth and mouth should
be something you would feel comfortable eating. Fluoride is toxic, and you
would not want it in your body even in small amounts.

Carrots, celery and apples are known to be good teeth cleansers, leaving
the mouth feeling refreshed. I recommend children take them along for lunch,
but still make sure they brush their teeth twice a day with a soft toothbrush.
It's essential for raw foodists to be informed of dental hygiene rules. Putting
them into practice will enable raw foodists to raise their children to avoid
dental problems while eating health promoting foods.

Unfortunately, too many raw foodists have experienced tooth decay and
gum disease, especially after having abandoned dental hygiene while embracing the mindset: "If it's raw, how can it hurt my teeth?" But dried fruits do

just that. Tooth-destroying bacteria feed on fruit sugars and make their home in the mouth, and only a dramatic dietary change toward alkaline-forming foods can stop the erosion. Many experienced raw foodists have reformed their ways after mistakenly believing themselves impervious to fruit sugars. They ate dried fruits, nuts and seeds to excess, not to mention sweet unripe fruits, dates and honey, without regularly brushing, flossing or rinsing. This resulted in painful and expensive dental problems.

After eating, the pH in the mouth drops to a more acid level, and it takes up to two hours for it to return to its ideal alkalinity. Frequent snacking keeps the mouth pH acidic, providing just the right setting for bacteria to thrive and create tooth decay. Additionally, avoid regularly eating dried fruits, dehydrated cookies and crackers, nut and dried fruit combinations, and dehydrated patties. Nuts and seeds, best eaten frugally, and not directly from the bag, should be soaked, blended and eaten with large quantities of leafy green vegetables.

Much conventional and even some organically grown fruit is picked prior to achieving full ripeness on the plant. It is best to choose fruits that cannot be picked unless ripe or almost fully ripe. In northern climates, blueberries, apples, pears, and cherries are some of the more healthful choices. I enjoy watermelon from my local farmer in the summer. Ideally, eat ripe locally grown fruits. Unripe fruits are deficient in vital alkaline minerals—calcium and magnesium, necessary to maintaining strong enamel. Vegetables contain minerals necessary for strong teeth.

Rinse your mouth with water after eating, especially after eating fruits. Floss and rinse regularly, and after eating fruits, brush your teeth without toothpaste, and rinse with water without brushing after citrus. A small pinch of Celtic sea salt or aluminum-free baking soda in the rinse water restores alkalinity. It is not advisable to snack on fruits all day. Avoid constant dental contact with sugar. Eating greens following fruits and swishing water in the mouth diminish bacterial activity.

Dehydrating foods is an effort to make raw foods mimic old-fashioned cooking. It is simply a low temperature version of cooking—less harmful, but not healthful. The water in plants accounts for at least 70% or more of their composition. This perfectly filtered water is irreplaceable, and is the single most valuable aspect of raw foods. Simply eat fresh foods with their water intact for optimal health, including dental health.

Important vitamins and minerals must be present in the diet. Particularly important are calcium, magnesium, phosphorus, boron, and vitamins C, D and E complexes. Leafy greens are highest in the minerals, and organic fruits and vegetables are highest in the vitamins.

I recommend the Waterpik to remove bits of food neither brushing nor dental floss can reach. Whoever has the discipline to do it for two minutes every day, in the long run stands to save thousands in dental work. A thorough brushing with a soft brush takes two minutes to reach every area of the mouth. One or two such complete brushings, especially at night, plus flossing, should suffice to prevent problems.

Cavities are caused by acid-forming carbohydrates, especially bread and rice. Carbohydrate abuse, especially the refined variety, causes cavities and keeps dentists in business. When it comes to packaged cereals, 45 year raw foodist, Dr. Fred Bisci, says, "You'd be better off eating the box!"

A longtime raw foodist friend was thrilled when after years of gum and loose teeth problems, his gums healed and teeth became strong after switching from a high fruit diet to one still low in fat but high in green vegetables and sprouts.

Many people, including raw foodists, eat vinegar with their foods. Known chemically as acetic acid, vinegar is extremely acidic. When my kids were little, they enjoyed making "volcanoes" by adding just a little vinegar to the alkaline baking soda to cause a terrific explosion. This is happening to some degree in the stomachs of vinegar eaters, and any form of vinegar will do it.

As will be noted in the chapter on "Sun and Health," Vitamin D is absolutely necessary for calcium absorption, and therefore, vital for dental health. It is important to get sun on the skin daily without use of sunscreen.

In an article titled "Critical Situations in the Mineral Metabolism of Human Beings and Domestic Animals" by E.B. Forbes in the September 1933 Ohio Journal of Science, the following information is presented on cooking food and its effect on the dentition:

> ...cooking renders food pasty, so it sticks to the teeth, and undergoes acid fermentation. Furthermore, the cooking of food greatly diminishes the need for use of the teeth; and thus tends to diminish the circulation of blood to the jaws and teeth, and to produce underdevelopment of the maxillary and contiguous bones— thus leading to contracted dental arches, and to malocclusion and impaction of the teeth, with complications of great seriousness.

For further study on dental health, the following resources will help:

The Tooth Truth by Frank Jerome, D.D.S
The Root Canal Coverup by George E. Meinig, D.D.S
It's All in Your Head by Hal Huggins, D.D.S
Elements of Danger: Protect Yourself against the Hazards of Modern Dentistry by Morton Walker, D.P.M.
The Raw Food Diet and Your Compromised Teeth by Tonya Zavasta (www.beautifulonraw.com)

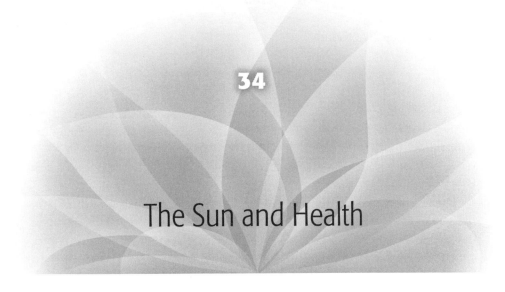

The Sun and Health

"Babies should be born in the spring."
DR. HERBERT SHELTON

Investigative reporter, Mike Adams, interviewed Dr. Michael Holick, author of *The UV Advantage*. He compiled "Fifteen Facts You Probably Never Knew about Vitamin D and Sunlight Exposure": "Vitamin D prevents osteoporosis, depression, prostate cancer, breast cancer, and even affects diabetes and obesity; Vitamin D is produced by your skin in response to natural sunlight; sunlight cannot penetrate glass; it is almost impossible to get vitamin D from your diet; the further you live from the equator, the longer exposure you need to the sun in order to generate vitamin D; people with dark skin pigmentation may need 20–30 times as much exposure to sunlight as fair-skinned people to generate the same amount of vitamin D; sufficient levels of vitamin D are crucial for calcium absorption in the intestines (the body cannot absorb calcium without vitamin D, therefore calcium supplements are useless); even weak sunscreens block the body's ability to absorb vitamin D (sunscreen lotions actually cause disease by creating a serious vitamin D deficiency); the sunscreen industry doesn't want you to know your body needs sunlight; if it hurts to press firmly on your sternum, you may be suffering from chronic vitamin D deficiency right now; and even though vitamin D is one of the most powerfully healing chemicals in your body, your body makes it absolutely free." This important article may be read in its entirety at: http://www.naturalnews.com/003069.html

In an article titled "Sunlight and Cancer," presented in the Moss Reports, "A growing number of dissenters within the medical profession and biological sciences believe avoidance of sunlight may actually contribute to the development of several diseases, including multiple sclerosis and certain cancers, such as non-Hodgkin's lymphoma, indicating vitamin D most likely plays an important role in preventing cancer." A report from the University of Sydney, Australia, reveals sunlight may provide protection from non-Hodgkin's lymphoma. Researcher William B. Grant found: "Not only is solar UVB radiation dose an important risk reduction factor, but city living is itself a risk factor, attributable to reduced UVB doses received by urban dwellers."

However, this does not mean you should go to the beach and bake in the sun until you turn bright red. It's best to avoid the intense sunlight in the afternoon hours, especially if at the beach or places where the sun is very strong. Get sun in the morning and late afternoon. For many years, I wanted a dark tan and sat in the sun for many hours at the beach in summer, sometimes coming home with sunburn. I now go out early and later in the day, but try to get sunlight as frequently as possible, even in mid-winter. Many living the raw food lifestyle, myself included, have observed naturally tanning more quickly, without burning, and have good skin color throughout the year.

Children raised outdoors in Nature often appear the brightest, the happiest and the most connected to the world around them. Children who stay indoors most of the time are more likely to get sick and become irritable, being deprived of oxygen and sunlight. They may be extremely deficient in vitamin D and calcium, even if supplements are taken. Vitamin D is essential to good health, but synthetic vitamin D added to milk and dairy products is dangerous. Dr. Brian Clement recommends fresh-water algae, sea vegetables and edible weeds as the vegetable sources highest in naturally-occurring vitamin D. For those staying indoors most of the time in cold winter climates, Dr. Fred Bisci recommends vitamin D supplements by the Innate Company. Those who don't take supplements and are aware of the importance of getting sunlight on the skin for creating vitamin D will make the extra effort to spend some time outdoors in the winter sun. If one doesn't live in a tropical setting, it's advisable to vacation in the winter. Our family vacations in a tropical setting each winter, usually in January, to receive needed sunlight and oxygen.

Four times in the last five years, we visited Costa Rica where we were so happy to awaken at 6:30 each morning under the beautiful sun and listen to the sounds of animals in Nature. Costa Rica is a beautiful country with many sunny days, and fresh ocean and mountain air.

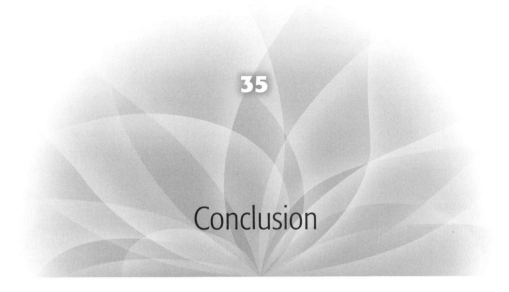

35

Conclusion

"Life, we learn too late, is in the living, the tissue of every day and hour."
STEPHEN B. LEACOOKE

Children today are targeted by much junk food advertising, and many countries have adopted fast foods with the accompanying use of vaccinations and medications. Consequently, children's level of health and nutrition worldwide is worse than ever. Many children consume only processed foods, without eating any fresh, enzyme and vitamin-mineral rich fruits and vegetables. I know children who have no idea what various fruits look like on the inside, nor what they're called. Many children have no idea where their food comes from. A nine year old girl disagreed with my daughter that bacon came from a pig, insisting instead it was made at the supermarket.

The pesticide industry and corporations owning genetically engineered seeds monopolize the conventional food market despite the fact the organic food industry in 2009 enjoys thirty times the sales volume it had in 1990. Most parents are unaware of the powerful benefits raw foods would offer their families. When illnesses occur, a "cure" for the symptoms is the immediate care sought instead of eliminating the cause of the problem, which almost always comes from what is eaten. Our long-term exclusive reliance on a medical system that focuses on disease and drugs rather than health has made most of us dependant and fearful, lacking the knowledge to be in control of our own health. Fear tactics result in our following advice which will cause harm to our bodies. Allowing dangerous shots to be given to our children, while believing we can consume whatever toxic foods are advertised, has shown disastrous results. It is illogical to think these foods and shots will not affect us negatively.

Once we gain confidence in the science of raw vegan foods and the related lifestyle principles, we will have the knowledge to take care of our family's health. This creates a freedom and joy of living beyond imagination.

Much can be learned by observing other species. Animals living in the wild follow their true biological instincts, whereas domesticated animals suffer the diseases similar to humans.

Each species instinctively provides care for its young, according to the maturation period of the particular species. Today, women are admired for returning to work soon after their babies are born because they can participate as bread-winners and compete with men in the workforce. However, there is a growing number of intuitive women who feel in their hearts and have faith in their powerful maternal instincts that bringing a child into this troubled world requires a strong maternal presence to build confidence and trust in the child. Long-term nursing is essential for the growing human child who takes longer to mature than any other species. A constant nurturing of the child's spirit is critical during growth throughout its stages.

I believe the children we bring into this difficult world deserve the best care to help them grow up to become healthy vibrant examplars of their true potential. It is our responsibility as parents to nourish them ideally, and to teach them to nourish themselves with Nature's superior foods. Our duty as parents is in every way to provide them with loving care and closeness throughout their growing years. By not following the standard processed food diet inexorably linked to medical treatment so acceptable in our society, children learn to listen to their bodies and to Nature; they will know it's all right to stand independently, and they will be empowered.

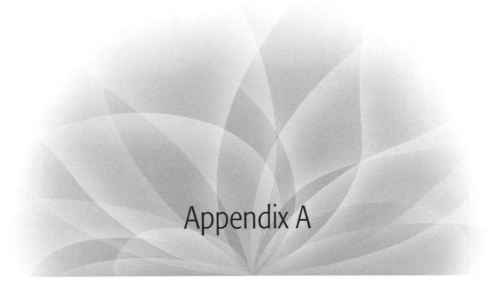

Appendix A

Healthy Lifestyle and Respect for Animals – Books for Children

The Fruit Bowl: A Contest among the Fruit and
  Vegetable Soup: The Nutritional ABC's [two books in one]
  by Diane Warren, Susan Smith Jones, and Amy Sorvaag Lindman

Born to Move—Nacido para Moverme by Dianne Warren

The Children's Health Food Book by Ron Seaborn

Brown BagWell & StayWell by Victoria Bidwell and Shirlene Lundskog

Doctor GetWell's Book of Nursery Rhymes by Victoria Bidwell

The Fruit & Vegetable Lovers' Coloring Book by Victoria Bidwell and Jaquelynn Mauvais

Doctor GetWell's "Apples to Zucchini" Coloring Book by Victoria Bidwell, Jaquelynn Mauvais,
  Kathy Rush, Larry Beeler and Teresa Gomez

I Eat Fruit by Hannah Tofts

I Eat Vegetables by Hanna Tofts

Victor the Vegetarian by Radha Vignola

'Twas the Night before Thanksgiving by Dav Pilkey

Fowl Play, Desdemona by Beverly Keller

Fruits and Vegetables of the World by Michel Viard

Saving Emily by Nicholas Read

Charlotte's Web by E.B. White

Everything Kid's Nature Book by Kathiann Kowalski

The Giving Tree by Shel Silverstein

The Lorax by Dr. Seuss

The *Anastasia* Books by Vladimir Megre

Replacing School Hatching Projects: Alternative Resources and How to Order Them by Karen Davis, Ph.D.

Animal Place: Where Magical Things Happen by Kim Sturla

Goosie's Story by Louise Van Der Merwe

Nature's Chicken, The Story of Today's Chicken Farms by Nigel Burroughs

A Boy, A Chicken and the Lion of Judah—How Ari Became a Vegetarian by Roberta Kalechofsky

The Pig Who Sang to the Moon: The Emotional World of Farm Animals by Jeffrey Moussaieff Masson

Benji Bean Sprout Doesn't Eat Meat! by Sarah Rudy

Pleasurable Kingdom: Animals and the Nature of Feeling Good by Jonathan Balcombe

That's Why We Don't Eat Animals by Ruby Roth

Children's books based on raw fruits and vegetables can be purchased through:
Karen Ranzi:
www.SuperHealthyChildren.com
or phone (201) 934-6778
Children's books based on raw fruits and vegetables by Victoria Bidwell can be purchased through: www.getwellstaywellamerica.com

Many of the books on animals can be purchased through the Farm Sanctuary
www.farmsanctuary.org
Watkins Glen, New York · (607) 583-2225
Orland, California · (530) 865-4617

Many books and videos for children on love of poultry and abuse of our feathered friends can be purchased through The United Poultry Concerns
www.upc-online.org
Machipongo, Virginia · (757) 678-7875

Videos and DVDs for Families

Breakthrough: A Raw Family Documentary
www.thegardendiet.com

Raising Children Raises Us
Contact Shannon Leone 1-866-LEONE.11 (53663) (toll free)

The Witness and *Peaceable Kingdom* – For older children to view: See www.tribeofheart.org

Diet for a New America by John Robbins

My Friends at the Farm
A humane education DVD narrated by Casey Affleck
Suitable for grades 3–6, 19 minutes
Can be purchased from The Farm Sanctuary

The Emotional World of Farm Animals by Animal Place
Can be purchased through United Poultry Concerns. This wonderful documentary is all about the thinking and feeling side of farmed animals. A PBS Primetime favorite.

Eating – For older children to view: See www.RaveDiet.com

Greens Can Save Your Life – with Victoria Boutenko
www.rawfamily.com

Interview with Sergei Boutenko
www.rawfamily.com

Reversing the Irreversible by Valya Boutenko

Overcoming the Food Imprint by Valya Boutenko
www.rawfamily.com

Raw for Life: The Ultimate Encyclopedia of the Raw Food Lifestyle
www.rawfor30days.com

Supercharge Me…30 Days Raw with Jenna Norwood
www.SuperchargeMe.com

The Adventures of Rawman & Green-Girl — a short animated film featuring the voice of Tonya Kay as Green-Girl and Steve Prussack of Raw Vegan Radio as the Chief. A new breed of Superhero has emerged to save us from our ecological shortsightedness, and those that would abuse our world for their own benefit. Running time: 10 minutes
www.gilmomedia.com/rawman/

Birth As We Know It by Elena Tonetti-Vladimirova
www.birthasweknowit.com

All Jacked Up: hungry for the truth? by Faerie Films, LLC.
"All Jacked Up will blow your mind. Its powerful and timely message is one that desperately needs to be heard. Your understanding of food is about to be rocked! Every family in America needs to see this film right now." —Mike Adams, Natural News
www.alljackedupmovie.com

Supersize Me
by Morgan Spurlock

The Future of Food
www.thefutureoffood.com

Food, Inc.
www.foodincmovie.com

CD: *Creating Healthy Children* with Karen Ranzi on "Hooked on Raw," New York Talk Radio, for purchase at www.superhealthychildren.com

CD: *Nurturing Peace: Healing Your Inner Child and Raising Your Little Cherub in Health and Happiness* with Professor Rozalind Graham
www.foodnsport.com

Raw Food Recipe Books

Raw 'n Delish Vibrant Recipes
Living Nutrition Publications, Edited by David Klein, Ph.D.
www.rawndelish.us

Hooked on Raw by Rhio
www.rawfoodinfo.com

The High Energy Diet Recipe Guide by Dr. Douglas Graham
www.foodnsport.com

Instant Raw Sensations by Frederic Patenaude
www.fredericpatenaude.com

The Raw Gourmet by Nomi Shannon
www.rawgourmet.com

Rainbow Green Live Food Cuisine by Gabriel Cousens, M.D.
www.treeoflife.nu

The Health Seeker's Yearbook by Victoria Bidwell
www.getwellstaywellamerica.com

Eating without Heating by Sergei and Valya Boutenko
www.rawfamily.com

Two e-books: *Sun-Sational Raw Baby Food* and *Sun-Sational Smoothies* by Melissa Gilbert
www.loverawlife.com

Rawsome by Brigitte Mars
www.brigittemars.com

Angel Foods: Healthy Recipes for Heavenly Bodies by Cherie Soria
www.rawfoodchef.com

Too Much Thinking, Not Enough Pooping/Instant Whole Food Raw Recipes by Dr. Ruza
Bogdanovich and Sean Bogdanovich
www.thecureisinthecause.com

The Healthy Lunchbox: Nutritious Meals Your Kids Won't Trade for a Lollipop by Shannon Leone
www.rawmom.com/HealthyLunchbox/

Healthy Halloween Treats: Quick, Nourishing and Delicious – Recipes and Rituals To Delight Children of All Ages
By Dr. Ritamarie Loscalzo
www.drritamarie.com

[There are numerous raw food recipe books available]

Some of these recipe books list salt and soy sauce as ingredients. Although I don't recommend these ingredients for health purposes, there may be a place for them in the beginning of the transition from cooked to raw foods. Without the use of salt or soy sauce, the recipes will still be delicious.

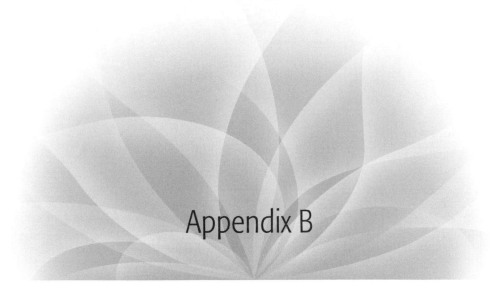

Appendix B

Equipment for Child Participation in Raw Food Preparation

Champion Juicer—Plastaket Manufacturing Co., Inc., Lodi, California, (209) 369-2154
    A fine juicer that also makes nut butters, patés, and fruit ice cream.

Vita-Mix - Cleveland, Ohio, (800) 848-2649
    The Vita-Mix is excellent for people wanting to add more fruits and vegetables to their diet. It's the best raw food preparation device I've ever purchased!

Braun MX2050 Blender
    The container is glass and is the best buy at $50 including $10 for shipping, from amazon.com. It is powerful enough to blend celery and dandelion, but is quieter than the Vita-Mix.

The Magic Bullet Blender
    This is a small compact travel blender. It can be purchased on amazon.com or from some department stores (available at Bed, Bath and Beyond). Excellent for trips and for use by children.

Saladacco
    This is excellent for making veggie pasta.

Veggie Spiralizer
    Also great for pasta shapes

The Healthy Juicer
    An inexpensive manual hand-powered auger juicer
    www.discountjuicers.com
    www.naturalzing.com

Krups Mini Juicer
    It most likely does not make as nutritious juices as some of the larger juicers, but this little juice machine was very useful when my kids were little—perfect for small hands. We bought it at Macy's.

Old-fashioned glass citrus-squeezer
I prefer squeezing orange juice the old-fashioned way using glass instead of plastic. The acid of oranges causes the plastic to erode into the juice over time.

Mini Food Processor

Small Utensils

Excalibur Dehydrator
Excalibur Products, Sacramento, California, (800) 875-4254 or (916) 381-4254
Dehydration of foods such as crackers, veggie burgers and cookies can be a fun treat especially at parties, but should not be the main part of the raw food diet as these foods, when dehydrated, become depleted of the water content which our bodies need, therefore dehydrating our systems which will then require increased amounts of free water to replenish us.

Coffee Grinder
For grinding seeds quickly, although this can also be done in a Vita-Mix or other heavy duty blender

Glass jars and sprout bags for sprouting

Decorating devices
Many of these can be purchased from Living Light Marketplace (www.rawfoodchef.com) or The Pampered Chef (www.pamperedchef.com).

Cookie cutters and designs to place in cakes to make them decorative
I purchase these at party stores.

Snow Cone Maker
Make fresh organic fruit juice ices. I bought my snow cone maker from a company called "The Pampered Chef," but I contacted them in 2006 to find out they discontinued sale of this excellent device. It can still be found on Ebay. Make fresh orange juice or other fruit juices (I've tried watermelon and strawberries, which were also delicious) and freeze them, then crank them out into ices. All kids love these! These delicious ices were served for birthday breakfasts for many years at our house.

Many products for raw food living can be ordered through well-known raw food sites:
www.livingnutrition.com
www.rawfoodinfo.com
www.rawlife.com
www.sunfood.com
www.living-foods.com
www.discountjuicers.com
www.rawfoodchef.com
www.hippocratesinst.org
www.naturalzing.com
www.highvibe.com
www.live-live.com

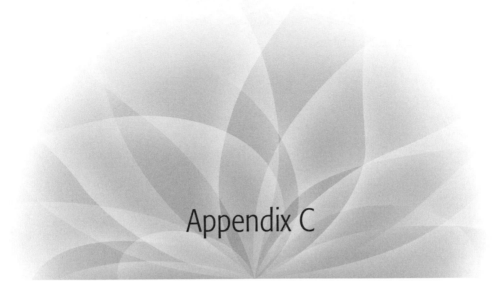

Appendix C

Periodicals and Raw Parenting Websites

www.superhealthychildren.com – Karen Ranzi

Vibrance
   www.livingnutrition.com, Publisher Dave Klein
   P.O. Box 256, Sebastopol, California 95473, (707) 829-0362

Get Fresh!
   A United Kingdom raw foods magazine, www.fresh-network.com
   Or call: +44 (0)845-833-7017
   Also available through One Source Distribution (800) 541-5542

The Raw Mom Times – from The Raw Divas, Tera Warner and Shannon Leone
   www.rawmom.com/blog – an informative website about healthy pregnancy, raising
   children on raw food, kid-pleasing recipes, uncluttering your home, and valuable
   articles about parenting.

Raw Foods News Magazine
   Judy Pokras, editor, www.rawfoodsnewsmagazine.com

The Raw Dish
   Stephen Parker, editor, www.rawdish.com

Pear Magazine and *Daily Raw Inspiration*
   www.pearmagazine.com, Info@thegardendiet.com

Juno Magazine, a natural approach to family life
   www.junomagazine.com

Boletin Crudivegano – A Spanish raw foods magazine
   Lista de Correos, 18960 Almunecar (Granada), Spain, 01-619-78-85-70

Purely Delicious Magazine
   www.PurelyDelicious.net

Sign up for rawpregnancy@yahoo.com, an informative discussion group:
   http://health.groups.yahoo.com/group/RawPregnancy/
   www.yahoogroups.com/groups/rawandpregnant - rawandpregnant yahoo group

There are also articles on raw parenting on www.vegetarianbaby.com.

www.rawfamily.com – The Boutenko family

www.raw-food-for-families.com – Raw recipes for the entire family

http://groups.google.com/group/raw-vegan-pregnancy-study – by Karen Rae Ferreira

www.rawfoodteens.com – largest forum for the young and raw

www.giveittomeraw.com/group/rawteenagers – a group for raw teenagers to talk raw

www.loverawlife.com/articles/interviewsrawteens.pdf – interview of raw teens by Melissa Gilbert

http://pullingdaisies.blogspot.com – Annelise's blog following a raw pregnancy, birth and child raising.

http://rawtoddleralex.blogspot.com – blog from raw mom Melissa Gilbert, raising her son Alex raw and tracking his progress online since birth.

www.TheRawfoodFamily.com – Ka Sundance and family

Mothering Magazine
  www.mothering.com

The Mother Magazine, the UK
  www.themothermagazine.co.uk

Fathering Magazine
  www.fathermag.com

Mother and Child Reunion Newsletter
  peacefulsimplicity@yahoo.com

Compleat Mother
  www.compleatmother.com

Alliance for Transforming the Lives of Children
  www.atlc.org

Organizations

Health Liberties Network – www.healthliberties.org
  A not-for-profit organization co-founded by Karen Ranzi and Rhio, the Health Liberties Network was set up in 2010 to address the issues of Health Choice in all areas of health care. The HLN plans to educate, advocate, aid, support and lobby on the issues of its mission, namely to come to the aid of individuals and families who are being persecuted due to their health care choices, and doctors and/or practitioners guiding those choices.

The Fruit Tree Planting Foundation (FTPF) – www.ftpf.org
  Founded by author David Wolfe, The Fruit Tree Planting Foundation is a nonprofit charity dedicated to planting edible, fruitful trees and plants to benefit the environment, human health, and animal welfare.

Mothers for Natural Law – Fairfield, IA, (515) 472-2809
  Call this organization to get the facts on genetically engineered foods.

National Vaccine Information Center (NVIC) – Vienna, VA. (703) 938-0342, www.NVIC.org
  Protecting the Health and Informed Consent Rights of Children since 1982

Turtle Lake Refuge, Durango, Colorado – www.turtlelakerefuge.org
  The Refuge is a non-profit organization whose mission is to celebrate the connection between personal health and wild lands.

Healing, Fasting, and Raw Food Retreats

TrueNorth Health Education and Water and Juice Fasting Center
   Dr. Alan Goldhamer, Dr. Douglas Lisle
   Santa Rosa, California, (707) 586-5555, www.healthpromoting.com

Dr. Douglas Graham—Water Fasting Retreats in Costa Rica
   Dr. Graham supervises fasting retreats in January and February, www.foodnsport.com

Scott's Natural Health Institute (Water Fasting Center)
   Dr. David Scott
   Strongsville, Ohio, (216) 671-5023

Tree of Life Rejuvenation Center
   Dr. Gabriel Cousens
   Patagonia, Arizona, (520) 394-006, www.treeoflife.nu
   The Tree of Life was founded by Dr. Gabriel Cousens. Dr. Cousens is an empowered spiritual teacher, yogi and rabbi. There are 10, 17, and 24 day green juice cleansing retreats. You can participate in Native American Sweat Lodges, Yoga, Kabbalah, and daily meditation and fire ceremonies.

Hippocrates Health Institute
   Directors Brian and Anna Maria Clement
   West Palm Beach, Florida, (800) 842-2125, www.hippocratesinst.org
   Guests on a quest for self-improvement come for health and nutritional counseling, non-invasive remedial and youth enhancing therapies, state of the art spa services, inspiring talks on life principles, and a daily buffet of fresh enzyme-rich organic meals. Life-giving juices from fresh organic vegetables and sprouts are served three times daily.

Optimum Health Institute
   Lemon Grove, California or Cedar Creek, Texas, (512) 303-4817
   www.optimumhealth.org
   OHI is a detoxification institute. They have 1, 2, 3, and 4 week programs.

Vida Clara Transformation Institute – Supervised Water Fasting Retreat
   Directed by Dr. Robert Sniadach, Located in Belize, Central America
   www.vidaclara.com, Email: heal@vidaclara.com

Ana Inez Matus –Water Fasting Director
   Pine Grove, Pennsylvania, www.beingwithvitalhealth.com

Creative Health Institute
   Union City, Michigan, (517) 278-6260, www.creativehealthinstitute.us
   CHI is a healing center offering 1–3 week cleansing and detoxification programs using wheatgrass and raw plant foods.

The Clohesy River Health Farm
   Cairns, Queensland, Australia, (617) 4093-7989, www.iig.com.au/anl
   Supervised fasting and detoxification programs
   John L. Fielder, DO, DC, ND, Osteopath and Lifestyle Consultant, Academy of Natural Living. www.johnfielder.com.au

Ann Wigmore Institute
   Rincon, Puerto Rico, (787) 868-6307, Email: wigmore@caribe.net
   The Ann Wigmore Foundation is a retreat and healing center that advocates enzyme-rich plant foods and fasting to heal the body.

The Living Centre and Living Arts Institute, Ontario, Canada
The Living Centre and Living Arts Institute, founded and co-directed by Shantree Walter Kacera and Lorenna Kacera, offers life-inspiring programs and services to thousands of people seeking greater health and vitality in their personal life and careers. www.livingcentre.com

The Raw Vegan Retreat Network Center – organized by Jingee and Storm Talifero, www.thegardendiet.com:

The Raw Vegan Retreat, Woodlands, Texas, with Joann Martin—Providing a variety of raw foods and juicing programs along with yoga and personal development.

The Raw Retreat, Ojai, CA, with Wyn Matthews and Cynthia Waring-Matthew, author of "Bodies Unbound"—Providing raw foods and juicing programs with creative workshops and body work.

Raw Retreat, Glendale, CA, with Revvell Revati, producer of Revvellations Radio— Unique raw food programs.

American Yogini
Director Mary McGuire-Wien, (631)-325-3492, www.americanyogini.com
Email: web@americanyogini.com
Juice fasting retreat and spa in luxurious Hamptons beach setting, New York

Manhattan Juice Cleansing Group
Led by Donna Perrone, www.donnaperrone.com
Juice cleanse meetings and supervision in Manhattan

Gentle Earth Retreat
Director: Katherine Croll 1-866-GentleE (436-8533) or (607) 339-9649
www.gentle-earth.com
Juice fasting retreat in Ithaca, New York

Body Mind Restoration
Spencer, New York 14883, (607) 277-7779, www.bodymindretreats.com

Raw Family Camps and Programs
Karen Ranzi offers her class "Raw Food Fun for Kids" www.SuperHealthyChildren.com

Sonja Watt organized a Raw Family Fun Camp in Austin, Texas and is now offering her program in Germany www.rawfunfamily.com

Dr. Douglas Graham's Health and Fitness Weeks—provide Olympic-class training and nutritional guidance to people of all fitness levels in beautiful settings around the world. www.foodnsport.com

Sergei Boutenko leads hikes through beautiful Oregon country. Hikers get to eat delicious raw meals with wild edibles and swim in pristine lakes and rivers. www.harmonyhikes.com

The Boutenko Family leads green smoothie retreats, and can be reached through their website: www.rawfamily.com.

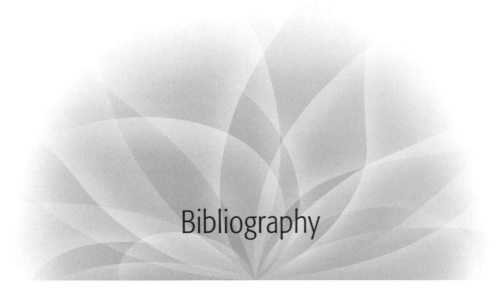

Bibliography

"Adoption of Genetically Engineered Crops in the U.S." USDA ERS, July 14, 2006.

Armstrong, Thomas. *Awakening Your Child's Natural Genius: Enhancing Curiosity, Creativity, and Learning Ability*. New York, NY: Putnam Publishing Group, 1991.

Baker-Laporte, Paula, Erica Elliot and John Banta. *Prescriptions for a Healthy House: a practical guide for architects, builders, and homeowners*. Gabriola Island, B.C.: New Society Publishers, 2001.

Barnard, Neal. *Food for Life*. New York, N.Y.: Harmony Books, 1993.

Baroody, Theodore A. *Alkalize or Die: superior health through proper alkaline-acid balance*. Waynesville, NC: Eclectic, 1991.

Bell, Eric. "Home and Lawn Pesticides More Dangerous than Previously Believed." Epidemiology, March 2001.

Benett, Don. *Avoiding Degenerative Disease: The Operation and Maintenance Manual for Human Beings*. KayLastima Publishing Company, 2006.

Blaylock, Russell. *Excitotoxins: The Taste That Kills*. Santa Fe, NM: Health Press, 1994.

Bogdanovich, Ruza. *The Cure is in the Cause*. Genoa, NV: Spirit Spring Foundation, Inc., 2001.

Boutenko, Sergei and Valya Boutenko. *Eating without Heating*. Ashland, OR: Raw Family Publishing, 2002.

Boutenko, Victoria. *12 Steps to Raw Foods: How to End Your Addiction to Cooked Food*. Ashland, OR: Raw Family Publishing, 2001.

Boutenko, Victoria, Igor Boutenko, Valya Boutenko, and Sergei Boutenko. *Raw Family*. Ashland, OR: Raw Family Publishing, 2000.

Boutenko, Victoria. *Green for Life*. Ashland, Oregon: Raw Family Publishing, 2005.

Bren, Linda. "Turning Up the Heat on Acrylamide." FDA Consumer Magazine, January-February 2003.

Brink, Susan. "Sleeplessness in America." U.S. News and World Report, October 16, 2000.

Campbell, T. Colin, and Thomas M. Campbell II. *The China Study*. Dallas, TX: BenBella Books, 2004, 2005.

Cohen, Jill. "Why Homebirth?" Midwifery Today, Issue 50, Summer 1999.

Cohen, Robert. *Milk: A to Z*. Englewood Cliffs, NJ: Argus Publishing, 2001.

Cohen, Robert. *Milk: The Deadly Poison*. Argus, 1998.

Cousens, Gabriel. *Conscious Eating*. Santa Rosa, CA: Vision Books International, 1992.

Cousens, Gabriel. *Rainbow Green Live-Food Cuisine*. Berkely, CA: North Atlantic Books, 2000.

Cousens, Gabriel. *Spiritual Nutrition*. Berkely, CA: North Atlantic Books, 2005.

Diamond, Harvey, and Marilyn Diamond. *Fit for Life*. New York, NY: Warner Books, Inc., 1985.

Dixon Lebeau, Mary. "The Serious Business of Play." The Parent Guide, November 2002.

Downey, Charles. "Donating Mother's Milk: The Gift of Life," (Web MD), Dec. 23, 1999.

Doubleday, Jock. *Spontaneous Creation: 101 Reasons Not to Have Your Baby in a Hospital*, Volume 1. www.spontaneouscreation.org.

Dzendzel, Joe. "Vaccination: Informed Consent." Vision Magazine, September 2005.

Ehret, Arnold. *Mucusless-Diet Healing System*. Yonkers, NY: Ehret Literature Publishing Co., Inc., 1953, 1981, 1983, 1989.

Eiger, M.S. *The Complete Book of Breastfeeding*. New York, NY: Workman Publishing Co., Inc., 1999.

Environmental Working Group. "High Levels of Toxic Rocket Fuel Found in Lettuce." April 29, 2003.

Epel, Elissa S. and Elizabeth H. Blackburn. "Accelerated Telomere Shortening in Response to Life Stress." The Proceedings of the National Academy of Sciences, Nov. 30, 2004.

Evans, Laurie. "Counseling Couples in Disagreement about Circumcision: A Jewish Perspective." The Journal of Prenatal and Perinatal Psychology and Health, (17) 1, Fall 2002, pp.85-94.

Forbes, E. B., "Critical Situations in the Mineral Metabolism of Human Beings and Domestic Animals," The Ohio Journal of Science. Vol. 33, No.5 (September, 1933), 389-406.

Fuhrman, Joel. *Disease-Proof Your Child: Feeding Kids Right*. New York, NY: St. Martin's Press, 2005.

Fuhrman, Joel. *Eat to Live*. Boston, New York, London: Little, Brown and Company, 2003.

Fry, T.C. and David Klein. *Your Natural Diet: Alive Raw Foods*. Sebastopol, CA: Living Nutrition Publications, 2004.

Gaskin, Ina May. *Spiritual Midwifery (3rd ed.)*. Summertown, TN: The Farm Publishing Co., 1990.

Grace, Matthew. *A Way Out: Dis-ease Deception and the Truth about Health*. Matthew Grace, 2000.

Graedon, Joe and Teresa Graedon. *Dangerous Drug Interactions: How to Protect Yourself from Harmful Drug/Drug, Drug/Food, Drug/Vitamin Combination*. New York: St. Martin's Paperbacks, 1999.

Graham, Douglas N. *The 80/10/10 Diet: Balancing Your Health, Your Weight, and Your Life One Luscious Bite at a Time*. Key Largo, FL: FoodnSport Press, 2006.

Graham, Douglas N. *Grain Damage: Rethinking the high starch diet*. Marathon, FL: FoodnSport Press, 1998.

Graham, Douglas N. *The High Energy Diet Recipe Guide*. Key Largo, FL: FoodnSport Press, 1998, 2007.

Gruben, Rozalind. "Sleep Your Way to Health." Living Nutrition Magazine. Sebastopol, CA: Vol.3, 2002.

Gruben-Graham, Rozalind. "Women's Health Empowerment." Living Nutrition Magazine. Sebastopol, CA: Vol. 16, 2005.

Halfmoon, Hygeia. *Primal Mothering in a Modern World*. San Diego, CA: Maul Brothers Publishing, 1998.

Hanchette, John. "Mountain Views: Precipitous Increase in Autism Cases May Be Tied to

Childhood Vaccines." Niagara Falls Reporter (www.niagarafallsreporter.com), Feb. 24, 2004.

Harper, Barbara. *Gentle Birth Choices*. Rochester, VT: Healing Arts Press, 1994, 2005.

Holick, Michael F. *The UV Advantage: The Medical Breakthrough That Shows How to Harness the Power of the Sun for Your Health*. New York, NY: Ibooks Inc., 2004.

Howell, Edward. *Enzyme Nutrition*. Wayne, NJ: Avery, 1985.

Hunt, Jan. *The Natural Child: Parenting from the Heart*. Gabriola Island, BC, Canada: New Society Publishers, 2001.

Idol, Olin. *Pregnancy, Children and the Hallelujah Diet*. Shelby, NC: Hallelujah Acres Publishing, 2002.

Joint WHO/FAO Press Release/51. "Additional Research on Acrylamide in Food Essential, Scientists Declare." June 27, 2002.

Jones, G., M. Riley and T. Dwyer. "Breastfeeding in Early Life and Bone Mass in Prepubertal Children: A Longitudinal Study." Osteoporosis Int 2000; 11:146-52.

Jones, Susan Smith. *The Healing Power of NatureFoods: 50 Revitalizing SuperFoods and Lifestyle Choices to Promote Vibrant Health*. Carlsbad, CA: Hay House, Inc., 2007.

Kamen, Betty, and Michael Rosenbaum. "Nutrition Hints," www.bettykamen.com.

Kashtan, Inbal. "Compassionate: Nonviolent Communication with Children." Mothering Magazine. Issue 110, Jan/Feb issue, 2002.

Kimmel, James. *Whatever Happened to Mother?—A Primer for Those Who Care about Children*. Tucson, AZ: Sweet & Simple Publishing, 1992.

Kohn, Alfie. *Punished by Rewards*. New York, NY: Houghton Mifflin Company, 1993.

Kurtz, Ellen. "The Bounce That Counts—Rebounding." Option Magazine. August 2002.

Leahy, Stephen. "New Studies Back Benefits of Organic Diet." Toronto, Canada: Inter Press Service, March 4, 2006.

Magaziner, Allan, Linda Bonvie and Anthony Zolezzi. *Chemical-Free Kids*. New York, NY: Kensington Publishing Corp., 2003.

Malina, Robert M. "Secular Changes in Size and Maturity: Causes and Effects." Monograph of the Society for Research in Child Development, volume 44 (ser 179): 59-102.

McClure, Vimala Schneider. *Infant Massage: A Handbook for Loving Parents, 3rd Edition*. New York, NY: Bantam Books, 2000.

McDougall, John A. "Energy to Grow a Healthy Baby." The McDougall Newsletter. March/April 1997.

McDougall, John A., and Mary McDougall. *The McDougall Plan*. Piscataway, NJ: New Century Publishers, Inc., 1983.

McDougall, John A. *The McDougall Program For Women: What Every Woman Needs to Know to Be Healthy for Life*. New York, NY: Dutton, Penquin Putnam, Inc., 1999.

Minshew, Brazos. "Get Energy from Good Fats." Trivita Weekly Wellness Newsletter. March 8, 2008.

Montgomery, Beth. *Transitioning to Health: A Step by Step Guide for You and Your Child*. Montgomery, 2001.

Nelson, Dennis. *Food Combining Simplified*. Santa Cruz, CA: Dennis Nelson Books, 1983.

Nison, Paul. *Raw Knowledge: Enhance the Powers of Your Mind, Body and Soul*. Brooklyn, NY: 343 Publishing Company, 2002.

Nison, Paul. *The Daylight Diet: Divine Eating for Superior Health and Digestion*. West Palm Beach, FL: 343 Publishing Company, 2009.

Nutritive Value of American Foods in Common Units. Agriculture Handbook No. 456,

Agriculture Research Service, U.S. Department of Agriculture. 1975.

Offit, Paul A., Jessica Quarles, Michael A. Gerber, Charles J. Hackett, Edgar K. Marcuse, Tobias R. Kollman, Bruce G. Gellin, and Sarah Landry. "Addressing Parent's Concerns…Do Multiple Vaccines Overwhelm or Weaken the Infant's Immune System?" Pediatrics. Vol. 109, No. 1, Jan. 2002, pp. 124-129.

Patenaude, Frederic. *Instant Raw Sensations*. Montreal (Quebec), Canada: Raw Vegan, 2005.

Patenaude, Frederic. *Raw Secrets: The Raw Vegan Diet in the Real World*. Montreal (Quebec), Canada: Raw Vegan, 2002.

Pizzi, William J. and June E. Barnhart. "MSG Greatly Reduces Pregnancy Success." Department of Psychology, Northeastern Illinois University, Chicago, Illinois, *Neurobehavioral Toxicology*. Vol. 2:1-4, 1979.

Price, Weston. *Nutrition and Physical Degeneration*. Los Angeles, CA: Keats, 1997.

Quackenbush, Thomas. *Relearning to See*. Berkeley, CA: North Atlantic Books, 1997, 1999.

O'Shea, Tim. *The Sanctity of Human Blood: Vaccination Is Not Immunization, 12th Edition*. San Jose, CA: The Doctor Within, 2008.

Ragnar, Peter. *Alive and Well with Wild Foods*. Asheville, NC: Roaring Lion Publishing, 2005.

Ranzi, Karen. "Discovery." Living Nutrition Magazine. Vol. 13, 2002, p. 9.

Ranzi, Karen. "Homeschooling: An Option That Makes Sense." *Raw Knowledge: Enhance the Powers of Your Mind, Body and Soul*. Brooklyn, NY: 343 Publishing Company, 2002.

Ratey, John J. *Spark: The Revolutionary New Science of Exercise and the Brain*. New York, NY: Little, Brown, and Company, 2008.

Rhio. *Hooked on Raw*. New York, NY: Beso Entertainment, 2000.

Rhio. "Genetically Engineered Foods Explained in Plain Language." Just Eat An Apple Magazine. Issue 22, Spring 2004.

Ring, Phyllis Edgerly. "The Vision Thing." Delicious Living Magazine. February 2005.

Robbins, John. *Diet for a New America*. Tiburon, CA: H.J. Kramer Inc., 1998.

Schenck, Susan. *The Live Food Factor: The Comprehensive Guide to the Ultimate Diet for Body, Mind, Spirit and Planet*. San Diego, CA: Awakening Publications, 2006, 2008.

Sears, William and Martha Sear. *The Attachment Parenting Book: A Commonsense Guide to Understanding and Nurturing Your Baby*. New York, NY: Little, Brown and Company, 2001.

Shelton, Herbert M. *The Science and Fine Art of Food and Nutrition*. Oldsmar, FL: Natural Hygiene Press, 1984.

Silverstein, Olga. *The Courage to Raise Good Men*. New York, NY: Viking Press, 1994.

Snedeker, Suzanne M. "Five Types of Parabens Detected Intact in Human Breast Tumors." Cornell University Sprecher Institute for Comparative Cancer Research. The Ribbon, Vol. 9, no.1, Winter 2004.

Stanchich, Lino. *The Power Eating Program*. Miami, FL: Healthy Products, Inc., 1989.

Sommers, Craig B. *Raw Foods Bible*. Guru Beant Press, 2004—2007.

The Department of Environmental Protection Water Quality Inventory Reports. 1995.

"The Role of Skin Absorption as a Route of Exposure for Volatile Organic Compounds," American Journal of Public Health, 1984.

Thevenin, Tine. *The Family Bed*. Wayne, NJ: Avery Publishing Group Inc., 1987.

Thompson, Athena. *Homes that Heal and those that don't: How your home may be harming your family's health*. Gabriola Island, BC, Canada: New Society Publishers, 2004.

Walker, Norman W. *Fresh Vegetable and Fruit Juices*. Prescott, AZ: Norwalk Press, 1970, 1978.

Weaver, Don. *To Love and Regenerate the Earth: Further Perspectives on the Survival of Civilization*. Woodside, CA: Earth Health Regeneration, 2002. Currently free online in the Agriculture Library of the Soil and Health website: www.soilandhealth.org.

Wolfe, David. *Eating For Beauty*. San Diego, CA: Maul Brothers Publishing, 2003.

Yaron, Ruth. *Super Baby Food*. Archbald, PA: F. J. Roberts Publishing Company, 1997.

Young, Robert O. and Shelley Redford Young. *The pH Miracle: Balance Your Diet, Reclaim Your Health*. New York, NY: Warner Books, 2002.

Zamm, Alfred V. *Why Your House May Endanger Your Health*. New York, NY: Simon & Schuster, 1980.

Zavasta, Tonya. *Quantum Eating: The Ultimate Elixir of Youth*. Cordova, TN: BR Publishing, 2007.

Zavasta, Tonya. *Your Right to be Beautiful: How to Halt the Train of Aging & Meet the Most Beautiful You*. Cordova, TN: BR Publishing, 2003.

Additional Resources to Assist with Raw/Vegetarian Parenting and Raising Healthy Children

Bauer, Gene. *Farm Sanctuary: Changing Hearts and Minds about Animals and Food*. New York, NY: Touchstone Publishing, 2008.

Bower, Lynn. *Creating a Healthy Household: The Ultimate Guide for Healthier, Safer, Less-Toxic Living*. Bloomington, IN: Healthy House Institute, 2000.

Braley, James and Ron Hoggam. *Dangerous Grains: Why Gluten Cereal Grains May Be Hazardous to Your Health*. Avery, 2002.

Bumgarner, Norma Jane. *Mothering Your Nursing Toddler*. Franklin Park, Ill: La Leche League International, Inc., 1980, 1982, 1986.

Clement, Anna Maria and Brian Clement. *Children: The Ultimate Creation*. West Palm Beach, FL: A. M. Press, 1994.

Dadd, Debra Lynn. *The Nontoxic Home: Protecting Yourself and Your Family from Everyday Toxics and Health Hazards*. Los Angeles, CA: Jeremy P. Tarcher, 1986.

Dadd, Debra Lynn. *Home Safe Home: Creating a Healthy Home Environment by Reducing Exposure to Toxic Household Products*. New York: Jeremy P. Tarcher/Penguin, 2004.

Davis, Karen. *Prisoned Chickens, Poisoned Eggs: An Inside Look at the Modern Poultry Industry*. Summertown, TN: Book Publishing Company, 1996. New Revised Edition, 2008.

Eisnitz, Gail A. *Slaughterhouse: The Shocking Story of Greed, Neglect, and Inhumane Treatment Inside the U.S. Meat Industry*. Amherst, NY: Prometheus Books, 1997.

Finn, Tom. *Dangers of Compulsory Immunizations: How to Avoid Them Legally*. New Port Richey, FL: Family Fitness Press, 1983.

Gallo, Roe and Stephen Zocchi. *Overcoming the Myths of Aging: Lose Weight, Look Great and Live a Happier, Healthier Life*. San Francisco, CA: Roe Gallo Publishing, 2007.

Gary Null Production. *Healing Autism Naturally* (DVD). Gary Null & Associates, Inc., 2006.

Gary Null Production. *Vaccine-Nation* (DVD). Gary Null & Associates, Inc. 2007.

Gary Null Production. *Autism: Made in the U.S.A.* (DVD). Gary Null & Associates, Inc. 2009.

Gorman, Carolyn and Marie Hyde. *Less-Toxic Alternatives*: DeKalb, TX: Optimum Publishing, 1997.

Jones, Susan Smith. *Be Healthy—Stay Balanced*. Camarillo, CA: DeVorss, 2008.

Kitzinger, Sheila. *Breastfeeding Your Baby*. New York: Alfred Knopf, 1998.

Kulvinskas, Viktoras. *Survival into the Twenty-First Century*. 21st Century Bookstore, 1975.

La Leche League, *The Womanly Art of Breastfeeding*. Franklin Park, Ilinois: La Leche League International, 1958, 1963, 1981.

Lieberman, Jacob. *Take Off Your Glasses and See*. Three Rivers Press, 1995.

Lyman, Howard. *Mad Cowboy: Plain Truth from the Cattle Rancher Who Won't Eat Meat*. New York: Scribner, 1998.

Lynn, Michaela and Michael Chrisemer. *Baby Greens: A Live-Food Approach for Children of All Ages*. Berkeley, CA: Frog, Ltd., 2004, 2005.

Mason, Jim and Peter Singer. *Animal Factories*. New York: Harmony Books, 1990.

Masson, Jeffrey Moussaieff. *The Pig Who Sang to the Moon: The Emotional World of Farm Animals*. New York, NY: Ballantine Books, 2003.

Moran, Victoria. *Shelter for the Spirit: How to Make Your Home a Haven in a Hectic World*. New York: Harper Collins Publishers, 1997.

Mountrose, Phillip and Jane Mountrose. *Getting Through to Kids: Problem Solving With Children Ages 6 to 18*. Sacramento, CA: Holistic Communications, 1997.

Olds, Sally and Marvin Eiger. *The Complete Book of Breastfeeding, 3rd Edition*. New York: Workman Publishing, 1999.

Presser, Janice and Gail Brewer. *Breastfeeding*. New York, NY: Alfred A. Knopf, 1983.

Rifkin, Jeremy. *Beyond Beef: The Rise and Fall of the Cattle Culture*. New York, NY: Dutton, 1992.

Robbins, John and Dean Ornish. *The Food Revolution: How Your Diet Can Help Save Your Life and the World*. Berkely, CA: Conan Press, 2001.

Rosenberg, Marshall B. *Nonviolent Communication: A Language of Compassion*. Encinitas, CA: PuddleDancer Press, 2002.

Rosenberg, Marshall B. *Nonviolent Communication: A Language of Life, 2nd Edition*. Encinitas, CA: PuddleDancer Press, 2003.

Sears, William. *Nighttime Parenting*. Franklin Park, Ill: La Leche League International, Inc., 1986.

Shanley, Laura Kaplan. *Unassisted Childbirth*. Westport, CT: Bergen & Garvey, 1994.

Shazzie. *Evie's Kitchen*. United Kingdom: Rawcreation Ltd, 2008.

Sturla, Kim. *Animal Place: Where Magical Things Happen*. Vacaville, CA: Animal Place, 1994.

Tansey, Geoff and Joyce DeSilva. *The Meat Business: Devouring a Hungry Planet*. New York: St. Martin's Press, 1999.

Viard, Michel. *Fruits and Vegetables of the World*. Ann Arbor, MI: Longmeadow Press, 1995.

Weaver, Don. *The Survival of Civilization*. Currently free online in the Agriculture Library of the Soil and Health website: www.soilandhealth.org.

Weed, Carol. "The Dandelion is a Healthful, Great Tasting Weed You Can Eat," *Back Woods Magazine*, Issue 44.

Wigmore, Ann. *Be Your Own Doctor*. Avery Publishing, 1982.

Wolfson, David J. *Beyond the Law: Agribusiness and the Systemic Abuse of Animals Raised for Food or Food Production*. Watkins Glen, NY: Farm Sanctuary, 1999.

Yntema, Sharon. *Vegetarian Baby*. Ithaca, NY: McBooks Press, 1991.

Yntema, Sharon. *Vegetarian Children*. Ithaca, NY: McBooks Press, 1995.

Resources on Homeschooling and Mindful Parenting

Armstrong, Thomas. *Awakening Your Child's Natural Genius: Enhancing Curiosity, Creativity, and Learning Ability*. New York, NY: Putnam Publishing Group, 1991.

Armstrong, Thomas. *In Their Own Way: Discovering and Encouraging Your Child's Personal Learning Style*. New York, NY: Tarcher/Putnam, 1987.

Dobson, Linda. *The Homeschooling Book of Answers: The 101 Most Important Questions Answered by Homeschooling's Most Respected Voices*. Roseville, CA: Prima Publishing, 2002.

Epstein, Robert. *The Case Against Adolescence: Rediscovering the Adult in Every Teen*. Sanger, CA:

Quill Driver Books/Word Dancer Press, 2007.

Gatto, John Taylor. *Dumbing Us Down: The Hidden Curriculum of Compulsory Schooling.* Philadelphia, PA: New Society Publishers, 1992.

Gatto, John Taylor. *The Underground History of American Education.* New York, NY: The Odysseus Group, 2000.

Griffith, Mary. *The Unschooling Handbook: How to Use the Whole World as Your Child's Classroom.* Rocklin, CA: Prima Publishing, 1998.

Heuer, Loretta. *The Homeschooler's Guide to Portfolios and Transcripts.* Arco Publishing, 2000.

Holt, John. *How Children Learn.* New York: Addison-Wesley Publishing Company, 1967, 1983.

Holt, John. *How Children Fail.* Reading, MA: Addison-Wesley Publishing Company, 1982.

Holt, John. *Teach Your Own: The John Holt Book of Homeschooling.* Cambridge, MA: Perseus Publishing, 2003.

Home Education Magazine—(800) 236-3278 or (907) 746-1336
http://www.home-ed-magazine.com

Kirshenbaum, Mira and Charles Foster. *Parent/Teen Breakthrough: The Relationship Approach.* New York, NY: Penguin Books USA Inc., 1991.

Kohn, Alfie. *Punished by Rewards: The Trouble with Gold Stars, Incentive Plans, A's, Praise, and Other Bribes.* New York, NY: Houghton Mifflin Company, 1993.

Kream, Rue. *Parenting a Free Child: An Unschooled Life.* Self-published, 2005.

Llewellyn, Grace. *The Teenage Liberation Handbook.* How to Quit School and Get a Real Life and Education. Rockport, MA: Element, 1997.

Liedloff, Jean. *The Continuum Concept.* Menlo Park, CA: Addison-Wesley Publishing Company, 1993.

Neufeld, Gordon and Gabor Mate. *Hold On To Your Kids: Why Parents Need to Matter More Than Peers.* New York: Ballantine Books, 2005.

Pearce, Joseph Chilton. *Magical Child.* New York, NY: Penguin Books, Inc., 1977.

Prensky, Marc. *Don't Bother Me Mom, I'm Learning: How Computer and Video Games Are Preparing Your Kids for Twenty-First Century Success and How You Can Help!* St. Paul, Minn: Paragon House, 2006.

Sheffer, Susannah. *A Sense of Self: Listening to Homeschooled Adolescent Girls.* Portsmouth, NH: Boynton/Cook Publishers, Inc. 1995.

Websites on homeschooling and mindful parenting

http://www.holtgws.com/index.html
http://home.earthlink.net/~fetteroll/rejoycing/
http://sandradodd.com/
http://learninfreedom.org/
http://www.livingjoyfully.ca/anneo/anne_o.htm

Unschooling Yahoo groups:

Always Learning – Learning All the Time, http://groups.yahoo.com/group/AlwaysLearning/
Consensual Living, http://groups.yahoo.com/group/Consensual-living/
Radical Unschoolers List (RUL), http://groups.yahoo.com/group/RUL/
Home Education Magazine—Unschooling, http://groups.yahoo.com/group/HEM-Unschooling/
Unschooling Basics,http://groups.yahoo.com/group/unschoolingbasis
shinewithunschooling@yahoogroups.com (Anne Ohman)

FamiliesUnschoolinginNY@yahoogroups.com
http://groups.yahoo.com/group/RadicalUNschoolersinNY/
http://groups.google.com/group/UnschoolingDiscussion
http://groups.yahoo.com/group/alwaysunschooled/

Website Resources

www.alljackedupthemovie.com – DVD by Mike Adams of Natural News
www.americanyogini.com – American Yogini
www.ams.usda.gov/farmersmarkets/ – Farmer's Markets around the USA
www.askdrsears.com – Dr. William Sears
www.AutismMadeInTheUSA.com – DVD by Gary Null
www.beautifulonraw.comTonya Zavasta
www.bestfed.com – breastfeeding, natural birth
www.birthasweknowit.com – film by Elena Tonetti-Vladimirova
www.birthpower.com
www.bodyandfitness.com/information/health/research/b12.htm – B12 information
www.brigittemars.com – Brigitte Mars
www.cancernomore.com – preventing or overcoming cancer
http://www.cdc.gov/nchs/products/pubs/pubd/hestats/obese03_04/overwght_child_03.htm
    – National Health and Nutrition Examination Survey
www.centerforfoodsafety.com – Center for Food Safety
www.cgcvt.org – Camp Commonground, Vermont
www.chidiet.com – Dr. James Carey and the Creative Health Institute
www.cnn.com/1999/HEALTH/women/12/12/breast.milk.angles.wmd/, Dec. 23, 1999.
    – "Donating Mother's Milk: The Gift of Life" by Charles Downey
www.cnvc.org – Nonviolent Communication
www.donnaperrone.com – Donna Perrone
www.drritamarie.com – Dr. Ritamarie Loscalzo
www.drfuhrman.com – Dr. Joel Fuhrman
www.drgreene.com/21_1904.html – Autism: New Evidence in Mercury-Autism Link
www.drgreger.org – DVDs: Latest in Clinical Nutrition by Dr. Michael Greger
www.drmcdougall.com – Dr. John A. McDougall
www.economads.com – Economads (Erika and Ofek)
www.elsonhaas.com – Dr. Elson Haas
www.fitday.com – to calculate daily nutrition
www.foodnsport.com – Dr. Douglas Graham, Professor Rozalind Graham
www.fredericpatenaude.com – Frederic Patenaude's website, sale of his books and other raw
    vegan lifestyle products
www.garynull.com – Gary Null
www.getwellstaywellamerica.com – Victoria Bidwell
www.ghlp.org – The Grassroots Healthy Lawn Plan (environmentalist Patti Wood)
www.grassrootsinfo.org – Grassroots Environmental Education
www.greenlifestylefilmfestival.com – organized in Los Angeles by Dorit
www.harmonyhikes.com – Hiking with Sergei Boutenko (Full day or extended hikes, foraging
    for wild edibles, and only raw food served)
www.healthpromoting.com – True North Health Education and Fasting Center
http://health.groups.yahoo.com/group/RawPregnancy/

www.hippocratesinst.org – Hippocrates Health Institute
www.home-ed-magazine.com – Home Education Magazine
www.howgreenismytown.org – environmentalists Patti and Doug Wood
www.jjvitalityfood.com – Jaylene Johnson
www.krispin.com/protein.html – Protein information
www.lalecheleague.org – La Leche League
www.lifesave.org/vitaminB12.htm. (part 2) – B12 information
www.livefoodenergy.com – Chrissy Gala, raw food chef (retreats in Sedona, AZ)
www.livefoodfactor.com – Susan Schenk
www.livingfoodsinstitute – Brenda Cobb
www.living-foods.com – John Kohler's website (largest raw food website)
www.livingnutrition.com – Dave Klein and Vibrance Magazine, sale of books, and other
    products
www.matthewgrace.com – Matthew Grace
www.mercola.com – Dr. Joseph Mercola, "New Research Supports the Link Between
    Cooking and Cancer"
www.milkshare.birthingforlife.com – Mothers donate breast milk
www.mothering.com – Mothering Magazine
www.naturalchild.org – The Natural Child Project – Psychologist Jan Hunt
www.naturallyhome.com/articles/parabens.shtml). Parabens and their relation to breast
    cancer tumors
www.newearthrecords.com – DVD *A Birth without Violence* by Frederick Leboyer, M.D.
www.notmilk.com – Research site detailing evidence against milk consumption
http://nov55.com/hea/food.html – Gary Novak, biologist and moral philosopher
www.nutridiary.com – To calculate daily nutrition
www.nvic.org – The National Vaccine Information Center
www.orgasmicbirth.com – Film "Orgasmic Birth"
www.paulnison.com – Paul Nison
www.pbs.org/tradesecrets – Bill Moyers' PBS exposé of the chemical industry, *Trade Secrets*
www.pcrm.org – The Physicians Committee for Responsible Medicine
www.permaculture.com – scientist David Blume
www.quest.tv – Kevin Shuker and Eric Czoka – raw food lifestyle and health programs
www.ravediet.com – The film *Eating*
www.rawdish.com – Stephen Parker
www.rawfamily.com – The Boutenko Family
www.rawfoodchef.com—Cherie Soria and The Living Light Culinary Arts Institute
www.rawfoodeducation.com – Dr. Rick Dina
www.rawfoodinfo.com – Rhio's Raw Energy: information, books and products
www.rawfoodrevival.com – Raw food educators and chefs Jackie and Gideon Graff
www.rawfoodsbible.com – Dr. Craig Sommers
www.rawfoodsnewsmagazine.com – Judy Pokras
www.rawfunfamily.com – Sonya Watt – Raw Fun Family Camp
www.rawgourmet.com – Nomi Shannon
www.rawlife.com – Paul Nison
www.rawtism.com – Autism and Raw Foods, Sunshine Boatright
www.remineralize.org – Don Weaver, Earth Health Regeneration
www.rawmom.com – Tera Warner and Shannon Leone
www.rense.com/general26/milk.htm – "The Truth about Milk" by Dave Rietz

www.shazzie.com - Shazzie and *Evie's Kitchen*
www.soilandhealth.org – The Agriculture Library and free books by Don Weaver
www.spontaneouscreation.org – Jock Doubleday
www.sunfood.com – David Wolfe
www.superhealthychildren.com – Karen Ranzi and *Creating Healthy Children*
www.susansmithjones.com – Susan Smith Jones, Ph.D.
www.thebusinessofbeingborn.com – film produced by Ricki Lake and directed by
    Abby Epstein
www.thechinastudy.com – The China Study website – Dr. T. Colin Campbell and Thomas M.
    Campbell II
www.thecureisinthecause.com – Dr. Ruza Bogdanovich
www.thedoctorwithin.com – Dr. Tim O'Shea (vaccinations)
www.thegardenbaby.com – Julie Pitcher – Raw Vegan Pregnancy
www.thegardendiet.com – Jingee and Storm Talifero and family
www.themothermagazine.co.uk – The Mother Magazine, UK
www.therawfoodfamily.com – Ka Sunshine and Family
www.thewelltoexcell.com – raw food chefs and educators Cheryll Lynn and Scott McNabb
www.thinktwice.com/laws.htm – state laws regarding vaccination and a sample exemption
    letter
www.treeoflife.nu – Dr. Gabriel Cousens and The Tree of Life Rejuvenation Center
www.turtlelakerefuge.com – Turtle Lake Refuge, Katrina Blair – founder
www.unassistedbirth.com – articles about unassisted home birthing
www.vaccinenation.net – Film Vaccine-Nation
www.veganhealth.org/b12/ – "Vitamin 12: Are You Getting It?" by Jack Norris
www.veganoutreach.org – Vegan information
www.vegetarianbaby.com – vegetarian baby and child online magazine—also includes articles
    on raw vegan babies and children. Article by Karen Ranzi.
www.vegetarianteen.com – Teen vegetarian and vegan site, with articles by raw vegan teens
http://vetrano.cjb.net – Dr. Vivian V. Vetrano
http://www.vibrancy.homestead.com/pageone.html – Dr. Gina Shaw, UK
www.vidaclara.com – Vida Clara Transformation Institute, Dr. Robert Sniadach
www.VivaLaRaw.org – Eric Rivkin, raw food chef and educator
www.waterbirth.org/spa – Barbara Harper
www.westonaprice.org – The Weston A. Price Organization
www.womengoraw.com – *Women Go Raw* by Dr. Ariel Policano

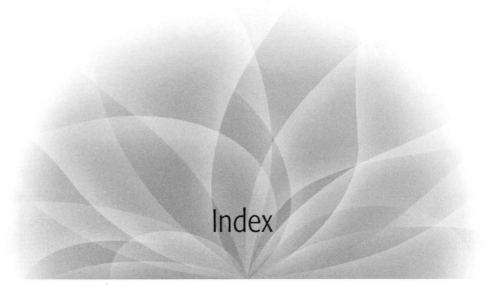

Index

Index by Tamar Raum, M.A., M.L.S., H.H.C.
Comprehensive Indexing Services: Email contact: tammyraum@gmail.com
Excerpts of the index may be used or copied only with express permission of the indexer.

NOTE: Authors are included in the index. For complete information, this index coordinates with the author's bibliography, webliography, and additional appendices.

O

P

About the Author

Karen Ranzi is an author, lecturer and raw food consultant. Karen has been working in the natural health movement for over 15 years in the field of nutrition, health, and child development. Her many activities include: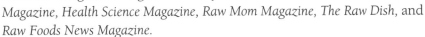

Author – *Creating Healthy Children: Through Attachment Parenting and Raw Foods.*

Articles written for – *Living Nutrition Magazine, Vibrance Magazine, Vegetarian Baby and Child Magazine, Health Science Magazine, Raw Mom Magazine, The Raw Dish,* and *Raw Foods News Magazine.*

Coordinator and Lecturer – New Jersey Raw Food Support Network 2006 to present.

Leader – Accent on Wellness raw lifestyle support group in Manhattan 1996 to 2006.

Interviewed on TV and radio on the topics of vegetarian and raw food parenting, and homeschooling.

Lecturer – Portland International Raw Food Festival, Portland, OR, 2003; Creative Health Institute, Union City, MI, 2004; Raw Passion Seminar, Philadelphia, PA, 2004; Living Now Festival, Buffalo, NY, 2004; The Raw Spirit Festival, Sedona, AZ, 2007 and 2008; Yoga/Raw Foods New Life Expo, New York, NY, 2008; Optimum Health Solution, Waltham, MA, 2009.

461

Director – children's program, Raw Spirit Festival, Sedona, AZ, 2007.

Teacher – her class "Creating Healthy Children" for eleven years throughout the United States.

Karen and Rhio (author of *Hooked on Raw* and www.rawfoodinfo.com) have established a non-profit organization, Health Liberties Network, to protect the freedoms of individuals and families in their health care choices (www.healthliberties.org).

Karen and her husband Harvey have successfully homeschooled their children, Gabriela and Marco, in New Jersey and abroad. Gabriela is passionate about Global Environmental Studies, while Marco is attracted to Sports Broadcasting.

In addition to her background in nutrition, Karen holds a Masters Degree in Speech Pathology and is a speech therapist, working with children, ages 3–21, for over thirty years, specializing with autistic children for the past eight years. She holds a Bachelor's Degree from Montclair State University and a Master's Degree from New York University.

Her father's powerful influence had a profound effect on her, leading her toward a passion for living a life of health and truth.

Karen found the natural path that enabled her son to heal from asthma, chronic ear infections and allergies. The dietary and lifestyle improvements she learned removed the causes of disease, bringing about her own healing from digestive, gynecological and skin problems. She has maintained a 100% raw vegan diet since 1994. By means of her education, life-changing personal experiences, and sincere desire to share her message, Karen has guided thousands toward developing excellent health.

Karen gives lectures all over the U.S., and is interested in presenting internationally. She is available for workshops, seminars and radio shows. If you would like Karen to speak to your group, please call: **(201) 934-6778**, or contact her through her website: **www.superhealthychildren.com** to set up a class, lecture, or private consultation. You can also contact Karen and to receive her free monthly e-newsletter, "Creating Healthy Children," by emailing her at: **karen@superhealthychildren.com**.

Quick Order Form

Order additional copies of *Creating Healthy Children* directly from
Super Healthy Children Publishing:

online: www.SuperHealthyChildren.com
or by telephone: (201) 934-6778
Mail Orders (please photocopy form):

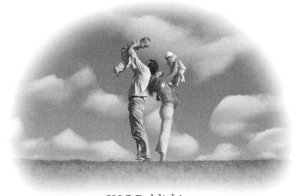

SHC Publishing
P.O. Box 13
Ramsey, NJ 07446-0013

Please send me _____ copies of Creating Healthy Children @ $24.95 each.

_____
NAME

_____
ADDRESS

_____
CITY   STATE   ZIP

_____
EMAIL ADDRESS

Please add $5 for each book for shipping.
To order up to 4 books, the cost is $10.35 shipping.
For reduced shipping costs on larger orders, and for international rates,
please email: karen@superhealthychildren.com or call: (201) 934-6778.

Payment: ☐ Check   ☐ Money Order